Microbiome in Gastrointestinal Cancer

Jun Yu
Editor

Microbiome in Gastrointestinal Cancer

Springer

Editor
Jun Yu
Department of Medicine & Therapeutics
The Chinese University of Hong Kong
Hong Kong, China

ISBN 978-981-19-4494-9 ISBN 978-981-19-4492-5 (eBook)
https://doi.org/10.1007/978-981-19-4492-5

This Springer imprint is published by the registered company Springer Nature Singapore Pte Ltd.
The registered company address is: 152 Beach Road, #21-01/04 Gateway East, Singapore 189721, Singapore

Contents

Chapter 1
Introduction

Jun Yu

Keywords Gastrointestinal cancer · Gut microbiome · Basic research · Clinical research

Gastrointestinal cancers account for over a third of new cancer cases globally, and represent a major public health burden. Colorectal cancer (CRC), gastric cancer (GC), and liver cancer are the most common gastrointestinal cancers in most parts of the world. Accumulating evidence has documented a rising trend in gastrointestinal cancers over the past 5–10 years, and thus is a serious health threat to humans. Multiple international genetic and transcriptomic sequencing projects over the past decade have established the role of genetic and epigenetic determinants of cancer. Nevertheless, environmental factors, such as smoking, diet, alcohol consumption, obesity, and more, are proposed to play predominant roles in the development of sporadic gastrointestinal cancers. In this context, a unique feature of gastrointestinal cancers, such as CRC and GC, is their close proximity to our gut microbiota. Gut microbiota consists of a collection of trillions of microorganisms encompassing bacteria, viruses, fungi, and archaea. Our gut microbes could interact with host cells in a variety of ways to modulate cancer initiation and progression.

Over the past decade, the investigation of gut microbiome in GI carcinogenesis has flourished—facilitated by major technological advances. First, metagenomic sequencing efforts have enabled rapid and comprehensive profiling of the gut microbiota, which clearly demonstrated that the gut microbiota is dysregulated in gastrointestinal cancers including CRC, GC, and liver cancer. On the other hand, molecular and cell biology studies have resulted in great strides in our understanding of the functional role and mechanism of action of gut microbiota in gastrointestinal cancers. Accumulating evidence indicates that gut microbiota can be harnessed for cancer prevention as well as to modulate the efficacy of chemotherapy and

J. Yu (✉)
Institute of Digestive Disease and Department of Medicine and Therapeutics, State Key Laboratory of Digestive Disease, Li Ka Shing Institute of Health Sciences, The Chinese University of Hong Kong, Hong Kong, China
e-mail: junyu@cuhk.edu.hk

J. Yu (ed.), *Microbiome in Gastrointestinal Cancer*,
https://doi.org/10.1007/978-981-19-4492-5_1

immunotherapy. Against this backdrop, we believe that it is timely to propose this series "Microbiome in Gastrointestinal Cancer" to cover state-of-the-art topics covering these major areas, including (1) characterization of the dysregulated microbiome in gastrointestinal cancers (Chaps. 1–6); (2) the molecular mechanism of action of gut microbiota via microbial metabolites and direct interaction with host cancer or immune cells (Chaps. 7–11); (3) key methodologies for studying the role of gut microbiota in cancers (Chaps. 12 and 13); and (4) the potential application of gut microbes for the prevention and treatment of gastrointestinal cancers (Chaps. 14–17).

To open our discussion on the gut microbiome, Lau et al. provide an overview of the role of gut microbiome in health and disease (Chap. 2). This is followed by detailed review and discussion on the phenomenon of microbial dysbiosis in specific gastrointestinal cancers, such as colorectal cancer (Chap. 3), gastric cancer (Chap. 4), and liver cancer (Chap. 5), major GI cancers worldwide. These chapters provide succinct description of the changing gut microbiome landscape in tumorigenesis, highlight their potential molecular mechanisms, and briefly discuss potential clinical implications. In earlier studies, our evaluation of the gut microbiome is largely restricted to bacteria. Nevertheless, accumulating data have shown that microbial dysregulation in cancer also extends to the gut viruses, fungi, and even archaea, the latter of which are thought to exist only in extreme environments. In this regard, Chap. 6 is devoted to these emerging microbes, their dysregulation and potential contributions to tumorigenesis of GI cancers. Collectively, these chapters consolidate the view that gut microbiome is dysregulated in GI cancers, and is critically involved in disease initiation and progression.

Studying the underlying molecular mechanisms of gut microbiome is essential to establishing the causality of dysregulated gut microbiome in GI cancers. To this end, Chaps. 7–11 mainly dealt with the molecular mechanisms by which gut microbiota could interact with the host and alter host physiology. In Chap. 7, Lee provides a detailed discussion of the role of microbial metabolome as the link between a dysregulated microbiome and host disease. Particular focus is placed on the gut–liver axis as an important mediator of fatty liver disease. This followed by Chap. 8 describing how gut microbiome–liver axis and metabolite transfer contribute to the pathogenesis of NAFLD and its associated liver cancer. Diet has a significant influence on the gut microbiota. Chapter 9 attempts to extend the notion of "you are what you eat" to the gut microbiome by exploring studies highlighting 3-way crosstalk between diet, gut microbiome, and GI tumorigenesis. Chapters 10 and 11 then provide in-depth review of the mechanisms of host–microbiome interactions in GI cancers, with a focus on signaling pathways modulated by gut microbiome (Chap. 10) and influence of the gut microbiome on antitumor immune response (Chap. 11). Complementing these reviews, Chaps. 12 and 13 are dedicated summaries to state-of-the-art tools in studying the gut microbiome in GI cancers. Animal models, especially germ-free mice, are vital tools to studying gut microbiome and they summarized in Chap. 12. Chapter 13 describes the bioinformatic tools that are fundamental to metagenome analysis, and potential applications of artificial intelligence in microbiome analysis.

Given the close association between gut microbiome and GI cancers, how we can harness the power of microbes in clinical translation has become a subject of intensive investigations. Accumulating evidence has indicated that beneficial commensals are depleted in tumorigenesis, thus providing the biological basis of restoring a health microbiome for disease prevention or treatment. Au-Doung et al. review the evidence in support of application of probiotics and prebiotics in GI cancer management in Chap. 14. Chapters 15 and 16 cover the impact of gut microbiome in affecting treatment efficacy in GI cancers, including chemotherapy and immune checkpoint blockade (ICB) therapy. Chapter 17 outlines the strategies that could be used for targeting the gut microbiome in GI cancers, including probiotics, prebiotics, diet, and fecal microbial transplantation (FMT). These chapters collectively demonstrate the tremendous potential in the clinical translation of gut microbiome in GI cancers. Last but not least, Lau et al. provide an interesting and timely review on COVID-19 and gut microbiota, their potential interaction and biological significance.

This series is unique in that we will bring together a group of experts to provide their perspectives on the subject from the viewpoint of basic, translational, and clinical research. We are grateful to all our contributors, including international experts in molecular biology, microbiology, metabolomics, bioinformatics, and physician scientists to provide in-depth review of this subject. We hope that this book will offer a rich resource of information on this important topic for graduate students, basic researchers as well as physicians.

Conflict of Interest All authors declare no conflict of interest.

Chapter 2
Gut Microbiome in Health and Gastrointestinal Cancer

Harry Cheuk-Hay Lau

Abstract Human gastrointestinal tract harbours trillions of microbes including bacteria, fungi, and viruses to form the gut microbiome. The recent advance in both bioinformatic analyses and functional investigations has greatly improved understandings of the complex host–microbe interactions. The gut microbiome has shown their impacts across a variety of physiological functions. Whereas dysbiosis or alterations in the gut microbiome is correlated with pathogenesis and progression of numerous diseases including cancer. In this chapter, the contribution of a healthy gut microbiome to digestion and immunity of the host is discussed. The association of a dysbiotic microbiome with the development of common gastrointestinal cancers (colorectal cancer, gastric cancer, and hepatopancreatic cancer) is also explored. The article is summarised with highlight of the current limitations and opportunities to advance this line of research.

Keywords Gut microbiome · Healthy microbiome · Digestion · Immunity · Dysbiosis · Gastrointestinal cancer

2.1 Introduction

The surface barriers of the human body are inhabited by trillions of microbes including bacteria, fungi, viruses, archaea, and protozoa (Lloyd-Price et al. 2016). Together, these microbes form complex microbial communities to make up the human microbiota, whilst the genomes of these microbes collectively form the

H. C.-H. Lau (✉)
Institute of Digestive Disease and The Department of Medicine and Therapeutics, State Key Laboratory of Digestive Disease, Li Ka Shing Institute of Health Sciences, CUHK Shenzhen Research Institute, The Chinese University of Hong Kong, Hong Kong, China
e-mail: harrylau@link.cuhk.edu.hk

J. Yu (ed.), *Microbiome in Gastrointestinal Cancer*,
https://doi.org/10.1007/978-981-19-4492-5_2

human microbiome. Being considered as the second genome of humans, the microbiome has shown its great impacts across a broad spectrum of physiological functions such as regulation of host metabolism and maintenance of the immune system (Belkaid and Hand 2014; Martinez-Guryn et al. 2019).

High-throughput sequencing is fundamental for profiling microbial communities in different human habitats including the gastrointestinal tract, oral cavity, skin, and vagina (Human Microbiome Project Consortium 2012). From amplicon to shotgun metagenomic sequencing, these next-generation sequencing technologies have revolutionised understandings of the human microbiome by characterising microbes associated with health or diseases (Knight et al. 2018). Notably, although functional analysis can be performed using sequencing data, mechanistic investigations are necessary to validate the physiological roles of microbes in humans. The improvements in the methods of anaerobic culture have greatly enhanced the feasibility to isolate pure microbes that were previously unculturable in laboratory (Browne et al. 2016). Various animal experiments including germ-free mice and human microbiota-associated mouse models have also been popularised in mechanistic studies (Walter et al. 2020). Overall, the recent progression of both bioinformatic analyses and functional investigations has contributed to the elucidation of complex host–microbe interactions in health and disease conditions. In this chapter, the gut microbiome and its functional traits in health and gastrointestinal cancer are explored.

2.2 Digestive Roles of Healthy Gut Microbiome

The gastrointestinal tract harbours the greatest amount of commensal microbes among the human body. The abundance and diversity of commensal microbes are highly varied among different regions of the gastrointestinal tract. While several microbes from phyla *Actinobacteria, Bacteroidetes, Firmicutes,* and *Proteobacteria* are commonly present in the gut, others seem to be present in a region-specific manner (Martinez-Guryn et al. 2019). The microbial community in each region or organ is associated with host features such as pH, oxygen level, bile acids, and nutrient bioavailability (Friedman et al. 2018). Likewise, gut microbes are necessary for dietary digestion and nutrient absorption, thus the complex interplay between host and microbes lays the foundation for host survival. In this section, the microbiome in oesophagus, stomach, and intestines are explored with discussion on the correlation between microbes and digestive functions in healthy state (Table 2.1).

2.2.1 Oesophagus and Stomach

Given its proximity with the oral cavity, the composition of oesophageal microbiome is similar to the oral microbiome with *Streptococcus*, *Prevotella*, and *Veillonella* being the predominant species (May and Abrams 2018). In the stomach, the growth

Table 2.1 Digestive roles of healthy gut microbiome

Region	Dominant genus	Digestive role in healthy condition
Oesophagus	*Streptococcus, Prevotella, Veillonella*	Unclear, ethically inappropriate to study the microbiome in healthy subjects by endoscopy
Stomach	*Streptococcus, Prevotella, Lactobacillus, Helicobacter*	Unclear, ethically inappropriate to study the microbiome in healthy subjects by endoscopy Produce lipases to facilitate fat digestion
Duodenum	*Streptococcus, Prevotella*	Maintain bile acid metabolism by deconjugating primary bile acids
Jejunum	*Streptococcus, Prevotella, Veillonella, Fusobacterium, Lactobacillus*	Involved in lipid metabolism Produce lipases to facilitate lipid degradation
Ileum	*Streptococcus, Veillonella, Ruminococcus, Bacteroides, Clostridium*	Maintain bile acid metabolism by reabsorbing bile acids and transferring them to the liver for detoxification and recycle
Colon	*Bacteroides, Prevotella, Clostridium, Lactobacillus, Peptostreptococcus*	Mediate gut motility Maintain bile acid metabolism by conversing primary to secondary bile acids Produce SCFAs for regulating energy metabolism, insulin sensitivity, host immunity, intestinal homeostasis

of commensal microbes is heavily limited by gastric acidity, mucosal thickness, and peristalsis, hence the stomach harbours the least amount (about 10^1–10^3 colony-forming unit (CFU)/mL) and diversity of microbes along the gastrointestinal tract) (O'Hara and Shanahan 2006). Only a few microbes particularly *Streptococcus, Prevotella*, *Lactobacillus*, and *Helicobacter* can survive and colonise in such harsh conditions (May and Abrams 2018; Nardone and Compare 2015).

Like other gastrointestinal organs, diet is one of the most influential factors to the composition of gastroesophageal microbiome in healthy state. For instance, high dietary fibre intake promotes the abundance of phylum *Firmicutes* in the oesophageal microbiome, and low fibre intake is associated with enrichment of *Prevotella* and *Neisseria* (Nobel et al. 2018). An in vivo study reported that mice fed with natural source-derived food have higher gastric microbial loads and abundance of *Lactobacillus* than mice fed with refined food (Sahasakul et al. 2012). Interestingly, *Lactobacillus* enrichment was found to be inversely correlated with toll-like receptor (TLR)-2 expression in mice stomach (an innate receptor activated by gram-positive bacteria including *Lactobacillus* Rocha-Ramirez et al. 2017), suggesting that TLR2 in the stomach and intestines may have different sensitivity or tolerance towards commensal microbes.

As the oesophagus and stomach are distant from the large intestine, faecal samples which are commonly assessed in gut microbiome studies may not accurately represent the actual composition of microbiome in the upper gastrointestinal tract. Instead, invasive endoscopy is needed to collect mucosal specimens for examining the gastroesophageal microbiome. It is therefore challenging to study the gastroesophageal microbiome in non-pathological state due to the ethical inappropriateness to perform endoscopy in healthy subjects (Wen et al. 2021). Meanwhile, increasing evidence has highlighted the association of altered gastroesophageal microbiome and their related pathways with precancerous lesion and cancer. For example, energy generation and amino acid metabolism are upregulated in the gastric microbiome of patients with gastric inflammation (Sung et al. 2020). Whilst enrichment of gastric lactic acid bacteria including *Lactobacillus* and *Streptococcus* was observed in patients with gastric cancer of which these bacteria can produce lactate as a fuel source for tumour cells, thereby promoting inflammation, tumourigenesis, and immunomodulation (Vinasco et al. 2019). These findings suggest the potential association of gastroesophageal microbes with digestive functions in healthy host. It is reasonable to propose that certain lipase-producing microbes particularly *Lactobacillus* may facilitate the digestion of dietary fats in the stomach (Gupta et al. 2004; Ogawa et al. 2015; Manasian et al. 2020).

2.2.2 *Small Intestine*

The abundance and diversity of gut microbes increase in the small intestine. Numerous bacteria including *Bifidobacterium, Prevotella, Lactobacillus, Clostridium, Streptococcus, Enterococcus,* and *Escherichia* were reported to be the predominant species in the small intestine (Martinez-Guryn et al. 2019). Human small intestine can be divided into 3 regions—duodenum, jejunum, and ileum. The duodenum harbours a relatively low amount of microbes (about 10^1–10^3 CFU/mL) among the three regions with *Streptococcus* and *Prevotella* being the predominant species (O'Hara and Shanahan 2006). Such reduced bacterial abundance is attributed to the elevated pH and oxygen levels as well as the presence of antimicrobial bile acids and other digestive enzymes (Li et al. 2015). The duodenum is a major breakdown site of macronutrients including dietary fats and oils, and this process is mainly regulated by bile acids. Primary bile acids are first produced by the liver and then transferred into the duodenum. To enable their digestive activities, translocated primary bile acids need to be deconjugated by gut microbes particularly *Clostridium, Lactobacillus,* and *Bifidobacterium* (Jia et al. 2018). In turn, bile acids-mediated digestion involves oxidative chemical reactions which can change the luminal oxygen levels in mice, subsequently affecting the composition of duodenal microbiome (Friedman et al. 2018). Hence, duodenal microbes cooperate with host to maintain balanced lipid and carbohydrate metabolism.

The jejunum is a major site of lipid digestion and nutrient absorption. To date, there are limited investigations of the jejunal microbiome in healthy state, as endoscopic samples are the primary sources of information which could only be ethically collected from subjects with underlying condition (Wang and Yang 2013). A few studies reported that the jejunum harbours a denser microbial community than the duodenum (10^4–10^7 CFU/mL), mainly represented by *Streptococcus, Prevotella, Veillonella, Fusobacterium*, and *Lactobacillus* (O'Hara and Shanahan 2006; Sundin et al. 2017). Comparing to the gastric and duodenal microbiome, the jejunal microbiome has higher microbial stability indicating that the indigenous microbes residing in more distal regions of the gastrointestinal tract may be less affected by environmental factors (Seekatz et al. 2019). Notably, diet is still the major factor affecting the jejunal microbiome, as exemplified by an in vivo study reporting the altered microbiome in the jejunum of mice fed with high-fat diet (Martinez-Guryn et al. 2018). These microbial changes induced by high dietary fat intake can directly increase host lipid absorption. In addition, jejunal *Lactobacillus* was proposed to play a substantial role in lipid metabolism, given by its high abundance and ability to produce lipases and short-chain fatty acids (SCFAs) which are all essential for lipid degradation (Lema et al. 2020). Further investigation on lipid-degrading microbes is needed to unravel the functional role of jejunal microbiome in lipid metabolism or other digestive functions.

Digestion and absorption in the ileum are known to be distinct from the other regions of small intestine. Consistently, the ileum was found to harbour a different microbial community with an estimated microbial load of 10^3–10^8 CFU/mL (O'Hara and Shanahan 2006). Limited studies have reported the predominance of *Streptococcus, Veillonella, Ruminococcus, Bacteroides,* and *Clostridium* in the ileal microbiome (Booijink et al. 2010). Unlike the duodenum as aforementioned, both conjugated and unconjugated bile acids are reabsorbed in the ileum and transferred into the enterohepatic circulation to be detoxified and recycled by the liver (Jia et al. 2018). Specifically, ileal epithelial cells express nuclear receptors (e.g. farnesoid X receptor and bile acid-specific G-protein-coupled receptor 5) that can be activated by unconjugated bile acids for the downstream bile acid metabolism, whereas activities of these receptors are directly influenced by gut microbes particularly *Bacteroides* and *Clostridium* (Ridlon et al. 2016). Of note, the ileal microbiome can also be affected by bile acids, as exemplified by the inhibition of bacterial overgrowth by certain conjugated bile acids (Hegade et al. 2016). Collectively, the gut microbiome bidirectionally interacts with different host features to ensure normal digestion and nutrient absorption in healthy state.

2.2.3 Large Intestine

The abundance and diversity of gut microbes reach the peak in the large intestine with an estimated microbial load of 10^{11}–10^{12} CFU/mL (O'Hara and Shanahan 2006). A diverse microbial community is harboured in the large intestine, primarily represented by phyla *Bacteroidetes* (including genera *Bacteroides* and *Prevotella*) and *Firmicutes* (including genera *Clostridium, Lactobacillus,* and *Peptostreptococcus*) (Martinez-Guryn et al. 2019). Human large intestine can be divided into the proximal/right-sided and the distal/left-sided colon. The proximal colon is a major site of nutrient fermentation and microbes-mediated processes, while the distal colon is responsible for gut motility. Owing to the easier accessibility, several studies have reported the microbiome similarity between proximal and distal colon in healthy subjects but not in cancer patients (Wu et al. 2019). In the proximal colon, numerous bacterial SCFA producers including *Clostridium, Enterococcus,* and *Roseburia* are enriched (Martinez-Guryn et al. 2019). These bacteria ferment dietary carbohydrates and fibres that are indigestible by host enzymes to produce metabolites SCFAs (e.g. acetate, propionate, butyrate, and valerate) (Koh et al. 2016). SCFAs are crucial to a broad spectrum of physiological functions, ranging from maintenance of energy metabolism and insulin sensitivity, regulation of host immunity (Canfora et al. 2015; McCarville et al. 2020), and to epigenetic mediation of histone deacetylases to contribute intestinal homeostasis (Wu et al. 2020).

The large intestine is critically involved in conversion of primary to secondary bile acids via a variety of microbes-mediated processes (Ridlon et al. 2016). In brief, bile acid conversion requires bile salt hydrolase (BSH), an enzyme produced by gut anaerobes especially *Clostridium, Lactobacillus, Bifidobacterium,* and *Bacteroides* (Jia et al. 2018). The deconjugated bile acids are then processed by 7α-dehydroxylase mainly secreted by *Clostridium* and *Eubacterium* to form deoxycholic acid and lithocholic acids, which can be absorbed into the enterohepatic circulation and eventually detoxified and recycled by the liver. The high abundance of *Clostridium* and other BSH-producing bacteria in the large intestine thus facilitates reabsorption of bile acids and subsequently completes the bile acid metabolism for dietary lipid digestion.

The distal colon is responsible for gut motility which refers to the movement of ingested food across the gastrointestinal tract. Early studies reported the significant increased gastric emptying and gut transit time in germ-free mice, highlighting the vital role of gut microbiome in gut motility. Microbes mediate the gut motility mainly via their metabolites. For example, administration of SCFAs improves the gut motility by increasing the concentration of neurotransmitter 5-hydroxtryptamine to stimulate peristalsis in mice (Grider and Piland 2007), whereas the bacterial endotoxin lipopolysaccharides (LPS) could dysregulate motility (Rebollar et al. 2002). Given by its close association with commensal microbes, the gut motility can be readily influenced by diet as exemplified by an in vivo study showing that high dietary fibre intake leads to reduced motility in mice (Kashyap et al. 2013). Moreover, the gut microbiome can also indirectly affect the gut motility through TLRs or other microbes-associated immune responses (Dimidi et al. 2017). Altogether, the intricate interplay between host and gut microbes is essential for having a fully functional digestion system in humans.

2.3 Gut Microbiome and Immunity

Another important role of a healthy gut microbiome is to maintain intestinal homeostasis by interacting with the host immune system. The innate immunity is maintained by antigen-presenting cells (APCs) consisting of B cells and dendritic cells. These cells are key to initiate the immunity-microbiome crosstalk as they can detect and be provoked by microbe-associated molecular patterns such as peptidoglycans, and LPS using their germline-encoded pattern recognition receptors (e.g. extracellular TLRs and intracellular nod-like receptors) (Gaudino and Kumar 2019). Once activated, APCs trigger multiple signalling cascades that are crucial for host defence including production of antimicrobial peptides, cytokines, and chemokines (Rooks and Garrett 2016). To initiate the adoptive immunity, APCs present antigens on their surface via major histocompatibility complex to allow recognition from corresponding T cell receptor, thereby promoting T cell differentiation and effector functions (Gaudino and Kumar 2019). Meanwhile, metabolites also have distinct roles in manipulating the host immunity. For instance, butyrate promotes colonic regulatory T cells (T_{Reg}) differentiation and T cell-independent immunoglobulin A (IgA) response in mice by epigenetically inducing histone acetylation at the promoter and enhancer regions of *Foxp3* (a transcription factor of CD4+ T_{Reg} development) (Furusawa et al. 2013; Arpaia et al. 2013). Butyrate can also prolong the memory potential of CD8+ T cells by shifting their metabolic reliance on glycolytic substrates for tricarboxylic acid cycle to glutamine utilisation and fatty acid catabolism from oxidative phosphorylation (Bachem et al. 2019).

Early evidence from germ-free mice has reported the importance of gut microbiome in shaping the host immunity. Comparing to mice housed in standard condition, germ-free mice displayed higher susceptibility to bacterial infection and immunological deflects including impaired T_{Reg} development, lower IgA level, and poorer growth of gut-associated lymphoid tissues (Round and Mazmanian 2009). The immunomodulatory capabilities of individual microbes were then discovered. For example, *Bacteroides fragilis* directs the conversion of CD4+ naive T cells into Foxp3+ mature T_{Reg} to stimulate production of anti-inflammatory cytokines interleukin (IL)-10 through the TLR2 pathway (Round and Mazmanian 2010). Similarly, 17 *Clostridium* strains are also able to increase intestinal differentiated T_{Reg} and IL-10 level (Atarashi et al. 2013). In contrast, certain segmented filamentous bacteria of *Clostridia* modulate immunity by inducing a broad spectrum of pro-inflammatory responses including upregulation of T helper cells (T_H)-1, IL-17-producing T_H17, and T_{Reg} (Gaboriau-Routhiau et al. 2009; Ivanov et al. 2009). In 2017, Geva-Zatorsky et al. conducted a screen for immunomodulatory microbes in human gut microbiome with subsequent mono-colonisation into germ-free mice, generating 24,255 distinct immuno-phenotypes (Geva-Zatorsky et al. 2017). Several novel microbial immunomodulation was discovered including the augmentation of colonic IL-10-producing CD4+ T cells upon *Veillonella* colonisation. Conversely, the gut microbiome can also be altered by the host immunity. Previous studies have demonstrated that secretary IgA from gut plasma cells has reactivity to a broad subset of microbes, and these IgA could selectively enhance translocation of commensal bacteria into lymphoid tissues to facilitate antigen presentation, thereby maintaining microbiome diversity (Palm et al. 2014; Fransen et al. 2015; Bunker et al. 2017).

2.4 Gut Microbiome and Gastrointestinal Cancer

In healthy state, the gut microbiome stably and continuously interacts with host to contribute intestinal homeostasis (Lozupone et al. 2012). However, such equilibrium is hard to maintain since the microbiome is readily affected by host genetic background (Kurilshikov et al. 2021) and a variety of extrinsic factors especially dietary intake and antibiotic use (Cotillard et al. 2013; Rothschild et al. 2018). Once the stability of microbial community is constantly disrupted, dysbiosis, termed as the compositional and functional alteration in microbiome, can occur which may trigger numerous diseases including cancer (Lloyd-Price et al. 2016; Tamboli et al. 2004). Different pathogenic events including change in microbial diversity, decrease in probiotic commensals, and outgrowth of pathobionts are occurred in a dysbiotic microbiome which can potentially contribute to tumourigenesis locally in the gut or distantly in the liver and pancreas (Levy et al. 2017; Matson et al. 2021) (Fig. 2.1).

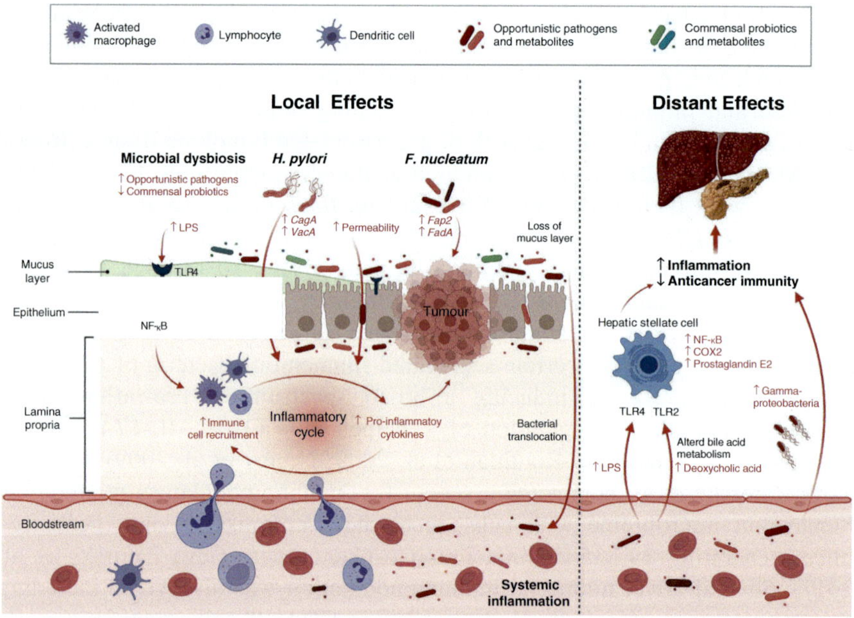

Fig. 2.1 The effects of gut microbiota in gastrointestinal tumourigenesis. Abnormal compositional and functional alterations in the gut microbiome are closely associated with gastrointestinal tumourigenesis. These changes involve the enrichment of opportunistic pathogens including *H. pylori* and *F. nucleatum*, which, respectively, promote GC and CRC by inducing chronic inflammation, as well as the depletion of commensal probiotics. A dysbiotic microbiome also impairs the gut barrier, thereby allowing the translocation of microbes and their metabolites into the bloodstream. These translocated microbial derivatives could reach the hepatopancreatic system, eventually inducing inflammation and weaking anticancer immunity in organs distant from the intestines

2.4.1 Local Effects of Gut Microbiome on Gastric and Colorectal Cancer

Chronic inflammation is a hallmark of gastric cancer (GC) and colorectal cancer (CRC), while its correlation with microbial dysbiosis has been demonstrated in accumulated studies. Early study reported the reduced colonic tumour growth in germ-free mice compared to mice housed in standard condition, implicating the necessity of microbial commensals in colorectal tumourigenesis (Uronis et al. 2009). Enrichment of pathobionts in the dysbiotic microbiome is closely associated with cancer development, as exemplified by a multi-cohort analysis revealing the correlation between enriched bacteria in CRC patients and increased LPS expression (Dai et al. 2018). LPS is the most abundant antigen on gram-negative bacteria, and it can stimulate host toll-like receptor (TLR)-4 signalling to promote survival, proliferation, and migration of tumour cells (Hsu et al. 2011). Activated TLR4 also upregulates reactive oxygen species to promote colorectal tumourigenesis in mice with intact microbiome but not in germ-free mice (Burgueno et al. 2021). Moreover, the activated TLR4 pathway can initiate NF-$_{\kappa}$B signalling cascade to promote production of pro-inflammatory cytokines, most notably IL-23 which regulates expression of downstream cancer-promoting inflammatory cytokines including IL-17A and IL-6 (Grivennikov et al. 2012). Altogether, a dysbiotic microbial community plays crucial roles in cancer development by promoting oxidative stress and chronic inflammation.

Certain bacterial species are highly enriched in the gut microbiome of cancer patients, and functional investigations have uncovered their mechanistic roles in driving tumourigenesis. For instance, *Helicobacter pylori* is one of the most infamous bacteria associated with cancer. About half of the world's population is infected with *H. pylori* which can cause chronic inflammation and increase the risk of gastritis and progression to GC (Wroblewski et al. 2010). Whereas eradication of *H. pylori* could significantly reduce the progression to metachronous GC in patients with high-grade adenoma, hence further confirming the pro-tumourigenic role of *H. pylori* in humans (Choi et al. 2018). In general, *H. pylori* produces a variety of virulence factors (e.g. *CagA* and *VacA*) that can cause oxidative stress and autophagy in the gastric epithelium to promote chronic inflammation and gastritis (Wang et al. 2014). Of note, recent work on gastric microbiome revealed the constant decrease of *H. pylori* abundance in GC patients, suggesting a potential link between *H. pylori* depletion and gastric tumourigenesis (Ferreira et al. 2018). A hypothesis is that *H. pylori* may undergo a "suicidal" journey in GC progression by reducing gastric acidity to facilitate colonisation of pathobionts from the oral cavity, which were found to be greatly enriched in GC patients from multiple studies (Ferreira et al. 2018; Coker et al. 2018; de Assumpcao et al. 2019).

The microbiome alteration in CRC has been comprehensively studied with identification of numerous pro-tumourigenic bacterial species (Yachida et al. 2019). Particularly, enrichment of *Fusobacterium nucleatum* in the colon mucosa of CRC patients has been consistently reported (Allali et al. 2015; Flemer et al. 2017; Liu et al. 2021), and patients with high abundance of *F. nucleatum* are correlated with shorter survival (Mima et al. 2015). *F. nucleatum* can suppress anticancer immunity by binding to immunoinhibitory receptor TIGIT on T cells through its adhesive protein *Fap2* (Kostic et al. 2013) and induce inflammatory response by activating E-cadherin/β-catenin signalling through its another adhesive protein *FadA* (Rubinstein et al. 2013). *F. nucleatum* was also found to have central roles in mediating chemoresistance by orchestrating a molecular network of TLR4-dependent immune response to activate autophagy (Yu et al. 2017). Interestingly, *F. nucleatum* enrichment was identified in tumours of breast and other non-gastrointestinal organs, suggesting that *F. nucleatum* may also be pro-tumourigenic in tumours distant from the gastrointestinal tract (Nejman et al. 2020). Recent evidence reported that *F. nucleatum* could promote metastasis by stimulating tumour cells to secrete exosomes carrying oncogenic microRNAs to infect normal cells (Guo et al. 2020). In addition, *F. nucleatum* enrichment is accompanied by increased abundance of various CRC-associated pathobionts including *Peptostreptococcus anaerobius* (Yachida et al. 2019). Similar to *F. nucleatum*, *P. anaerobius* also contributes CRC progression via immunomodulation of which its surface protein PCWBR2 could directly interact with epithelial cell receptor α2/β1-integrin to initiate oncogenic and inflammatory PI3K-AKT-NF-$_{\kappa}$B signalling cascade (Long et al. 2019).

Apart from direct interplays between microbial virulent factors and host cells, several bacteria promote tumourigenesis by producing toxins. For example, enterotoxigenic *Bacteroides fragilis* can secrete enterotoxin to accelerate colonic tumour growth in mice through activating STAT3- and T_H17-dependent inflammatory response (Wu et al. 2009). These signalling pathways in turn induce CXC chemokines to recruit polymorphonuclear immature myeloid cells, creating a pro-inflammatory microenvironment in mice colon (Chung et al. 2018). Another example of toxigenic CRC-associated bacteria is *Escherichia coli*. A strain of *E. coli* with expression of the *pks* genomic island can secrete genotoxic metabolite colibactin to cause immunosuppression (Dalmasso et al. 2014) and promote oncogenic mutation (Pleguezuelos-Manzano et al. 2020).

2.4.2 Distant Effects of Gut Microbiome on Liver and Pancreatic Cancer

Given that human liver and pancreas are anatomically connected to the intestines, they are readily influenced by the gut microbiome. The association of gut dysbiosis with cancer in liver (e.g. hepatocellular carcinoma (HCC)) and pancreas (e.g. pancreatic ductal adenocarcinoma (PDAC)) has been increasingly acknowledged (Yu and Schwabe 2017; Thomas and Jobin 2020). In general, dysbiosis can damage the gut barrier to enhance intestinal permeability, allowing more bacterial endotoxins particularly LPS to enter the circulation (Gabele et al. 2011). LPS is classically recognised by the pattern recognition receptor TLR4 which is widely present in multiple hepatic cell types. For instance, high circulating LPS level could activate TLR4 on hepatocytes and hepatic stellate cells to promote fibrogenesis and hepatocarcinogenesis through upregulating NF-$_{\kappa}$B signalling cascade (Dapito et al. 2012). Activation of the LPS-TLR4 signalling pathway in Kupffer cells could also lead to TNF- and IL-6-dependent compensatory hepatocyte proliferation as well as reduced apoptosis to accelerate HCC development (Yu et al. 2010).

Besides microbial components, the entire microbes can be migrated from the intestine to the pancreas, as evidenced by gavaging mice with fluorescently labelled bacteria (Pushalkar et al. 2018). Indeed, a clinical study reported the presence of *Gammaproteobacteria* in PDAC tumours, whereas these intratumoural bacteria could metabolise the active form of chemotherapeutic drug gemcitabine to decrease its efficacy and promote drug resistance (Geller et al. 2017). Two subsequent studies in 2018 investigated the role of pancreatic microbiome in PDAC progression using transgenic mouse models, yet inconsistent results were reported (Pushalkar et al. 2018; Thomas et al. 2018). Pushalkar et al. revealed that alteration in pancreatic microbiome composition is stage-specific and could drive tumourigenesis by suppressing CD8+ T cell activation and other anticancer immune responses (Pushalkar et al. 2018). While Thomas et al. found that only microbes indigenous to the gut but not the pancreas have immunoinhibitory capacity to promote pancreatic tumourigenesis (Thomas et al. 2018). Similarly, there has been controversy over the existence of microbiome in the liver tissue. Although a recent study identified that patients with non-alcoholic fatty liver disease (a risk factor of HCC) contain bacterial DNA in their liver, it remains uncertain whether these DNA signatures are attributed to live bacteria or bacterial debris from immune cells (Sookoian et al. 2020).

Gut dysbiosis can also interrupt the bile acid metabolism. Secondary bile acids are normally derived from *Clostridium*-mediated 7α-dehydroxylation (Jia et al. 2018). Yet, under dysbiotic condition induced by high-fat diet, *Clostridium* was found to be enriched in mice, leading to overproduction of deoxycholic acid (Loo et al. 2017). Accumulation of deoxycholic acid then stimulates the TLR2 pathway and causes COX2 overexpression and prostaglandin E2 overproduction in hepatic stellate cells, thereby suppressing anticancer immunity and accelerating HCC development. In another mice study, *Clostridium* depletion by antibiotics could increase CXCL16 expression in liver sinusoidal endothelial cells, resulting in accumulation of interferon-γ-producing natural killer T cells which contributes to inhibition of liver tumour growth (Ma et al. 2018). Moreover, increased level of deoxycholic acid in the gut could disrupt the intestinal barrier, allowing more pathobionts and their components to enter the circulation and reach the hepatopancreatic system (Liu et al. 2018).

2.5 Current Limitations and Future Perspective

Although being extensively studied, to date there is still no universally accepted definition of a "healthy" gut microbiome. Health is a relative condition of which a microbiome could be normal in one person but pathogenic in another person. More work is therefore suggested to decipher how the gut microbiome varies among apparently healthy people, how it changes with age, and the effects of different environmental factors including diet, medications, ethnicity, and lifestyle (Shanahan et al. 2021). Meanwhile, given the substantial number of publications, inconsistent results are inevitably reported which could be attributed by the differences in sample collection, sequencing technology, and bioinformatic pipelines among studies (Knight et al. 2018; Costea et al. 2017). To reduce inter-study variations and ensure reproducibility, an expert consensus in 2019 stated the necessity of standardisation and transparency in reporting microbiome research (Scott et al. 2019). On the other hand, a systematic review in 2020 reported the unrealistic high rate of pathologies being transferred from human gut microbiome to rodents among publications (95%), hence the authors expressed their concerns as current mechanistic findings may overstate the role of microbiome in human diseases (Walter et al. 2020). In general, a more rigorous approach of both bioinformatic analysis and functional investigation is required worldwide to avoid false concepts.

Apart from bacteria, the gut microbiome contains microbes from other taxonomic kingdoms including fungi and viruses. However, research on these non-bacterial microbes has been heavily obstructed due to their relatively low abundance in human gut and lack of well-characterised reference genomes for aligning sequencing reads (Underhill and Iliev 2014; Shkoporov et al. 2019). Recent studies have revealed their crucial roles in health and disease. For example, the fungal community in human gut is closely associated with the host metabolic health through regulating gut bacterial functions and metabolites (Shuai et al. 2022). Whereas translocation of gut fungi to the pancreas could promote PDAC development (Aykut et al. 2019). Currently, various approaches of microbiome modulation particularly faecal microbiota transplantation (FMT) receive increasing attention which have shown their therapeutic potential against cancer (Cheng et al. 2020; Lau et al. 2021). Of note, FMT not only transfers bacteria but also other microbes including fungi and viruses from donors to recipients, yet their roles and effects to host remain unclear which may bring safety concerns. In conclusion, while there are still many challenges on the horizon, great promise lies ahead to advance the field through extensive investigations with next-generation bioinformatic and experimental technologies.

References

Allali I, Delgado S, Marron PI, Astudillo A, Yeh JJ, Ghazal H, et al. Gut microbiome compositional and functional differences between tumor and non-tumor adjacent tissues from cohorts from the US and Spain. Gut Microbes. 2015;6(3):161–72.

Arpaia N, Campbell C, Fan X, Dikiy S, van der Veeken J, deRoos P, et al. Metabolites produced by commensal bacteria promote peripheral regulatory T-cell generation. Nature. 2013;504(7480):451–5.

Atarashi K, Tanoue T, Oshima K, Suda W, Nagano Y, Nishikawa H, et al. Treg induction by a rationally selected mixture of Clostridia strains from the human microbiota. Nature. 2013;500(7461):232–6.

Aykut B, Pushalkar S, Chen R, Li Q, Abengozar R, Kim JI, et al. The fungal mycobiome promotes pancreatic oncogenesis via activation of MBL. Nature. 2019;574(7777):264–7.

Bachem A, Makhlouf C, Binger KJ, de Souza DP, Tull D, Hochheiser K, et al. Microbiota-derived short-chain fatty acids promote the memory potential of antigen-activated CD8(+) T cells. Immunity. 2019;51(2):285–297.e5.

Belkaid Y, Hand TW. Role of the microbiota in immunity and inflammation. Cell. 2014;157(1):121–41.

Booijink CC, El-Aidy S, Rajilic-Stojanovic M, Heilig HG, Troost FJ, Smidt H, et al. High temporal and inter-individual variation detected in the human ileal microbiota. Environ Microbiol. 2010;12(12):3213–27.

Browne HP, Forster SC, Anonye BO, Kumar N, Neville BA, Stares MD, et al. Culturing of 'unculturable' human microbiota reveals novel taxa and extensive sporulation. Nature. 2016;533(7604):543–6.

Bunker JJ, Erickson SA, Flynn TM, Henry C, Koval JC, Meisel M, et al. Natural polyreactive IgA antibodies coat the intestinal microbiota. Science. 2017;358(6361):eaan6619.

Burgueno JF, Fritsch J, Gonzalez EE, Landau KS, Santander AM, Fernandez I, et al. Epithelial TLR4 signaling activates DUOX2 to induce microbiota-driven tumorigenesis. Gastroenterology. 2021;160(3):797–808.e6.

Canfora EE, Jocken JW, Blaak EE. Short-chain fatty acids in control of body weight and insulin sensitivity. Nat Rev Endocrinol. 2015;11(10):577–91.

Cheng WY, Wu CY, Yu J. The role of gut microbiota in cancer treatment: friend or foe? Gut. 2020;69(10):1867–76.

Choi IJ, Kook MC, Kim YI, Cho SJ, Lee JY, Kim CG, et al. Helicobacter pylori therapy for the prevention of metachronous gastric cancer. N Engl J Med. 2018;378(12):1085–95.

Chung L, Thiele Orberg E, Geis AL, Chan JL, Fu K, DeStefano Shields CE, et al. Bacteroides fragilis toxin coordinates a pro-carcinogenic inflammatory cascade via targeting of colonic epithelial cells. Cell Host Microbe. 2018;23(2):203–214.e5.

Coker OO, Dai Z, Nie Y, Zhao G, Cao L, Nakatsu G, et al. Mucosal microbiome dysbiosis in gastric carcinogenesis. Gut. 2018;67(6):1024–32.

Costea PI, Zeller G, Sunagawa S, Pelletier E, Alberti A, Levenez F, et al. Towards standards for human fecal sample processing in metagenomic studies. Nat Biotechnol. 2017;35(11):1069–76.

Cotillard A, Kennedy SP, Kong LC, Prifti E, Pons N, Le Chatelier E, et al. Dietary intervention impact on gut microbial gene richness. Nature. 2013;500(7464):585–8.

Dai Z, Coker OO, Nakatsu G, Wu WKK, Zhao L, Chen Z, et al. Multi-cohort analysis of colorectal cancer metagenome identified altered bacteria across populations and universal bacterial markers. Microbiome. 2018;6(1):70.

Dalmasso G, Cougnoux A, Delmas J, Darfeuille-Michaud A, Bonnet R. The bacterial genotoxin colibactin promotes colon tumor growth by modifying the tumor microenvironment. Gut Microbes. 2014;5(5):675–80.

Dapito DH, Mencin A, Gwak GY, Pradere JP, Jang MK, Mederacke I, et al. Promotion of hepatocellular carcinoma by the intestinal microbiota and TLR4. Cancer Cell. 2012;21(4):504–16.

de Assumpcao PP, Araujo TMT, de Assumpcao PB, Barra WF, Khayat AS, Assumpcao CB, et al. Suicide journey of H. pylori through gastric carcinogenesis: the role of non-H. pylori microbiome and potential consequences for clinical practice. Eur J Clin Microbiol Infect Dis. 2019;38(9):1591–7.

Dimidi E, Christodoulides S, Scott SM, Whelan K. Mechanisms of action of probiotics and the gastrointestinal microbiota on gut motility and constipation. Adv Nutr. 2017;8(3):484–94.

Ferreira RM, Pereira-Marques J, Pinto-Ribeiro I, Costa JL, Carneiro F, Machado JC, et al. Gastric microbial community profiling reveals a dysbiotic cancer-associated microbiota. Gut. 2018;67(2):226–36.

Flemer B, Lynch DB, Brown JM, Jeffery IB, Ryan FJ, Claesson MJ, et al. Tumour-associated and non-tumour-associated microbiota in colorectal cancer. Gut. 2017;66(4):633–43.

Fransen F, Zagato E, Mazzini E, Fosso B, Manzari C, El Aidy S, et al. BALB/c and C57BL/6 mice differ in polyreactive IgA abundance, which impacts the generation of antigen-specific IgA and microbiota diversity. Immunity. 2015;43(3):527–40.

Friedman ES, Bittinger K, Esipova TV, Hou L, Chau L, Jiang J, et al. Microbes vs. chemistry in the origin of the anaerobic gut lumen. Proc Natl Acad Sci U S A. 2018;115(16):4170–5.

Furusawa Y, Obata Y, Fukuda S, Endo TA, Nakato G, Takahashi D, et al. Commensal microbe-derived butyrate induces the differentiation of colonic regulatory T cells. Nature. 2013;504(7480):446–50.

Gabele E, Dostert K, Hofmann C, Wiest R, Scholmerich J, Hellerbrand C, et al. DSS induced colitis increases portal LPS levels and enhances hepatic inflammation and fibrogenesis in experimental NASH. J Hepatol. 2011;55(6):1391–9.

Gaboriau-Routhiau V, Rakotobe S, Lecuyer E, Mulder I, Lan A, Bridonneau C, et al. The key role of segmented filamentous bacteria in the coordinated maturation of gut helper T cell responses. Immunity. 2009;31(4):677–89.

Gaudino SJ, Kumar P. Cross-talk between antigen presenting cells and T cells impacts intestinal homeostasis, bacterial infections, and tumorigenesis. Front Immunol. 2019;10:360.

Geller LT, Barzily-Rokni M, Danino T, Jonas OH, Shental N, Nejman D, et al. Potential role of intratumor bacteria in mediating tumor resistance to the chemotherapeutic drug gemcitabine. Science. 2017;357(6356):1156–60.

Geva-Zatorsky N, Sefik E, Kua L, Pasman L, Tan TG, Ortiz-Lopez A, et al. Mining the human gut microbiota for immunomodulatory organisms. Cell. 2017;168(5):928–43.e11.

Grider JR, Piland BE. The peristaltic reflex induced by short-chain fatty acids is mediated by sequential release of 5-HT and neuronal CGRP but not BDNF. Am J Physiol Gastrointest Liver Physiol. 2007;292(1):G429–37.

Grivennikov SI, Wang K, Mucida D, Stewart CA, Schnabl B, Jauch D, et al. Adenoma-linked barrier defects and microbial products drive IL-23/IL-17-mediated tumour growth. Nature. 2012;491(7423):254–8.

Guo S, Chen J, Chen F, Zeng Q, Liu WL, Zhang G. Exosomes derived from Fusobacterium nucleatum-infected colorectal cancer cells facilitate tumour metastasis by selectively carrying miR-1246/92b-3p/27a-3p and CXCL16. Gut. 2020.

Gupta R, Gupta N, Rathi P. Bacterial lipases: an overview of production, purification and biochemical properties. Appl Microbiol Biotechnol. 2004;64(6):763–81.

Hegade VS, Speight RA, Etherington RE, Jones DE. Novel bile acid therapeutics for the treatment of chronic liver diseases. Ther Adv Gastroenterol. 2016;9(3):376–91.

Hsu RY, Chan CH, Spicer JD, Rousseau MC, Giannias B, Rousseau S, et al. LPS-induced TLR4 signaling in human colorectal cancer cells increases beta1 integrin-mediated cell adhesion and liver metastasis. Cancer Res. 2011;71(5):1989–98.

Human Microbiome Project Consortium. Structure, function and diversity of the healthy human microbiome. Nature. 2012;486(7402):207–14.

Ivanov II, Atarashi K, Manel N, Brodie EL, Shima T, Karaoz U, et al. Induction of intestinal Th17 cells by segmented filamentous bacteria. Cell. 2009;139(3):485–98.

Jia W, Xie G, Jia W. Bile acid-microbiota crosstalk in gastrointestinal inflammation and carcinogenesis. Nat Rev Gastroenterol Hepatol. 2018;15(2):111–28.

Kashyap PC, Marcobal A, Ursell LK, Larauche M, Duboc H, Earle KA, et al. Complex interactions among diet, gastrointestinal transit, and gut microbiota in humanized mice. Gastroenterology. 2013;144(5):967–77.

Knight R, Vrbanac A, Taylor BC, Aksenov A, Callewaert C, Debelius J, et al. Best practices for analysing microbiomes. Nat Rev Microbiol. 2018;16(7):410–22.

Koh A, De Vadder F, Kovatcheva-Datchary P, Backhed F. From dietary fiber to host physiology: short-chain fatty acids as key bacterial metabolites. Cell. 2016;165(6):1332–45.

Kostic AD, Chun E, Robertson L, Glickman JN, Gallini CA, Michaud M, et al. Fusobacterium nucleatum potentiates intestinal tumorigenesis and modulates the tumor-immune microenvironment. Cell Host Microbe. 2013;14(2):207–15.

Kurilshikov A, Medina-Gomez C, Bacigalupe R, Radjabzadeh D, Wang J, Demirkan A, et al. Large-scale association analyses identify host factors influencing human gut microbiome composition. Nat Genet. 2021;53(2):156–65.
Lau HCH, Sung JJ, Yu J. Gut microbiota: impacts on gastrointestinal cancer immunotherapy. Gut Microbes. 2021;13(1):1–21.
Lema I, Araujo JR, Rolhion N, Demignot S. Jejunum: the understudied meeting place of dietary lipids and the microbiota. Biochimie. 2020;178:124–36.
Levy M, Kolodziejczyk AA, Thaiss CA, Elinav E. Dysbiosis and the immune system. Nat Rev Immunol. 2017;17(4):219–32.
Li G, Yang M, Zhou K, Zhang L, Tian L, Lv S, et al. Diversity of duodenal and rectal microbiota in biopsy tissues and luminal contents in healthy volunteers. J Microbiol Biotechnol. 2015;25(7):1136–45.
Liu L, Dong W, Wang S, Zhang Y, Liu T, Xie R, et al. Deoxycholic acid disrupts the intestinal mucosal barrier and promotes intestinal tumorigenesis. Food Funct. 2018;9(11):5588–97.
Liu W, Zhang X, Xu H, Li S, Lau HC, Chen Q, et al. Microbial community heterogeneity within colorectal neoplasia and its correlation with colorectal carcinogenesis. Gastroenterology. 2021;160(7):2395–408.
Lloyd-Price J, Abu-Ali G, Huttenhower C. The healthy human microbiome. Genome Med. 2016;8(1):51.
Long X, Wong CC, Tong L, Chu ESH, Ho Szeto C, Go MYY, et al. Peptostreptococcus anaerobius promotes colorectal carcinogenesis and modulates tumour immunity. Nat Microbiol. 2019;4(12):2319–30.
Loo TM, Kamachi F, Watanabe Y, Yoshimoto S, Kanda H, Arai Y, et al. Gut microbiota promotes obesity-associated liver cancer through PGE2-mediated suppression of antitumor immunity. Cancer Discov. 2017;7(5):522–38.
Lozupone CA, Stombaugh JI, Gordon JI, Jansson JK, Knight R. Diversity, stability and resilience of the human gut microbiota. Nature. 2012;489(7415):220–30.
Ma C, Han M, Heinrich B, Fu Q, Zhang Q, Sandhu M, et al. Gut microbiome-mediated bile acid metabolism regulates liver cancer via NKT cells. Science. 2018;360(6391):eaan5931.
Manasian P, Bustos AS, Palsson B, Hakansson A, Penarrieta JM, Nilsson L, et al. First evidence of acyl-hydrolase/lipase activity from human probiotic bacteria: Lactobacillus rhamnosus GG and Bifidobacterium longum NCC 2705. Front Microbiol. 2020;11:1534.
Martinez-Guryn K, Hubert N, Frazier K, Urlass S, Musch MW, Ojeda P, et al. Small intestine microbiota regulate host digestive and absorptive adaptive responses to dietary lipids. Cell Host Microbe. 2018;23(4):458–469.e5.
Martinez-Guryn K, Leone V, Chang EB. Regional diversity of the gastrointestinal microbiome. Cell Host Microbe. 2019;26(3):314–24.
Matson V, Chervin CS, Gajewski TF. Cancer and the microbiome-influence of the commensal microbiota on cancer, immune responses, and immunotherapy. Gastroenterology. 2021;160(2):600–13.
May M, Abrams JA. Emerging insights into the esophageal microbiome. Curr Treat Options Gastroenterol. 2018;16(1):72–85.
McCarville JL, Chen GY, Cuevas VD, Troha K, Ayres JS. Microbiota metabolites in health and disease. Annu Rev Immunol. 2020;38:147–70.
Mima K, Sukawa Y, Nishihara R, Qian ZR, Yamauchi M, Inamura K, et al. Fusobacterium nucleatum and T cells in colorectal carcinoma. JAMA Oncol. 2015;1(5):653–61.
Nardone G, Compare D. The human gastric microbiota: is it time to rethink the pathogenesis of stomach diseases? United Eur Gastroenterol J. 2015;3(3):255–60.
Nejman D, Livyatan I, Fuks G, Gavert N, Zwang Y, Geller LT, et al. The human tumor microbiome is composed of tumor type-specific intracellular bacteria. Science. 2020;368(6494):973–80.
Nobel YR, Snider EJ, Compres G, Freedberg DE, Khiabanian H, Lightdale CJ, et al. Increasing dietary fiber intake is associated with a distinct esophageal microbiome. Clin Transl Gastroenterol. 2018;9(10):199.

O'Hara AM, Shanahan F. The gut flora as a forgotten organ. EMBO Rep. 2006;7(7):688–93.
Ogawa A, Kobayashi T, Sakai F, Kadooka Y, Kawasaki Y. Lactobacillus gasseri SBT2055 suppresses fatty acid release through enlargement of fat emulsion size in vitro and promotes fecal fat excretion in healthy Japanese subjects. Lipids Health Dis. 2015;14:20.
Palm NW, de Zoete MR, Cullen TW, Barry NA, Stefanowski J, Hao L, et al. Immunoglobulin A coating identifies colitogenic bacteria in inflammatory bowel disease. Cell. 2014;158(5):1000–10.
Pleguezuelos-Manzano C, Puschhof J, Rosendahl Huber A, van Hoeck A, Wood HM, Nomburg J, et al. Mutational signature in colorectal cancer caused by genotoxic pks(+) E. coli. Nature. 2020;580(7802):269–73.
Pushalkar S, Hundeyin M, Daley D, Zambirinis CP, Kurz E, Mishra A, et al. The pancreatic cancer microbiome promotes oncogenesis by induction of innate and adaptive immune suppression. Cancer Discov. 2018;8(4):403–16.
Rebollar E, Arruebo MP, Plaza MA, Murillo MD. Effect of lipopolysaccharide on rabbit small intestine muscle contractility in vitro: role of prostaglandins. Neurogastroenterol Motil. 2002;14(6):633–42.
Ridlon JM, Harris SC, Bhowmik S, Kang DJ, Hylemon PB. Consequences of bile salt biotransformations by intestinal bacteria. Gut Microbes. 2016;7(1):22–39.
Rocha-Ramirez LM, Perez-Solano RA, Castanon-Alonso SL, Moreno Guerrero SS, Ramirez Pacheco A, Garcia Garibay M, et al. Probiotic Lactobacillus strains stimulate the inflammatory response and activate human macrophages. J Immunol Res. 2017;2017:4607491.
Rooks MG, Garrett WS. Gut microbiota, metabolites and host immunity. Nat Rev Immunol. 2016;16(6):341–52.
Rothschild D, Weissbrod O, Barkan E, Kurilshikov A, Korem T, Zeevi D, et al. Environment dominates over host genetics in shaping human gut microbiota. Nature. 2018;555(7695):210–5.
Round JL, Mazmanian SK. The gut microbiota shapes intestinal immune responses during health and disease. Nat Rev Immunol. 2009;9(5):313–23.
Round JL, Mazmanian SK. Inducible Foxp3+ regulatory T-cell development by a commensal bacterium of the intestinal microbiota. Proc Natl Acad Sci U S A. 2010;107(27):12204–9.
Rubinstein MR, Wang X, Liu W, Hao Y, Cai G, Han YW. Fusobacterium nucleatum promotes colorectal carcinogenesis by modulating E-cadherin/beta-catenin signaling via its FadA adhesin. Cell Host Microbe. 2013;14(2):195–206.
Sahasakul Y, Takemura N, Sonoyama K. Different impacts of purified and nonpurified diets on microbiota and toll-like receptors in the mouse stomach. Biosci Biotechnol Biochem. 2012;76(9):1728–32.
Scott AJ, Alexander JL, Merrifield CA, Cunningham D, Jobin C, Brown R, et al. International Cancer Microbiome Consortium consensus statement on the role of the human microbiome in carcinogenesis. Gut. 2019;68(9):1624–32.
Seekatz AM, Schnizlein MK, Koenigsknecht MJ, Baker JR, Hasler WL, Bleske BE, et al. Spatial and temporal analysis of the stomach and small-intestinal microbiota in fasted healthy humans. mSphere. 2019;4(2):e00126–19.
Shanahan F, Ghosh TS, O'Toole PW. The healthy microbiome-what is the definition of a healthy gut microbiome? Gastroenterology. 2021;160(2):483–94.
Shkoporov AN, Clooney AG, Sutton TDS, Ryan FJ, Daly KM, Nolan JA, et al. The human gut virome is highly diverse, stable, and individual specific. Cell Host Microbe. 2019;26(4):527–41 e5.
Shuai M, Fu Y, Zhong HL, Gou W, Jiang Z, Liang Y, et al. Mapping the human gut mycobiome in middle-aged and elderly adults: multiomics insights and implications for host metabolic health. Gut. 2022;71(9):1812–20.
Sookoian S, Salatino A, Castano GO, Landa MS, Fijalkowky C, Garaycoechea M, et al. Intrahepatic bacterial metataxonomic signature in non-alcoholic fatty liver disease. Gut. 2020;69(8):1483–91.
Sundin OH, Mendoza-Ladd A, Zeng M, Diaz-Arevalo D, Morales E, Fagan BM, et al. The human jejunum has an endogenous microbiota that differs from those in the oral cavity and colon. BMC Microbiol. 2017;17(1):160.

Sung JJY, Coker OO, Chu E, Szeto CH, Luk STY, Lau HCH, et al. Gastric microbes associated with gastric inflammation, atrophy and intestinal metaplasia 1 year after Helicobacter pylori eradication. Gut. 2020;69(9):1572–80.

Tamboli CP, Neut C, Desreumaux P, Colombel JF. Dysbiosis in inflammatory bowel disease. Gut. 2004;53(1):1–4.

Thomas RM, Jobin C. Microbiota in pancreatic health and disease: the next frontier in microbiome research. Nat Rev Gastroenterol Hepatol. 2020;17(1):53–64.

Thomas RM, Gharaibeh RZ, Gauthier J, Beveridge M, Pope JL, Guijarro MV, et al. Intestinal microbiota enhances pancreatic carcinogenesis in preclinical models. Carcinogenesis. 2018;39(8):1068–78.

Underhill DM, Iliev ID. The mycobiota: interactions between commensal fungi and the host immune system. Nat Rev Immunol. 2014;14(6):405–16.

Uronis JM, Muhlbauer M, Herfarth HH, Rubinas TC, Jones GS, Jobin C. Modulation of the intestinal microbiota alters colitis-associated colorectal cancer susceptibility. PLoS One. 2009;4(6):e6026.

Vinasco K, Mitchell HM, Kaakoush NO, Castano-Rodriguez N. Microbial carcinogenesis: lactic acid bacteria in gastric cancer. Biochim Biophys Acta Rev Cancer. 2019;1872(2):188309.

Walter J, Armet AM, Finlay BB, Shanahan F. Establishing or exaggerating causality for the gut microbiome: lessons from human microbiota-associated rodents. Cell. 2020;180(2):221–32.

Wang ZK, Yang YS. Upper gastrointestinal microbiota and digestive diseases. World J Gastroenterol. 2013;19(10):1541–50.

Wang F, Meng W, Wang B, Qiao L. Helicobacter pylori-induced gastric inflammation and gastric cancer. Cancer Lett. 2014;345(2):196–202.

Wen J, Lau HC, Peppelenbosch M, Yu J. Gastric microbiota beyond H. pylori: an emerging critical character in gastric carcinogenesis. Biomedicine. 2021;9(11):1680.

Wroblewski LE, Peek RM Jr, Wilson KT. Helicobacter pylori and gastric cancer: factors that modulate disease risk. Clin Microbiol Rev. 2010;23(4):713–39.

Wu S, Rhee KJ, Albesiano E, Rabizadeh S, Wu X, Yen HR, et al. A human colonic commensal promotes colon tumorigenesis via activation of T helper type 17 T cell responses. Nat Med. 2009;15(9):1016–22.

Wu Y, Shi L, Li Q, Wu J, Peng W, Li H, et al. Microbiota diversity in human colorectal cancer tissues is associated with clinicopathological features. Nutr Cancer. 2019;71(2):214–22.

Wu SE, Hashimoto-Hill S, Woo V, Eshleman EM, Whitt J, Engleman L, et al. Microbiota-derived metabolite promotes HDAC3 activity in the gut. Nature. 2020;586(7827):108–12.

Yachida S, Mizutani S, Shiroma H, Shiba S, Nakajima T, Sakamoto T, et al. Metagenomic and metabolomic analyses reveal distinct stage-specific phenotypes of the gut microbiota in colorectal cancer. Nat Med. 2019;25(6):968–76.

Yu LX, Schwabe RF. The gut microbiome and liver cancer: mechanisms and clinical translation. Nat Rev Gastroenterol Hepatol. 2017;14(9):527–39.

Yu LX, Yan HX, Liu Q, Yang W, Wu HP, Dong W, et al. Endotoxin accumulation prevents carcinogen-induced apoptosis and promotes liver tumorigenesis in rodents. Hepatology. 2010;52(4):1322–33.

Yu T, Guo F, Yu Y, Sun T, Ma D, Han J, et al. Fusobacterium nucleatum promotes chemoresistance to colorectal cancer by modulating autophagy. Cell. 2017;170(3):548–563.e16.

Chapter 3
Microbiome in Colorectal Cancer

Pingmei Huang and Chi Chun Wong

Abstract Colorectal cancer (CRC) is one of the most common cancer worldwide. A vast majority of CRC are sporadic in nature and heavily influenced by environmental factors. The gut microbiome forms an essential part of the colonic microenvironment and contributes to gut homeostasis. Recent work has highlighted the important role of the gut microbiome in modulating CRC initiation and progression. Gut dysbiosis, characterized by enriched pathogenic bacteria, promotes colorectal tumorigenesis by inducing cell proliferation and eliciting an inflammatory microenvironment. Counteracting these pro-tumorigenic effects are the beneficial commensals, which secrete antitumor metabolites or proteins, restore gut barrier function, and suppress colonic inflammation. Molecular mechanisms involved in gut microbiome-host interplay are diverse, including interaction via surface receptors, generation of bacterial metabolites/proteins, regulation of host immunity, and modulation of gut microbial communities. The further characterization of gut microbial species involved in CRC could lead to the development of novel microbial biomarkers for CRC diagnosis and microbial-based therapy for CRC prevention and treatment. In this book chapter, we will provide an overview on the role of bacterial, viral, and fungal species in CRC pathogenesis, their underlying molecular mechanisms and translational applications.

Keywords Colorectal cancer · Microbiome · Cancer diagnosis · Cancer therapy

---

P. Huang
Institute of Digestive Disease and Department of Medicine and Therapeutics, State Key Laboratory of Digestive Disease, Li Ka Shing Institute of Health Sciences, The Chinese University of Hong Kong, Hong Kong, China

C. C. Wong (✉)
Institute of Digestive Disease and Department of Medicine and Therapeutics, State Key Laboratory of Digestive Disease, Li Ka Shing Institute of Health Sciences, The Chinese University of Hong Kong, Hong Kong, China

Department of Medicine and Therapeutics, Prince of Wales Hospital, The Chinese University of Hong Kong, Hong Kong, China
e-mail: chichunwong@cuhk.edu.hk

J. Yu (ed.), *Microbiome in Gastrointestinal Cancer*,
https://doi.org/10.1007/978-981-19-4492-5_3

3.1 Introduction

Due to accumulating evidence indicating that microorganisms have a major influence on human physiology, scientists are now paying much more attention to the underlying role of gut microbiome in tumorigenesis, especially for colorectal cancer (CRC). The colonization of microbiota begins at the newborn gastrointestinal tract on early life and coevolves concomitantly with the host throughout development (Dominguez-Bello et al. 2019; Backhed et al. 2015). Establishment and maintenance of a dynamic and stable gut microbiota are believed to be beneficial for human health (Sommer et al. 2017). On the other hand, the disruption of this ecosystem, which is termed dysbiosis, could become a threat to the health of the host, as it is associated with various diseases ranging from gastrointestinal disorders to neurologic, respiratory, metabolic, hepatic, and cardiovascular illnesses (Lynch and Pedersen 2016). Given the intimate interaction of the colonic epithelium with the gut microbiota, it is perhaps unsurprising that the gut microbiome has a central role in promotion or suppression of CRC development. In this chapter, we will first provide a brief overview of microbial function in host biology and then dissect the role of microbial dysbiosis in colorectal tumorigenesis. Finally, we will discuss the potential clinical applications of microbiome in CRC prevention and treatment.

3.2 Microbiota in Human Biology

The microbiome encompasses the genes and genomes of microbiota, including bacteria, archaea, fungi, virus, and algae, and their products such as structural elements, secreted proteins and metabolites, which form an ecosystem together with the host environment (Berg et al. 2020; Whiteside et al. 2015). An enormous number of microbes resides in the human gut, and the bacteria cells and genomes are approximately outnumbered the humans by an estimated 10-fold and 150-fold, respectively (Wu and Lewis 2013). Despite remarkable individual variety in human microbiota composition and distribution (Human Microbiome Project Consortium 2012; Manor et al. 2020), the gut microflora residing in the gastrointestinal tract plays similar roles in maintaining host homeostasis. For instance, representative bacteria inhabiting in our body, like the *Bacteroidetes*, *Firmicutes,* and *Proteobacteria*, involved in biological processes of the host, which include non-digestible carbohydrate fermentation (Louis and Flint 2017), energy harvest and utilization (Turnbaugh et al. 2006), nutrient absorption and vitamin biosynthesis (Hooper et al. 2001; Funabashi et al. 2020; LeBlanc et al. 2013), xenobiotic and drug metabolization (Collins and Patterson 2020), immunity construction and regulation (Schirmer et al. 2016; Belkaid and Hand 2014). Apart from bacteria, other microorganisms including archaea, fungi, and viruses, as part of the microbial community, might also contribute to the well-being of host.

3.3 Association of Microbiome and CRC

Colorectal cancer (CRC) is one of the most prevalent malignant carcinomas around the world. CRC is the third most common cancer, and is the second in terms of mortality in 2020 (Sung et al. 2021). Overall incidence rates in CRC are higher in proximal colon as compared to distal colon (Siegel et al. 2020). Classically, risk factors for sporadic CRC include a high frequency of genetic mutations (e.g., *KRAS*, *TP53*, and *APC*) (Kudryavtseva et al. 2016) and environmental factors such as smoking, an unhealthy diet, high alcohol consumption, physical inactivity, obesity, etc. (Siegel et al. 2020). Alterations in gut bacteria communities have been documented by metagenomic studies, and such changes are stage- and location-specific. Compositional alterations in the microbiota are already present in the adenoma samples and they continue to evolve in the progression to cancer stage. Apart from gut bacteria, emerging evidence suggests that the enteric mycobiome and virome dysbiosis are also present in CRC (Coker et al. 2019; Nakatsu et al. 2018). The causality of gut dysbiosis in colorectal tumorigenesis was recently established, as fecal microbiota transplantation (FMT) from cancer patients could promote pro-tumorigenic response in conventional mice and germ-free mice (Wong et al. 2017a). Taken together, gut dysbiosis is an important contributing factor to CRC initiation and progression.

3.4 Role of Individual Gut Bacteria in CRC

Major CRC microbiome characterization efforts using 16S ribosomal RNA (rRNA) and shotgun metagenomic sequencing in stool and tumor samples have strongly linked the microbial dysbiosis to CRC. This is reflected by reduction in bacterial diversity in CRC patients and healthy subjects, associated with (1) the enrichment of pathogenic bacteria (Fig. 3.1) and (2) depletion of probiotics (Fig. 3.2).

3.4.1 Opportunistic Pathogens in Promoting CRC

Recently, several pathogenic bacteria, *F. nucleatum*, *Peptostreptococcus anaerobius* (*P. anaerobius*), enterotoxigenic *Bacteroides fragilis* (ETBF), *pks*$^{+}$ *Escherichia coli* (*E. coli*), *Porphyromonas gingivalis* (*P. gingivalis*) have been reported to promote CRC by diverse mechanisms (Fig. 3.1), as detailed below:

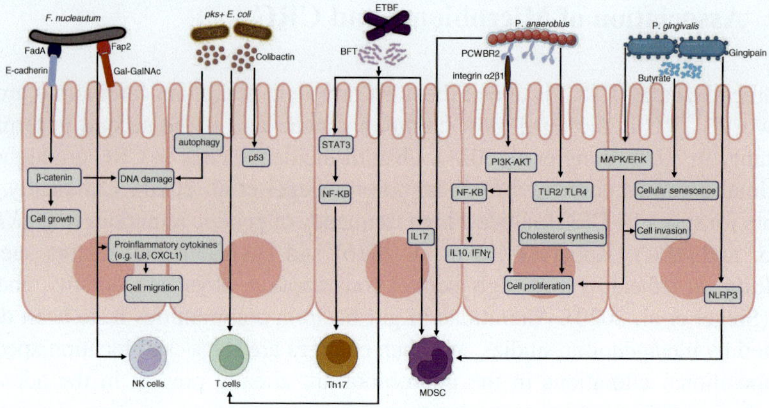

Fig. 3.1 Opportunistic pathogens in promoting CRC. Several reported pathogenic bacteria have been reported to promote CRC, which involved the direct interaction of bacterial surface proteins with CRC cell receptors, production of virulence factors that trigger DNA damage, promotion of an inflammatory microenvironment, and secretion of toxins or oncogenic metabolites. *FadA* Fusobacterium nucleatum adhesin A, *Fap2* F. nucleatum autotransporter protein 2, *IL8* interleukin 8, *BFT* Bacteroides fragilis toxin, *Th17* T helper cell 17, *IL17* interleukin 17, *MDSC* myeloid-derived suppresser cell, *PCWBR2* putative cell wall binding repeat 2, *IL10* interleukin 10, *IFNγ* interferon γ, *TLR2/TLR4* toll-like receptor 2/toll-like receptor 4, *NLRP3* nucleotide-binding oligomerization domain receptor and pyrin domain containing 3

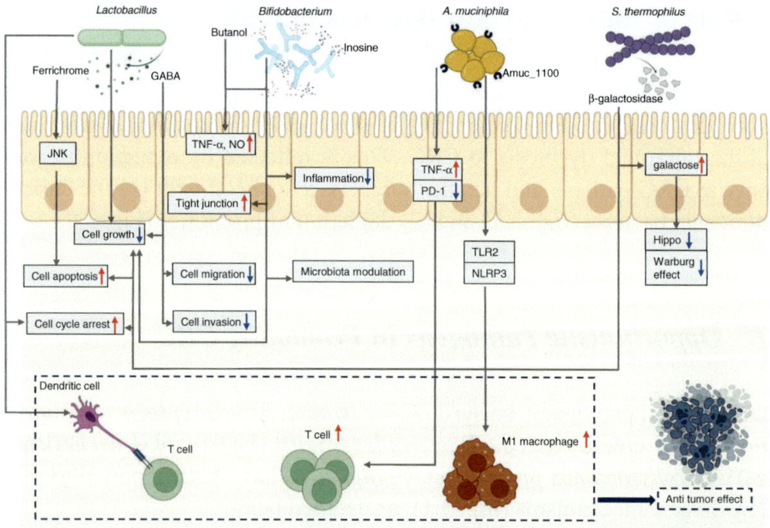

Fig. 3.2 Probiotics that are protective against CRC. Probiotics have been shown to exert tumor suppression by the secretion of tumor suppressive metabolites or proteins, the restoration of gut barrier function, modulation of the gut immune response, as well as by antagonizing pathogenic bacteria and their communities. *GABA* γ-aminobutyric acid, *JNK* c-Jun N-terminal kinase, *NLRP3* NLR family pyrin domain containing 3, *NO* nitric oxide, *PD-1* programmed cell death protein 1, *TLR2* toll-like receptor 2, *TNF-α* tumor necrosis factor-α

3.4.1.1 *Fusobacterium nucleatum*

F. nucleatum, an oral pathogen, is recognized early on as a key oncogenic bacterium in CRC. *F. nucleatum* abundance was elevated in CRC tissues, and its fecal levels could distinguish CRC patients from healthy subjects (Castellarin et al. 2012). It has also been reported that *F. nucleatum* levels in the tumor tissue were significantly associated with proximal tumors and higher depth of invasion (de Carvalho et al. 2019). Functionally, in vitro and in vivo studies have shown that *F. nucleatum* promotes colorectal tumorigenesis (Nakatsu et al. 2015), implying the involvement of *F. nucleatum* in the transformation process. *F. nucleatum* is reported to exert a direct effect on colonic epithelial cells and other host cells through protein–protein interaction. A unique membrane protein on *F. nucleatum* is FadA adhesin (Rubinstein et al. 2013, 2019; Guo et al. 2020). It has been shown that FadA exerts a pro-tumorigenic effect in CRC by binding to E-cadherin on colonic cells, which in turn activates β-catenin signaling, inflammatory and oncogenic response. Mechanistically, FadA-E-cadherin binding up-regulates Annexin A1 to induce nuclear translocation of β-catenin and cyclin D1 expression, thereby promoting CRC growth. FadA-E-cadherin-β-catenin axis also induces DNA damage in $Apc^{Min/+}$ mice model via chk2overexpression. Apart from FadA, Fap2 is another *F. nucleatum* adhesin identified that functions as a Gal-GalNAc lectin that interact with tumor-expressed Gal-GalNAc, leading to the homing of *F. nucleatum* to CRC (Abed et al. 2016). Fap2 has been shown to facilitate *F. nucleatum* invasion into CRC cells, resulting the secretion of CRC-associated pro-inflammatory cytokines IL8 and CXCL1 (Casasanta et al. 2020). Besides colonic cells, Fap2 also interacts directly interact with human TIGIT to inhibit NK cell-mediated cytotoxicity (Gur et al. 2015). Taken together, *F. nucleatum* mediates its effect via direct interaction with host cell receptors to modulate tumor cell growth while concomitantly repressing antitumor immunity.

3.4.1.2 *pks*$^+$ *Escherichia coli*

Mounting evidence demonstrates that *pks*$^+$ *Escherichia coli* could generate virulence factors that modulate CRC initiation and progression. A cancer-related pathogen found frequently in CRC patients, polyketide synthase (pks) gene expressing *Escherichia coli* encodes a peptide-polyketide hybrid cytotoxin compound named colibactin that causes DNA double-strand breaks and the activation of DNA damage checkpoint pathway in eukaryotic cells (Nougayrede et al. 2006). Recent work has uncovered the role of colibactin in CRC. Even short exposure of *pks*$^+$ *E. coli*-induced DNA damage response in mammalian epithelial cells, as evidenced by formation of phosphorylated H2AX foci, G2/M cell cycle arrest, anaphase bridge, chromosome aberration, and instability (Cuevas-Ramos et al. 2010; Arthur et al. 2012; Iftekhar et al. 2021). Interestingly, colonic organoids recovered from short-term infection with *pks*$^+$ *E. coli* revealed characteristics of Wnt-independence, an oncogenic feature that is driven by mutational changes in p53 signaling cascade (Iftekhar et al. 2021). In addition, monocolonization with the genotoxin-producing *E. coli* promoted colon tumor invasion in AOM-treated interleukin-10-deficient mice (Arthur et al. 2012). On the other hand, Cougnoux, et al. demonstrated that *pks*$^+$ *E. coli* accelerates AOM-DSS-induced CRC by promoting emergence of growth factor-secreting senescent cells via alteration of p53 SUMOylation, which in turn, induces proliferation of uninfected cells (Cougnoux et al. 2014). Colonic cells limit *pks*$^+$ *E. coli*-induced DNA damage by inducing autophagy, suggesting that strategies that promote autophagy might be a therapeutic approach for *pks*$^+$ *E. coli* (Lucas et al. 2020). In addition to their DNA damaging effects, colibactin-producing *E. coli* also modulates immune microenvironment by impairing antitumor T-cell response and leading to immunotherapy resistance (Lopes et al. 2020).

3.4.1.3 Enterotoxigenic *Bacteroides fragilis*

Another key pathogen that secretes virulence factor to promote CRC is enterotoxigenic *Bacteroides fragilis* (ETBF), owing to its production of *B. fragilis* toxin or fragilysin that can elicit an inappropriate immune response. ETBF-treated mice showed a strong selective colonic Stat3 activation with colitis characterized by a selective Th17 response (Wu et al. 2009). Of note, a report by Chung et al. further supported the fact that BFTs target the colonic epithelium to trigger a mucosal immune response and multi-step inflammatory cascade, which requires IL-17, NF-kB, and Stat3 activation (Chung et al. 2018). Additional work from others defined molecular mechanisms of ETBF-induced adaptive immunity alteration in CRC. Geis et al. demonstrated that regulatory T cells limited the availability of IL2 in the local microenvironment, thus allowing Th17 development necessary to promote ETBF-induced CRC (Geis et al. 2015). Exosome miR-149-3p secreted by ETBF-treated colon cells also facilitates Th17 differentiation (Cao et al. 2021). Long-term ETBF infection with inflammation has oncogenic consequences. An animal study revealed that ETBF infection promoted AOM/DSS-induced CRC by enhancing colonic inflammation, an effect dependent on BFT (Hwang et al. 2020a). Thiele et al., identified a IL-17-driven monocytic-MDSC-dominant immune signature associated with ETBF-triggered CRC, suggesting that ETBF infection promotes MDSC-mediated immune suppression (Thiele Orberg et al. 2017). In a BRAF^{V600E}-driven CRC model, ETBF colonization is necessary to induce right-sided serrated CRC, similar to BRAF-mutant CRC in humans (DeStefano Shields et al. 2021). Interestingly, ETBF-colonized BRAF^{V600E} tumors exhibited an altered immune landscape with increased IFN-γ producing CD8$^+$ T cells, thus rendering these tumors sensitive to anti-PD1 therapy. Emerging evidence indicate that ETBF, at least in part, also promotes CRC by epigenetic deregulation in CRC cells, such as CpG methylation (DeStefano Shields et al. 2021), *Bacteroides fragilis*-associated lncRNA1 (BFAL1) (Bao et al. 2019), and histone modifications (Liu et al. 2020) to promote cancer cell growth and stemness.

3.4.1.4 *Peptostreptococcus anaerobius*

P. anaerobius is an anerobic bacterium that normally resides in the oral cavity. Notably, shotgun metagenomic sequencing of fecal samples and16S ribosomal RNA sequencing of mucosal samples both validated that *P. anaerobius* as a novel bacterium enriched in CRC as compared to healthy subjects (Feng et al. 2015; Yu et al. 2017a). Subsequent functional studies revealed that *P. anaerobius* induced CRC cell proliferation by inducing cholesterol biosynthesis via TLR2/TLR4 signaling and also accelerated AOM-induced colorectal (Tsoi et al. 2017). Long et al. further elucidated the underlying molecular mechanism of *P. anaerobius* through a novel surface protein named putative cell wall binding repeat 2 (PCWBR2). PCWBR2 expressed by *P. anaerobius* could directly interact with integrin α2β1 and subsequently induce the activation of the PI3K-AKT pathway, leading to increased cell proliferation. PI3K-AKT also activated NF-κB, followed by induction of pro-inflammatory cytokines such as interleukin-10 and interferon γ (Long et al. 2019). Consequently, *P. anaerobius* could modify the tumor microenvironment by increasing myeloid-derived suppressor cells (MDSCs), tumor-associated macrophages (TAMs), and tumor-associated neutrophils (TANs), that shapes a pro-tumorigenic immune microenvironment.

3.4.1.5 *Porphyromonas gingivalis*

An oral pathogen that causes periodontitis, *P. gingivalis* has been shown to associate with CRC. *P. gingivalis* secretes multiple virulence factors such as fimbriae, gingipain hemagglutinin, capsule, and lipopolysaccharides. Gingipain, a cysteine endopeptidase located on the outer membranes of *P. gingivalis*, is found to be responsible for invasion and proliferation capability of *P. gingivalis* in CRC cells by activating the MAPK/ERK signaling pathway (Mu et al. 2020). *P. gingivalis* invasion in CRC tissues coincided with elevated butyrate and signs of senescence-associated inflammatory phenotypes, suggesting a causal relationship between *P. gingivalis* and CRC which may be attributed to butyrate-induced senescence (Okumura et al. 2021). Recent work also demonstrated that *P. gingivalis* could impact the immune response including upregulating the programmed death-ligand-1 (PD-L1) through NOD1/2-dependent activation of RIP2 and MAPK signaling pathways (Adel-Khattab et al. 2021), as well as recruitment of tumor-infiltrating MDSC by stimulating NLRP3 inflammasome formation (Wang et al. 2021).

3.4.2 Probiotics that Are Protective Against CRC

Accumulating evidence has established that probiotic bacteria from *Lactobacillus*, *Bifidobacterium*, *Akkermansia,* and *Streptococcus* families have a promising role in the prevention of CRC. The probiotics have been shown to exert tumor suppressive effects by secretion of tumor suppressive metabolites, regulation of gut barrier and gut immune response, as well as by antagonizing pathogenic bacteria and their communities (Fig. 3.2).

3.4.2.1 *Lactobacillus* Family

Lactobacillus species are a significant component of the human gut microbiota and is a common probiotic found in food such as yogurt. They are characterized by fermentation of glucose into lactate as the predominant product. Individual *Lactobacillus* strains are associated with protective effects on CRC. For example, *Lactobacillus casei* (*L. casei*) was shown to secrete ferrichrome, a siderophore, and tumor suppressive molecule that induced apoptosis via JNK signaling pathway (Konishi et al. 2016). Interestingly, the suppressive effect of ferrichrome was comparable to that of cisplatin and 5-fluorouracil, and had a lesser effect on colonic non-cancerous cells compared to CRC cells. *Lactobacillus salivarius* may act as a prophylactic agent for CRC prevention by suppressing tumor formation in a dimethylhydrazine (DMH)-induced CRC model by inhibiting cell growth, arresting cell cycle, and inducing cell apoptosis in vitro (Dong et al. 2020). Similarly, gamma-aminobutyric acid (GABA)-producing *Lactobacillus plantarum* exerted anti-proliferative, anti-migration, and anti-invasion effects against 5-FU-resistant HT-29 cells, implicating its potential to be a therapeutic agent in combination with chemotherapeutic drugs (An et al. 2021). On the other hand, Ovens et al. showed that *Lactobacillus rhamnosus GG* (LGG) activated colonic $CD8^+$ T cells through a TLR2/dendritic cell axis, and LGG attenuated AOM-induced CRC in a $CD8^+$ T-cell dependent fashion. Heat-killed LGG is also effective, suggesting that heat-resistant LGG molecular patterns might stimulate dendritic cells. These data supported potential use of LGG to augment antitumor immunity in CRC (Owens et al. 2021).

3.4.2.2 *Bifidobacterium* Family

Bifidobacterium species are an important component of our gut microbiota and are also commonly used as probiotics. Several *Bifidobacterium* have demonstrated antitumor effect in vitro and in AOM-DSS models of colitis-associated CRC (Asadollahi et al. 2020; Liao et al. 2021) by inhibiting CRC cell proliferation and suppressing inflammation in the colon epithelium. Several studies have indicated that *Bifidobacterium* species generate beneficial metabolites to exert antitumor effects. For instance, butanol extract of *Bifidobacterium adolescentis* isolated from healthy individuals showed an anti-proliferation capability and increased activity of the host immune system by elevating production of tumor necrosis factor-α (TNF-α) and nitric oxide (NO) (Lee et al. 2008). Recently, it was also identified that *Bifidobacterium pseudolongum* secretes the metabolite inosine, which in turn enhanced immunotherapy response through promoting Th1 activation and antitumor immunity (Mager et al. 2020). The secreted metabolites of *Bifidobacterium infantis*, on the other hand, protected gut barrier through tight junction modulation

(Guo et al. 2017). In addition, *Bifidobacterium* species could promote gut microbiota homeostasis. A clinical trial showed that symbiotic supplementation with *Bifidobacterium lactis* (*B. lactis*) and resistant starch induced unique changes in fecal microflora (Worthley et al. 2009). Probiotic cocktails of *Lactobacillus* and *Bifidobacterium* are currently undergoing clinical trials for the treatment of cancers.

3.4.2.3 *Akkermansia muciniphila*

A. muciniphila is a highly abundant commensal bacterium that is inversely associated with obesity and inflammatory conditions such as inflammatory bowel disease. Recent work has revealed the protective role of *A. muciniphila* in AOM-DSS model of colitis-associated CRC in mice. Mechanistically, it was found that an outer membrane protein, Amuc_1100 blunted tumorigenesis by expanding cytotoxic T lymphocytes (CTLs) in colon and mesenteric lymph nodes (MLN) via induction of TNF-α and down-regulation of PD-1 (Wang et al. 2020). Besides, *A. muciniphila* was found to suppress colorectal pathogenesis by facilitating the enrichment of M1-like macrophages in a TLR2/NLRP3-dependent manner (Fan et al. 2021). Consistently, Shi et al. also showed that the antitumor immune response elicited by *A. muciniphila* was partially mediated by Amuc through activating TLR2 signaling pathway (Shi et al. 2020). *A. muciniphila* thus suppresses CRC development through the modulation of immune response through its membrane protein.

3.4.2.4 *Streptococcus thermophilus*

S. thermophilus is a probiotic bacterium widely used in the dairy products and is present in fermented milk products and yogurt. Metagenome sequencing efforts revealed significant depletion of *S. thermophilus* in CRC patients. *S. thermophilus* was found to suppressed CRC cell growth in vitro and colorectal tumorigenesis in $Apc^{Min/+}$ mice and AOM mice model (Li et al. 2021). Mechanistically, it was shown that *S. thermophilus* mediates its effect, at least in part, through the secretion of β-galactosidase. *S. thermophilus* derived β-galactosidase could inhibit cell viability and induce cell cycle arrest and cell apoptosis by generating galactose, which functions as a glucose antagonist to suppress Warburg effect and down-regulate Hippo pathway signaling (Li et al. 2021). *S. thermophilus* is thus a novel prophylactic for CRC prevention.

3.4.3 *Role of Gut Fungi in CRC*

Compared to bacteria, much less is known with regard to the role of the gut fungi in the pathogenesis of CRC. Analysis of shotgun metagenomic sequencing dataset from biopsy samples from adenomas and adjacent tissues revealed decreased fungal diversity of in subjects with adenomas (Luan et al. 2015). Fecal shotgun metagenomics from a larger cohort identified CRC-associated fungal dysbiosis with higher Basidiomycota:Ascomycota ratio, an increase in Malasseziomycetes, together with a decrease in Saccharomycetes and Pneumocystidomycetes, suggesting that gut fungi are potential biomarkers in CRC diagnosis (Coker et al. 2019). The molecular mechanism of gut fungi in CRC is understudied. While it is known that fungi could produce toxic metabolites, such as aflatoxins, ochratoxins, fumonisins, deoxynivalenol, secreted from some fungi can promote carcinogenesis (De Ruyck et al. 2015), their functional relevance in the context of fungi dysbiosis remains unclear (Sobral et al. 2018).

Several lines of evidence suggest that fungi could modulate host immune response. Zhu, et al. found that an exopolysaccharide (EPS) from *Rhizopus nigricans* suppressed the tumor growth in CT26 allograft models. The antitumor effects might be partly due to immune activation via increasing the expression of IL-2 and TNF-α and $CD8^+$ cytotoxic T cells (Zhu et al. 2016). To further elucidate the role of commensal fungi in CRC, two groups used CARD9 deficient mice model, with increased susceptibility of fungi infection. In both studies, it was shown that CARD9 deficient mice have increased tumor load following AOM-DSS treatment, concomitant with the accumulation of MDSCs (Wang et al. 2018; Malik et al. 2018). Wang et al. revealed fungi dysbiosis with higher fungal load and *C. tropicalis*. *C. tropicalis* was shown to promote MSDC-like features in bone marrow cells in vitro and promote CRC in germ-free mice. Finally, antifungal fluconazole inhibited AOM-DSS-induced CRC in CARD9 deficient mice, and was associated with decreased MDSC. In contrast. Malik et al. showed that gut fungi-mediated inflammasome activation helped to restrict colitis and CRC via SKY-CARD9 signaling. More recently, *Candida albicans* was shown to promote colitis-associated CRC by driving crosstalk between macrophages and innate lymphoid cells by enhancing IL-22 secretion in intestine, thereby triggering glycolysis and pro-inflammatory IL-7 secretion in macrophages (Zhu et al. 2021). These data suggest that the role of gut fungi might be species specific and context dependent.

Interkingdom interactions between fungi and bacteria can occur via physical interaction, metabolites, biofilm, etc. Ecological analysis of fecal microbiota revealed the co-occurrence interactions between fungi (*Ascomycota*) and bacteria (*Proteobacteria*) in control subjects, which then reverted into co-exclusive interaction in CRC samples (Coker et al. 2019). Nevertheless, the exact functional role of gut fungi–bacteria interactions in colorectal tumorigenesis awaits further investigation.

3.4.4 Role of Gut Viruses in CRC

Little is known about the potential role of viruses in CRC. Aiming to identify the viral component of CRC-associated microbiome, Nakatsu et al. analyzed viral sequences in healthy subjects and CRC patients, and devised a 22 viral taxa panel that discriminated CRC from controls; as well as a combination of four taxonomic markers that correlated with the poor survival of CRC patients independently of other clinical parameters (Nakatsu et al. 2018). Likewise, a study used various types of sequencing datasets to evaluate the differences in human colorectal cancer virus and bacterial community composition and provided evidence that bacteriophage communities were associated with CRC and may influence CRC progression by altering the bacterial communities (Hannigan et al. 2018).

3.5 Clinical Application and Challenge of Microbiome in CRC

3.5.1 Biomarkers for CRC Diagnosis and Prevention

Numerous studies have clearly demonstrated that gut dysbiosis as a cardinal feature of CRC and changes in gut microbiome is evident beginning from the earliest stage of malignant transformation. In our group, we have focused on the development of fecal bacterial marker panels that enables simple, non-invasive detection of CRC and adenomas. From our metagenomic efforts, we identified 20 bacterial markers that potentially distinguish between CRC patient and healthy subjects, including *F. nucleatum*, *Bacteroides clarus*, *Roseburia intestinalis*, *Clostridium hathewayi*, *P. anaerobius,* and *Parvimonas micra*. We have further developed PCR-based detection of these markers, and verified utility of *F. nucleatum*, "m3" (*Lachnoclostridium* sp) and four other markers for the diagnosis of CRC (Liang et al. 2017, 2020; Wong et al. 2017b), among which *F. nucleatum* and m3 perform best in distinguishing CRC and adenoma, respectively, with superior sensitivity to fecal immunochemical test (FIT). The combination of FIT with bacterial markers further improved the test performance. Other studies have reported consistent alterations of fecal bacterial biomarkers in CRC (Shah et al. 2018; Dai et al. 2018; Thomas et al. 2019; Yang et al. 2020; Wu et al. 2021). In addition to microbial abundance, alterations of gut bacteria-derived fecal and serum metabolome also showed potential for CRC and adenoma detection (Yachida et al. 2019; Chen et al. 2022).

Targeting these markers may also help to prevent from CRC development. However, there are still some limitations of microbial markers remaining for CRC detection (DeSantis et al. 2017). The number one reason is that they do not necessarily perform as well in the detection of polyps, adenomas, and other early-stage lesions as they do in the detection of more advanced disease. Secondly, it may be difficult for such a test to screen CRC in high-risk groups already carrying aberrant microbiota, such as those who with irritable bowel disease (IBD), type 2 diabetes, etc. What's more, validating potential microbial markers in the general population represents a critical step in confirming the accuracy and utility of microbial features in the diagnosis of CRC in the general public. Thus, the marker-based test must include those indicators that are robust to the influences of common lifestyle factors.

3.5.2 Modulation of Microbiota in CRC

Given to the crucial role of gut microbiota in CRC, modulation of gut dysbiosis for the prevention or treatment of CRC is an area of intensive investigations. Several strategies have been proposed, including FMT, dietary intervention, and antibiotic administration. A successful case of FMT has been made for recurrent *Clostridium difficile* infection; however, FMT for CRC prevention or treatment is limited to animal work at this stage (Wong et al. 2017a; Li et al. 2019; Shao et al. 2021). Nevertheless, usefulness of FMT in a prevention setting is limited. Dietary intervention is a more probable approach for modulating microbiota for CRC control. The diet-microbiome interplay in CRC development has been recently unraveled (O'Keefe 2016). For example, a significant shift in the gut microbiota composition, along with impaired gut barrier function was exhibited in high fat diet-fed mice, supporting that high fat drives CRC by promoting microbial dysbiosis (Yang et al. 2022). On the contrary, dietary fiber can promote outgrowth of beneficial commensals and leading to the production of metabolites such as short-chain fatty acids, which are associated with tumor suppressive effects (Makki et al. 2018). Interestingly, high salt diet was found to suppress ETBF-induced CRC in AOM-DSS mice models, implying the effect of diet can be context dependent (Hwang et al. 2020b). The greatest challenge for prebiotics or dietary approach is the translation of experimental results into real world effects in humans, given the complexities of the human diet and difficulties in standardizing prebiotic formulations that generate persistent impacts on the human microbiome across populations. Several studies have suggested that frequent antibiotics use increase the risk of CRC (Dik et al. 2016). Animal work also indicates that long-term antibiotic exposure mediates the selected depletion of gut microbial communities and concomitant thinning of the protective mucus layer, thereby promoting colorectal tumorigenesis (Kaur et al. 2018). Hence, non-selective depletion of microbiota is unlikely to yield benefit for CRC.

3.5.3 Effect of Microbiota on Cancer Therapy in CRC

Recent work implicates that the gut microbiota might influence host response in cancer treatments, including chemotherapy and immune checkpoint blockade (ICB) therapy. A comparison of *F. nucleatum* in untreated and post-neoadjuvant chemoradiotherapy (nCRT) samples from locally advanced rectal cancer demonstrated that *F. nucleatum* persistence post-nCRT is associated with high relapse rates that is linked to suppression of immune cytotoxicity (Serna et al. 2020). Consistently, it has been reported that *F. nucleatum* was more abundant in CRC patients with recurrence post-chemotherapy, and *F. nucleatum* targeted TLR4 and MYD88 innate immune signaling and microRNAs to activate the protective autophagy pathway and antagonize chemotherapeutic response (Yu et al. 2017b). These results suggest that pathogenic bacteria could promote therapeutic resistance in addition to their effect on colorectal tumorigenesis. Moreover, pathogenic bacteria are associated with immune suppressive effect in the tumor microenvironment, including inhibition of $CD8^+$ T and NK cells infiltration and activity (Gur et al. 2015, 2019; Lopes et al. 2020), recruitment of MDSC (Kostic et al. 2013), and enrichment of tumor-associated macrophages (Fan et al. 2021). In contrast, considerable evidence has also emerged showing that gut commensal bacteria can boost ICB therapy via the activation of antitumor T cells (DeStefano Shields et al. 2021; Owens et al. 2021; Mager et al. 2020). The combination of ICB therapy and probiotics holds great promise in improving therapeutic response in CRC patients.

3.6 Conclusion

It is now clear that gut microbes are critical determinants in CRC. Understanding the interaction between gut microbes and CRC pathogenesis will aid in disease diagnosis and treatment. Until now, most human studies are based on descriptive analysis of the gut microbiome in single populations. Further investigation in multiple geographically and ethnically diverse cohorts will be key to contextualize microbiome as a diagnostic and therapeutic biomarker. Moreover, longitudinal studies are required to assess if use of microbial biomarkers hold promise of identifying individuals at risk for CRC, and to determine the impact of gut microbiome modulation on cellular and molecular immune signatures in humans over time. For mechanistic studies, we have gained tremendous knowledge on individual bacteria on CRC by monocolonization. Nevertheless, the role of complex microbial communities including bacteria, fungi, or virus tip the balance toward CRC tumorigenesis. A multidisciplinary strategy incorporating metagenomics, metabolomics, and host genomics/proteomics is necessary to elucidate the mechanism of gut microbiota communities in mediating CRC initiation and progression.

Author Contributions PH and CCW contributed to writing and editing. Both authors approved the final version.

Conflict of Interest All authors declare no conflict of interest.

References

Abed J, et al. Fap2 mediates Fusobacterium nucleatum colorectal adenocarcinoma enrichment by binding to tumor-expressed Gal-GalNAc. Cell Host Microbe. 2016;20(2):215–25.

Adel-Khattab D, et al. Porphyromonas gingivalis induced up-regulation of PD-L1 in colon carcinoma cells. Mol Oral Microbiol. 2021;36(3):172–81.

An J, Seok H, Ha EM. GABA-producing Lactobacillus plantarum inhibits metastatic properties and induces apoptosis of 5-FU-resistant colorectal cancer cells via GABAB receptor signaling. J Microbiol. 2021;59(2):202–16.

Arthur JC, et al. Intestinal inflammation targets cancer-inducing activity of the microbiota. Science. 2012;338(6103):120–3.

Asadollahi P, et al. Anti-cancer effects of Bifidobacterium species in colon cancer cells and a mouse model of carcinogenesis. PLoS One. 2020;15(5):e0232930.

Backhed F, et al. Dynamics and stabilization of the human gut microbiome during the first year of life. Cell Host Microbe. 2015;17(5):690–703.

Bao Y, et al. Long noncoding RNA BFAL1 mediates enterotoxigenic Bacteroides fragilis-related carcinogenesis in colorectal cancer via the RHEB/mTOR pathway. Cell Death Dis. 2019;10(9):675.

Belkaid Y, Hand TW. Role of the microbiota in immunity and inflammation. Cell. 2014;157(1):121–41.

Berg G, et al. Microbiome definition re-visited: old concepts and new challenges. Microbiome. 2020;8(1):103.

Cao Y, et al. Enterotoxigenic Bacteroides fragilis promotes intestinal inflammation and malignancy by inhibiting exosome-packaged miR-149-3p. Gastroenterology. 2021;161:1552–1566.e12.

Casasanta MA, et al. Fusobacterium nucleatum host-cell binding and invasion induces IL-8 and CXCL1 secretion that drives colorectal cancer cell migration. Sci Signal. 2020;13(641):eaba9157.

Castellarin M, et al. Fusobacterium nucleatum infection is prevalent in human colorectal carcinoma. Genome Res. 2012;22(2):299–306.

Chen F, et al. Integrated analysis of the faecal metagenome and serum metabolome reveals the role of gut microbiome-associated metabolites in the detection of colorectal cancer and adenoma. Gut. 2022;71(7):1315–25.

Chung L, et al. Bacteroides fragilis toxin coordinates a pro-carcinogenic inflammatory Cascade via targeting of colonic epithelial cells. Cell Host Microbe. 2018;23(2):203–214.e5.

Coker OO, et al. Enteric fungal microbiota dysbiosis and ecological alterations in colorectal cancer. Gut. 2019;68(4):654–62.

Collins SL, Patterson AD. The gut microbiome: an orchestrator of xenobiotic metabolism. Acta Pharm Sin B. 2020;10(1):19–32.

Cougnoux A, et al. Bacterial genotoxin colibactin promotes colon tumour growth by inducing a senescence-associated secretory phenotype. Gut. 2014;63(12):1932–42.

Cuevas-Ramos G, et al. Escherichia coli induces DNA damage in vivo and triggers genomic instability in mammalian cells. Proc Natl Acad Sci U S A. 2010;107(25):11537–42.

Dai Z, et al. Multi-cohort analysis of colorectal cancer metagenome identified altered bacteria across populations and universal bacterial markers. Microbiome. 2018;6(1):70.

de Carvalho AC, et al. Microbiota profile and impact of Fusobacterium nucleatum in colorectal cancer patients of Barretos cancer hospital. Front Oncol. 2019;9:813.

De Ruyck K, et al. Dietary mycotoxins, co-exposure, and carcinogenesis in humans: short review. Mutat Res Rev Mutat Res. 2015;766:32–41.

DeSantis TZ, et al. Microbial markers in the diagnosis of colorectal cancer: the promise, reality and challenge. Future Microbiol. 2017;12:1341–4.

DeStefano Shields CE, et al. Bacterial-driven inflammation and mutant BRAF expression combine to promote murine colon tumorigenesis that is sensitive to immune checkpoint therapy. Cancer Discov. 2021;11(7):1792–807.

Dik VK, et al. Frequent use of antibiotics is associated with colorectal cancer risk: results of a nested case-control study. Dig Dis Sci. 2016;61(1):255–64.

Dominguez-Bello MG, et al. Role of the microbiome in human development. Gut. 2019;68(6):1108–14.

Dong Y, et al. Probiotic Lactobacillus salivarius Ren prevent dimethylhydrazine-induced colorectal cancer through protein kinase B inhibition. Appl Microbiol Biotechnol. 2020;104(17):7377–89.

Fan L, et al. A. muciniphila suppresses colorectal tumorigenesis by inducing TLR2/NLRP3-mediated M1-like TAMs. Cancer Immunol Res. 2021;9(10):1111–24.

Feng Q, et al. Gut microbiome development along the colorectal adenoma-carcinoma sequence. Nat Commun. 2015;6:6528.
Funabashi M, et al. A metabolic pathway for bile acid dehydroxylation by the gut microbiome. Nature. 2020;582(7813):566–70.
Geis AL, et al. Regulatory T-cell response to enterotoxigenic Bacteroides fragilis colonization triggers IL17-dependent colon carcinogenesis. Cancer Discov. 2015;5(10):1098–109.
Guo S, et al. Secretions of Bifidobacterium infantis and Lactobacillus acidophilus protect intestinal epithelial barrier function. J Pediatr Gastroenterol Nutr. 2017;64(3):404–12.
Guo P, et al. FadA promotes DNA damage and progression of Fusobacterium nucleatum-induced colorectal cancer through up-regulation of chk2. J Exp Clin Cancer Res. 2020;39(1):202.
Gur C, et al. Binding of the Fap2 protein of Fusobacterium nucleatum to human inhibitory receptor TIGIT protects tumors from immune cell attack. Immunity. 2015;42(2):344–55.
Gur C, et al. Fusobacterium nucleatum suppresses anti-tumor immunity by activating CEACAM1. Oncoimmunology. 2019;8(6):e1581531.
Hannigan GD, et al. Diagnostic potential and interactive dynamics of the colorectal cancer virome. mBio. 2018;9(6):e02248–18.
Hooper LV, et al. Molecular analysis of commensal host-microbial relationships in the intestine. Science. 2001;291(5505):881–4.
Human Microbiome Project Consortium. Structure, function and diversity of the healthy human microbiome. Nature. 2012;486(7402):207–14.
Hwang S, et al. Enterotoxigenic Bacteroides fragilis infection exacerbates tumorigenesis in AOM/DSS mouse model. Int J Med Sci. 2020a;17(2):145–52.
Hwang S, et al. Dietary salt administration decreases enterotoxigenic Bacteroides fragilis (ETBF)-promoted tumorigenesis via inhibition of colonic inflammation. Int J Mol Sci. 2020b;21(21):8034.
Iftekhar A, et al. Genomic aberrations after short-term exposure to colibactin-producing E. coli transform primary colon epithelial cells. Nat Commun. 2021;12(1):1003.
Kaur K, et al. Antibiotic-mediated bacteriome depletion in Apc(Min/+) mice is associated with reduction in mucus-producing goblet cells and increased colorectal cancer progression. Cancer Med. 2018;7(5):2003–12.
Konishi H, et al. Probiotic-derived ferrichrome inhibits colon cancer progression via JNK-mediated apoptosis. Nat Commun. 2016;7:12365.
Kostic AD, et al. Fusobacterium nucleatum potentiates intestinal tumorigenesis and modulates the tumor-immune microenvironment. Cell Host Microbe. 2013;14(2):207–15.
Kudryavtseva AV, et al. Important molecular genetic markers of colorectal cancer. Oncotarget. 2016;7(33):53959–83.
LeBlanc JG, et al. Bacteria as vitamin suppliers to their host: a gut microbiota perspective. Curr Opin Biotechnol. 2013;24(2):160–8.
Lee DK, et al. Anti-proliferative effects of Bifidobacterium adolescentis SPM0212 extract on human colon cancer cell lines. BMC Cancer. 2008;8:310.
Li L, et al. Gut microbiota from colorectal cancer patients enhances the progression of intestinal adenoma in Apc(Min/+) mice. EBioMedicine. 2019;48:301–15.
Li Q, et al. Streptococcus thermophilus inhibits colorectal tumorigenesis through secreting beta-galactosidase. Gastroenterology. 2021;160(4):1179–1193.e14.
Liang QY, et al. Fecal bacteria act as novel biomarkers for noninvasive diagnosis of colorectal cancer. Clin Cancer Res. 2017;23(8):2061–70.
Liang JQ, et al. A novel faecal Lachnoclostridium marker for the non-invasive diagnosis of colorectal adenoma and cancer. Gut. 2020;69(7):1248–57.
Liao W, et al. Bifidobacterium animalis: the missing link for the cancer-preventive effect of Gynostemma pentaphyllum. Gut Microbes. 2021;13(1):1847629.
Liu QQ, et al. Enterotoxigenic Bacteroides fragilis induces the stemness in colorectal cancer via upregulating histone demethylase JMJD2B. Gut Microbes. 2020;12(1):1788900.

Long X, et al. Peptostreptococcus anaerobius promotes colorectal carcinogenesis and modulates tumour immunity. Nat Microbiol. 2019;4(12):2319–30.

Lopes A, et al. Colibactin-positive Escherichia coli induce a procarcinogenic immune environment leading to immunotherapy resistance in colorectal cancer. Int J Cancer. 2020;146(11):3147–59.

Louis P, Flint HJ. Formation of propionate and butyrate by the human colonic microbiota. Environ Microbiol. 2017;19(1):29–41.

Luan C, et al. Dysbiosis of fungal microbiota in the intestinal mucosa of patients with colorectal adenomas. Sci Rep. 2015;5:7980.

Lucas C, et al. Autophagy of intestinal epithelial cells inhibits colorectal carcinogenesis induced by colibactin-producing Escherichia coli in Apc(Min/+) mice. Gastroenterology. 2020;158(5):1373–88.

Lynch SV, Pedersen O. The human intestinal microbiome in health and disease. N Engl J Med. 2016;375(24):2369–79.

Mager LF, et al. Microbiome-derived inosine modulates response to checkpoint inhibitor immunotherapy. Science. 2020;369(6510):1481–9.

Makki K, et al. The impact of dietary fiber on gut microbiota in host health and disease. Cell Host Microbe. 2018;23(6):705–15.

Malik A, et al. SYK-CARD9 signaling axis promotes gut fungi-mediated inflammasome activation to restrict colitis and colon cancer. Immunity. 2018;49(3):515–530.e5.

Manor O, et al. Health and disease markers correlate with gut microbiome composition across thousands of people. Nat Commun. 2020;11(1):5206.

Mu W, et al. Intracellular Porphyromonas gingivalis promotes the proliferation of colorectal cancer cells via the MAPK/ERK Signaling pathway. Front Cell Infect Microbiol. 2020;10:584798.

Nakatsu G, et al. Gut mucosal microbiome across stages of colorectal carcinogenesis. Nat Commun. 2015;6:8727.

Nakatsu G, et al. Alterations in enteric virome are associated with colorectal cancer and survival outcomes. Gastroenterology. 2018;155(2):529–541 e5.

Nougayrede JP, et al. Escherichia coli induces DNA double-strand breaks in eukaryotic cells. Science. 2006;313(5788):848–51.

O'Keefe SJ. Diet, microorganisms and their metabolites, and colon cancer. Nat Rev Gastroenterol Hepatol. 2016;13(12):691–706.

Okumura S, et al. Gut bacteria identified in colorectal cancer patients promote tumourigenesis via butyrate secretion. Nat Commun. 2021;12(1):5674.

Owens JA, et al. Lactobacillus rhamnosus GG orchestrates an antitumor immune response. Cell Mol Gastroenterol Hepatol. 2021;12(4):1311–27.

Rubinstein MR, et al. Fusobacterium nucleatum promotes colorectal carcinogenesis by modulating E-cadherin/beta-catenin signaling via its FadA adhesin. Cell Host Microbe. 2013;14(2):195–206.

Rubinstein MR, et al. Fusobacterium nucleatum promotes colorectal cancer by inducing Wnt/beta-catenin modulator annexin A1. EMBO Rep. 2019;20(4):e47638.

Schirmer M, et al. Linking the human gut microbiome to inflammatory cytokine production capacity. Cell. 2016;167(4):1125–1136 e8.

Serna G, et al. Fusobacterium nucleatum persistence and risk of recurrence after preoperative treatment in locally advanced rectal cancer. Ann Oncol. 2020;31(10):1366–75.

Shah MS, et al. Leveraging sequence-based faecal microbial community survey data to identify a composite biomarker for colorectal cancer. Gut. 2018;67(5):882–91.

Shao X, et al. Bacteroides fragilis restricts colitis-associated cancer via negative regulation of the NLRP3 axis. Cancer Lett. 2021;523:170–81.

Shi L, et al. Combining IL-2-based immunotherapy with commensal probiotics produces enhanced antitumor immune response and tumor clearance. J Immunother Cancer. 2020;8(2):e000973.

Siegel RL, et al. Colorectal cancer statistics, 2020. CA Cancer J Clin. 2020;70(3):145–64.

Sobral MMC, et al. Toxicological interactions between mycotoxins from ubiquitous fungi: impact on hepatic and intestinal human epithelial cells. Chemosphere. 2018;202:538–48.

Sommer F, et al. The resilience of the intestinal microbiota influences health and disease. Nat Rev Microbiol. 2017;15(10):630–8.
Sung H, et al. Global cancer statistics 2020: GLOBOCAN estimates of incidence and mortality worldwide for 36 cancers in 185 countries. CA Cancer J Clin. 2021;71(3):209–49.
Thiele Orberg E, et al. The myeloid immune signature of enterotoxigenic Bacteroides fragilis-induced murine colon tumorigenesis. Mucosal Immunol. 2017;10(2):421–33.
Thomas AM, et al. Metagenomic analysis of colorectal cancer datasets identifies cross-cohort microbial diagnostic signatures and a link with choline degradation. Nat Med. 2019;25(4):667–78.
Tsoi H, et al. Peptostreptococcus anaerobius induces intracellular cholesterol biosynthesis in colon cells to induce proliferation and causes dysplasia in mice. Gastroenterology. 2017;152(6):1419–1433.e5.
Turnbaugh PJ, et al. An obesity-associated gut microbiome with increased capacity for energy harvest. Nature. 2006;444(7122):1027–31.
Wang T, et al. The adaptor protein CARD9 protects against colon cancer by restricting mycobiota-mediated expansion of myeloid-derived suppressor cells. Immunity. 2018;49(3):504–514 e4.
Wang L, et al. A purified membrane protein from Akkermansia muciniphila or the pasteurised bacterium blunts colitis associated tumourigenesis by modulation of CD8(+) T cells in mice. Gut. 2020;69(11):1988–97.
Wang X, et al. Porphyromonas gingivalis promotes colorectal carcinoma by activating the hematopoietic NLRP3 inflammasome. Cancer Res. 2021;81(10):2745–59.
Whiteside SA, et al. The microbiome of the urinary tract—a role beyond infection. Nat Rev Urol. 2015;12(2):81–90.
Wong SH, et al. Gavage of fecal samples from patients with colorectal cancer promotes intestinal carcinogenesis in germ-free and conventional mice. Gastroenterology. 2017a;153(6):1621–1633.e6.
Wong SH, et al. Quantitation of faecal fusobacterium improves faecal immunochemical test in detecting advanced colorectal neoplasia. Gut. 2017b;66(8):1441–8.
Worthley DL, et al. A human, double-blind, placebo-controlled, crossover trial of prebiotic, probiotic, and synbiotic supplementation: effects on luminal, inflammatory, epigenetic, and epithelial biomarkers of colorectal cancer. Am J Clin Nutr. 2009;90(3):578–86.
Wu GD, Lewis JD. Analysis of the human gut microbiome and association with disease. Clin Gastroenterol Hepatol. 2013;11(7):774–7.
Wu S, et al. A human colonic commensal promotes colon tumorigenesis via activation of T helper type 17 T cell responses. Nat Med. 2009;15(9):1016–22.
Wu Y, et al. Identification of microbial markers across populations in early detection of colorectal cancer. Nat Commun. 2021;12(1):3063.
Yachida S, et al. Metagenomic and metabolomic analyses reveal distinct stage-specific phenotypes of the gut microbiota in colorectal cancer. Nat Med. 2019;25(6):968–76.
Yang J, et al. Establishing high-accuracy biomarkers for colorectal cancer by comparing fecal microbiomes in patients with healthy families. Gut Microbes. 2020;11(4):918–29.
Yang J, et al. High-fat diet promotes colorectal tumorigenesis through modulating gut microbiota and metabolites. Gastroenterology. 2022;162(1):135–149.e2.
Yu J, et al. Metagenomic analysis of faecal microbiome as a tool towards targeted non-invasive biomarkers for colorectal cancer. Gut. 2017a;66(1):70–8.
Yu T, et al. Fusobacterium nucleatum promotes chemoresistance to colorectal cancer by modulating autophagy. Cell. 2017b;170(3):548–563.e16.
Zhu L, et al. Anti-tumor and immunomodulatory activities of an exopolysaccharide from Rhizopus nigricans on CT26 tumor-bearing mice. Int Immunopharmacol. 2016;36:218–24.
Zhu Y, et al. Fungal-induced glycolysis in macrophages promotes colon cancer by enhancing innate lymphoid cell secretion of IL-22. EMBO J. 2021;40(11):e105320.

Chapter 4
Microbiome in Gastric Cancer

Elke Burgermeister and Matthias P. Ebert

Abstract Gastric Cancer (GC) belongs to the malignant diseases with one of the highest mortality rates despite declining incidences worldwide. The rapid advance of gene sequencing methodologies proposed at least four consensus molecular subtypes (CMS) which can be in part be reconciled with the traditional histomorphological classifications in individual patients, revealing causal relationships to oncogenic driver mutations and infection by pathogens. Therein, *Helicobacter pylori* (HP) and Epstein–Barr Virus (EBV) promote gastric carcinogenesis via defined virulence factors. In this context, both oral and intestinal microbiota have been suggested to compete for the ecological niche exposed by an HP colonized stomach. However, the contribution of non-HP microbiota and their metabolites, including the associated viromes and fungomes, to the development of GC remains largely elusive. The identification of distinct bacteria species and their pathogenic modes of action on mucosal epithelia and the host immune response shall open new avenues for prevention, early diagnosis and therapy of GC. In this book chapter, we will summarize the current state of knowledge on the gastric microbiome with respect to the transition of inflammation to pre-malignant states and progression to adenocarcinoma. An overview on specific pathogenic mechanisms and potential modalities for microbiota intervention treatments will be given, with a focus on clinical therapies with immune checkpoint inhibitors in patients.

E. Burgermeister (✉)
Department of Medicine II, Medical Faculty Mannheim, Heidelberg University, Mannheim, Germany
e-mail: elke.burgermeister@medma.uni-heidelberg.de

M. P. Ebert
Department of Medicine II, Medical Faculty Mannheim, Heidelberg University, Mannheim, Germany

Clinical Cooperation Unit Healthy Metabolism, Center of Preventive Medicine and Digital Health, Medical Faculty Mannheim, Heidelberg University, Mannheim, Germany

Mannheim Institute of Innate Immunoscience (MI3), Medical Faculty Mannheim, Heidelberg University, Mannheim, Germany

J. Yu (ed.), *Microbiome in Gastrointestinal Cancer*,
https://doi.org/10.1007/978-981-19-4492-5_4

Keywords Gastric cancer · Microbiome · Microbiota · Dysbiosis · Helicobacter pylori

Abbreviations

BabA	Blood group antigen binding adhesin A
CagA	Cytotoxin-associated gene A
CD	Cluster of differentiation
CIN	Chromosomal instability
CMS	Consensus molecular subtype
CTLA4	Cytotoxic T-Lymphocyte Associated Protein 4
DC	Dendritic cell
EBV	Epstein–Barr virus
EMT	Epithelial-to-mesenchymal transition
FadA	Fusobacterium adhesin A
GC	Gastric cancer
GIST	Gastrointestinal stroma tumor
GS	Genomic stability
HP	*Helicobacter pylori*
IFN	Interferon
IL	Interleukin
IM	Intestinal metaplasia
IRAE	Immune-related adverse events
IRF	Interferon regulatory factor
LPS	Lipopolysaccharide
MALT	Mucosa-associated lymphoid tissue
MSI	Microsatellite instability
MSS	Microsatellite stability
NACT	Neoadjuvant chemotherapy
NFκB	Nuclear factor kappa B
NSAID	Nonsteroidal anti-inflammatory drug
NT	Non-tumor
OMP	Outer membrane protein
PAI	Pathogenicity island
PAMP	Pathogen-associated molecular pattern
PD-1/PD-L1	Programmed Cell Death-1/Ligand-1
PPI	Proton pump inhibitor
PRR	Pattern-recognition receptor
pTNM	Primary tumor staging system
RHO	Ras homologue small GTPase
RO/NS	Reactive oxygen/nitrogen species
SRCC	Signet-ring cell carcinoma
T4SS	Type IV secretion system
Th/c/reg	T helper/cytotoxic/regulatory (cells)

TLR	Toll-like receptor
TNF	Tumor necrosis factor
TU	Tumor/cancer
VacA	Vacuolating cytotoxin A
WHO	World Health Organization

4.1 Introduction

The human microbiome comprises a complex ecological super-network which surpasses the total number of cells we have in our body (Human Microbiome Project Consortium 2012). Several privileged niches and large-scale habitats exist such as the skin, the urogenital tract, the oral cavity, and cranial-to-caudal toward the colorectum. These organismal communities not only contain bacteria but also viruses, fungi, and common parasites like helminths. This ecosystem is indispensable for the maintenance of the physiologic homeostasis, and its perturbation leads to an imbalance between beneficial and harmful species, also termed "dysbiosis," and is associated with or causally contributes to pathologies, including organ dysfunction, inflammation, and cancer (Elinav et al. 2019). Due to the complex spatio-temporal interplay of organisms and their metabolites either by direct contact with epithelial "barriers" outside and inside the body and the host immune system, unraveling individual species and virulence mechanisms remains a challenge (Levy et al. 2017).

The recent advances in nucleic acid sequencing technologies accelerated research in the field which previously relied on traditional methods of bacteria isolation from tissue biopsies and "liquid" sources (gastric juice, saliva, blood, feces) and their ex vivo cultivation. These achievements were also met by the novel system of CMS classification of GC (Cancer Genome Atlas Research Network 2014), which is now increasingly coherent by matching of oncogenic driver mutations, immune scores, and infectious status of patients with respective histomorphologies. Hitherto, GC was seen as a step-wise progressive disease, termed Correa cascade (Correa 1992), initiated by HP infection of the gastric mucosa evoking local gastritis, followed by dyspepsia and atrophy, finally progressing to metaplasia, dysplasia and adenocarcinoma, and other HP-related diseases (e.g., gastric or duodenal ulcers and MALT lymphoma). Despite the fact that more than half of the world population is infected with HP and it was rated as type I carcinogen by the WHO, only 1–4% develop GC, proposing the contribution of other oncogenic drivers, be them either mutations in the host genome or non-HP microbiota (Tshibangu-Kabamba and Yamaoka 2021). Therefore, the four GC subtypes are now to be stratified according to their microbiota and host immune profiles to allow subtype-selective interventions in patients in the future (Cancer Genome Atlas Research Network 2014). The CIN subtype has been associated with intestinal, the GS subtype with diffuse histology, both can have a history of HP infection. The EBV subtype is characterized by high immune cell infiltration and signaling scores, similar to MSI which has a high mutational burden and neoantigen load, making the latter two GC subtypes responsive to therapies with blocking antibodies against immune checkpoints (e.g., PD1, PD-L1, CTLA4).

Several landmark publications demonstrated that the gastrointestinal microbiome impacts on efficacy (Matson et al. 2018) and toxicity (Andrews et al. 2021) of checkpoint therapy. However, the underlying bacterial strains and mechanisms in GC are unknown. Third to cancers of the lung and colorectum, GC is a leading cause of cancer-related mortality and accounts for up to a million deaths per year worldwide (Wong et al. 2021). Thus, urgent medical need exists to improve diagnosis, prevention, and treatments for GC.

4.2 Microbiota in the Healthy, Non-neoplastic Stomach

The acidic environment and low pH of the normal oxyntic (corpus) part of the human stomach prevent overgrowth of the gastric mucosa by commensals and potentially harmful pathogens deriving both from the upper and lower GI tract, where the oral cavity and the small and large intestines harbor the majority of microbiota contained inside the body (Serrano et al. 2021). Therefore, the stomach has been regarded as a largely sterile organ. This false conclusion was also based on limited success of isolation and ex vivo cultivation of gastric microbiota, lack of serologic or rapid, non-invasive diagnostic tests, and was recently revolutionized by the technological advance in microarray and next-generation sequencing, with bacterial 16S ribosomal RNA (16S rRNA) as a prime target providing exact identifications for taxonomy and phylogeny (Elinav et al. 2019). Poor standardization of sampling (e.g., saliva/gastric juice vs. "depth" of biopsies) is an obstacle, and intra- and inter-individual variability of samples remains high, also due to multiple confounding effects ranging from age, gender, ethnicity to lifestyle (birth, diet, geography), and drug intake (e.g., NSAID, PPI, antibiotics) (Human Microbiome Project Consortium 2012). Contamination with oral and duodenal "passenger" bacteria adds to the complexity and calls for a clear definition of cut-off/threshold values for detection methods including PCR-based methods (Li and Yu 2020).

Marshall and Warren in 1982 discovered HP as the causative agent of gastritis and peptic ulcers and, thereby, drove the attention toward cancer as a consequence of infection of the stomach (Tshibangu-Kabamba and Yamaoka 2021). For decades, the research was occupied with the discovery of the virulence mechanisms of HP disregarding the physiological gastric non-HP microbiome. HP-induced loss of gastric acid secreting parietal cells is thought to enable outgrowth and/or colonization of non-HP bacteria, including intestinal and oral strains, under conditions of a rising pH. Likewise, routine eradication of HP by antibiotics now unveils the non-HP microbiome in patients worldwide.

Hence, diverse bacterial phylae were reported from both the human gastric juice and mucosa tissue dominated by **Firmicutes, Actinobacteria, Proteobacteria, and Bacteroidetes** (Noto and Peek Jr. 2017). Interestingly, the majority of the discovered families and species were actually either from environmental origin (e.g., soil, water, plants) or previously known as gut commensals from wild or domesticated mammals such as farm cattle and sewage (Table 4.1).

Table 4.1 The human gastric microbiome

NT Environmental / Commensals (Probiotics)		GC Environmental/Commensals (Pathogens)	
Fusobacteria **Leptotrichiaceae** Leptotrichia **Actinobacteria** **Actinomycetaceae** Actinomyces **Atopobiaceae** Olsenella, Atopobium **Bifidobacteriaceae** **Bifidobacterium**, Scardovia, Parascardovia **Brevibacteriaceae** Brevibacterium **Micrococcaceae** Rothia **Propionibacteriaceae** Tessaracoccus **Firmicutes** **Acidaminococcaceae** Phascolarctobacterium **Aerococcaceae** Abiotrophia **Bacillaceae** Anoxybacillus, Bacillus, Lentibacillus, Oceanobacillus **Bacillales (Family i.s.)** Gemella **Carnobacteriaceae** Granulicatella **Enterococcaceae** Enterococcus **Eubacteriaceae** Eubacterium **Erysipelotrichaceae** Solobacterium Bulleidia **Lactobacillaceae** **Lactobacillus** **Lachnospiraceae** Blautia, Lachnoclostridium, Catonella, Roseburia Lachnoanaerobaculum, Oribacterium, Stomatobaculum **Oscillospiraceae** Faecalibacterium, Oscillibacter **Peptostreptococcaceae** Filifactor **Selenomonadaceae** Megamonas **Staphylococcaceae** Staphylococcus **Streptococcaceae** **Lactococcus** **Thermoactinomycetaceae** Kroppenstedtia	**Bacteroidetes** **Bacteroidaceae** Bacteroides **Barnesiellaceae** Barnesiella **Chitinophagaceae** Sediminibacterium **Flavobacteriaceae** Flavobacterium **Prevotellaceae** Prevotella **Porphyromonadaceae** Porphyromonas **Tannerellaceae** Parabacteroides, Tannerella **Proteobacteria** **Bdellovibrionaceae** Bdellovibrio **Burkholderiaceae** Ralstonia, Burkholderia, Lautropia **Brucellaceae** Brucella/Ochrobactrum **Campylobacteraceae** Campylobacter **Comamonadaceae** Comamonas, Curvibacter **Desulfovibrionaceae** Desulfovibrio **Helicobacteraceae** Helicobacter **Legionellaceae** Legionella **Methylobacteriaceae** Methylobacterium **Neisseriaceae** Kingella, Bergeriella, Neisseria **Nitrobacteraceae** Bradyrhizobium **Pasteurellaceae** Haemophilu **Phyllobacteriaceae** Mesorhizobium **Pseudomonadaceae** Pseudomonas **Rhodanobacteraceae** Rudaea **Sphingomonadaceae** **Sphingobium**, Novosphingobium **Sterolibacteriaceae** Sulfuritalea **Vibrionaceae** Salinivibrio **Xanthomonadaceae** Stenotrophomonas, Pseudoxanthomonas **Yersiniaceae** Serratia **Zoogloeaceae** Thauera **Spirochaetes (phylum)** Treponema	**Fusobacteria** **Fusobacteriaceae** Fusobacterium **Actinobacteria** **Coriobacteriaceae** Collinsella **Corynebacteriaceae** Corynebacterium **Eggerthellaceae** Slackia **Gaiellaceae** Gaiella **Nocardiaceae** Rhodococcus **Propionibacteriaceae** Propionibacterium **Tsukamurellaceae** Tsukamurella **Firmicutes** **Clostridiaceae** Clostridium **Lachnospiraceae** Blautia Fusicatenibacter **Lactobacillaceae** Lactobacillus **Oscillospiraceae** Faecalibacterium Oscillospira **Peptoniphilaceae** Parvimonas **Peptostreptococcaceae** Peptostreptococcus Romboutsia **Streptococcaceae** Streptococcus **Selenomonadaceae** Selenomonas **Terrabacteria group** Intestinimonas **Veillonellaceae** Dialister Veillonella Megasphaera	**Bacteroidetes** **Flavobacteriaceae** Capnocytophaga **Porphyromonadaceae** Porphyromonas **Prevotellaceae** Prevotella Alloprevotella **Rikenellaceae** Alistipes **Weeksellaceae** Bergeyella **Proteobacteria** **Campylobacteraceae** Campylobacter **Enterobacteriaceae** Escherichia Shigella Klebsiella Citrobacter **Moraxellaceae** Acinetobacter **Neisseriaceae** Eikenella Uruburuella **Paraburkholderia** Burkholderia **Pasteurellaceae** Aggregatibacter **Rhodobacteraceae** Paracoccus Rhodospirillum **Xanthomonadaceae** Stenotrophomonas **Patescibacteria (candidate phyla)** **Acidobacteria (phyla)** **Nitrospirae (phyla)**

[a] Selection of bacteria detected in the healthy (NT, non-tumor) and neoplastic (GC, gastric cancer) human stomach including oral and intestinal microbiota originating from environmental sources (aquatic, soil, plants e.a.) and/or mucosa/skin commensals (farm cattle, sewage e.a.). Potential probiotics and pathogens (red) are detailed in Fig. 4.1

4.3 The Prime Pathogen: *Helicobacter pylori*

4.3.1 H. pylori-*Related Gastric Diseases*

Coexistence or symbiosis of HP with the human stomach has evolved over the last 50–100,000 years and resulted in adaptation and effective colonization of the world's population (Tshibangu-Kabamba and Yamaoka 2021). This gram-negative bacterium has a spiral shape and a flagellum which enables motility and adhesion to the gastric mucosa. A plethora of diseases have been associated with HP infections, including extra-gastrointestinal disorders.

The causal relationship between HP and the progressive sequence toward metaplasia (intestinal IM, pseudo/pyloric or spasmolytic polypeptide (TFF2)-expressing metaplasia (SPEM)) and adenocarcinoma has been well established together with the increased risks of ulcers and MALT lymphoma. The major driver of the Correa cascade (Correa 1992) is HP urease, besides other enzymes (catalase, oxidase) which cleave urea to ammonia to neutralize the gastric acid, leading to a pH rise and concomitant deterioration of gastric parietal, chief and endocrine cell functions and formation of a protective niche for its successful persistence in the organ.

Herein, HP also modulates the habitat of other resident microorganisms. Consistent with the general evidence, that abundance of HP in infected individuals decreases in the progression of the Correa cascade (Stewart et al. 2020), other non-HP strains can expand into and reconquer this "deserted" ecological niche (Coker et al. 2018). Accordingly, HP- individuals exhibited a higher alpha-diversity of the gastric microbiome than HP+ ones, indicative of a competitive microenvironment predominated by HP displacing other species in infected stomachs. Overall, there seems to be an inverse correlation between high HP abundance and low microbial diversity in the non-neoplastic stomach (Stewart et al. 2020). Vice versa, absence of HP is associated with increased abundance of non-HP species (Coker et al. 2018). Consistent with this, eradication of HP by antibiotics restores gastric microbial diversity (Sung et al. 2020). **Firmicutes, Actinobacteria, Proteobacteria, and Bacteroidetes** were among the major phyla detected in HP+ and HP- individuals (Stewart et al. 2020). No clear consensus was stated on the selective enrichment of certain non-HP strains in HP-infected vs. non-infected cases. Nonetheless, **Proteobacteria** were seemingly enriched in HP+ samples, whereas **Firmicutes, Actinobacteria, and Bacteroidetes** depleted (Noto and Peek Jr. 2017).

As for the normal healthy stomach, inconsistent data were obtained regarding the differential abundance of non-HP bacteria within the Correa cascade (Stewart et al. 2020). However, there is a general notion that the overall composition, given by the alpha-diversity of the gastric microbiome, changes in the course of transition from persistent inflammation of chronic gastritis with functional dyspepsia to gastric atrophy, peptic ulcer disease or metaplasia, a pre-malignant state for the development of GC (Li et al. 2017). Again, no consensus exists on the relative/selective enrichment vs. depletion of defined taxa (Noto and Peek Jr. 2017). As an overarching pattern one may conclude from the plethora of often contradicting reports, that along the proposed Correa cascade potentially pathogenic oral (Bakhti and Latifi-Navid 2021) and commensal gut bacteria (Chen et al. 2021) overtake the gastric niche at the expense of stomach-resident taxa often derived from "environmental" sources.

In chronic atrophic gastritis, disruption of the epithelial barrier (e.g., tight junctions), cell death, and inflammatory chemokines/cytokines (IL1/8, TNFα e.a.) promote a vicious cycle resulting in loss of organ function. For example, **Streptococcaceae, Prevotellaceae, and Fusobacteriaceae** were enriched compared with healthy controls (Parsons et al. 2017), as were in functional dyspepsia (Duran et al. 2021). HP infection and long-term drug intake (e.g., NSAIDs) cause peptic ulcers. Here, the injury of the gastric mucosa evoked by acid and peptic enzymes reaches outward into the submucosal tissue. Again, HP eradication reduces recurrence of the disease (Tshibangu-Kabamba and Yamaoka 2021) and non-HP bacteria were enriched in ulcers (Chen et al. 2018a).

In addition to the three predominant bacteria families mentioned above, intestinal metaplasia (IM) exhibits dysbiosis compared to healthy controls with a marked enrichment of strains encoding for type IV secretion system (**T4SS**) virulence transfer genes, enzymes for nitrate-to-nitrite reduction and N2-to-ammonia fixation (e.g., **Rhizobiales**) (Park et al. 2019a, b), which may be causally implicated in transition to GC from this pre-malignant state by producing N-nitroso-compounds. Vice versa, potentially protective nitrite-oxidizing bacteria (e.g., **Nitrospirae**) (Wang et al. 2020a) were reduced in IM. Hitherto, no studies were reported on the association of SPEM or MALT lymphoma with the gastric microbiome. Conclusively, early but persistent changes in microbiota composition and associated metabolic pathways may facilitate malignant transformation of an already challenged and susceptible gastric mucosa.

4.3.2 Pathogenic Mechanisms of H. pylori*: Virulence Factors*

HP employs multiple strategies to evade the host immune system and trigger formation of a protective niche for persistent colonization of the stomach (Salama et al. 2013). As a "side effect" of its own evolutionary success, HP evokes a sequential cascade of cell damaging and inflammatory events which ultimately leads to the above described step-wise Correa cascade and GC. In contrast to most non-HP strains, the virulence factors of HP have been well characterized (Yamaoka 2010). In addition, HP displays strong genetic diversity (e.g., mutation, recombination) and on the host side also relies on the genetic heterogeneity (e.g., polymorphisms in immune-related genes) for optimization of its life-long persistence in the body (Tshibangu-Kabamba and Yamaoka 2021).

For example, the outer membrane protein (OMP) **BabA** acts as an adhesion molecule for the ABO blood group antigens on host cells. Others are sialic acid binding adhesin (SabA), adherence-associated lipoprotein (AlpA/B), outer membrane inflammatory protein (OipA), and Hop proteins (Yamaoka 2010). These molecules enforce binding to the gastric mucosa and avoid shear forces to detach and flush the bacteria to the lower part of the digestive tract.

VacA is a pore forming toxin able to disrupt the plasma membrane and evoke vacuolization of the host epithelial cells by damaging intracellular traffic and mitochondrial permeability followed by cell death (Yamaoka 2010).

CagA has been robustly associated with GC pathogenesis (Yamaoka 2010). As such, CagA+ injection-proficient strains augment the risk to develop GC in humans (Huang et al. 2003) and animal models (Tshibangu-Kabamba and Yamaoka 2021). The CagA gene is located within the cag pathogenicity island (cag PAI), a region of the bacterial genome which also encodes a type IV secretion system (**T4SS**). This needle-like injection protein complex delivers CagA across the outer and inner bacterial membrane to the cytoplasm of the host cell. Upon translocation, CagA promotes rapid signaling events (e.g., phosphorylations) and rearrangement of the cytoskeleton (e.g., by the small GTPase RHO), culminating in disruption of cellular junctions, loss of polarity, and changes in cell proliferation and viability. Both VacA and CagA, via attacking the apical epithelial cell barrier of the host, once the epithelium is leaky, trigger multiple secondary effects on the immune cell repertoire in the lamina propria and submucosa. The release of "danger-associated molecular patterns" molecules (**DAMPs**) from stressed, damaged and dying cells further amplifies the tissue rearrangement ultimately leading to morphological (metaplasia) and malignant transformation of epithelial cells (Salama et al. 2013).

4.3.3 Pathogenic Mechanisms of **H. pylori***: Immunity*

Upon adherence and translocation of virulence factors into the gastric epithelial cells, disruption of this first front of defense, allows the bacterium to enter the next colonization phase by stimulating innate and adaptive immune responses in the host (Salama et al. 2013). Components of the bacterial cell wall, also termed microbial (**MAMPs**) or pathogen-associated molecular patterns (**PAMPs**), are recognized by host cells via pattern-recognition receptors (PRR). For example, toll-like receptors (TLR) bind lipopolysaccharide (LPS), various lipid compounds, nucleic acids, and flagellin derived from HP and propagate the signal transduction to transcription factors (NFκB, IRF) in the nucleus which trigger expression of proinflammatory genes (e.g., IFNγ, TNFα, IL1/6/8/12). These local events attract T effector (CD4+ Th1/2, CD8+ Tc, Th17) and Treg cells into the submucosa, amplifying the adaptive response followed by induction of immunosuppression and tolerance which results in a kind of "truce" allowing long-term survival of the bacteria in the colonized stomach and prevention of detrimental, severe inflammation, bacteria elimination, and overt tissue damage (Tshibangu-Kabamba and Yamaoka 2021). This delicate state of balance may also allow overgrowth of non-HP bacteria at the expense of HP.

4.4 Dysbiosis of Non-HP Microbiota in Gastric Cancer

For decades, HP has been regarded to be the dominant if not exclusively only bacterium which is able to survive in the acid environment of the stomach and promotes gastric carcinogenesis (Serrano et al. 2021). However, recent evidence from 16SrRNA sequencing collected evidence for the co-occurrence of non-HP strains in both HP+ and HP− individuals with GC (Li and Yu 2020). Accumulating data also delineates the term "**dysbiosis**" as most appropriate for a progressively altered microbiome during development of GC (Coker et al. 2018). However, no general consensus has been defined so far regarding a specific change of certain microbiota strains in association with progression (Stewart et al. 2020) or CMS (Cancer Genome Atlas Research Network 2014) of GC. Nonetheless, the occupation of the gastric niche upon a rising pH after HP infection by upward migration of commensal gut microbiota (caudal-to-cranial) (Chen et al. 2021) and downward migration of oral microbiota (cranial-to-caudal) (Bakhti and Latifi-Navid 2021) is an emerging theme (Fig. 4.1).

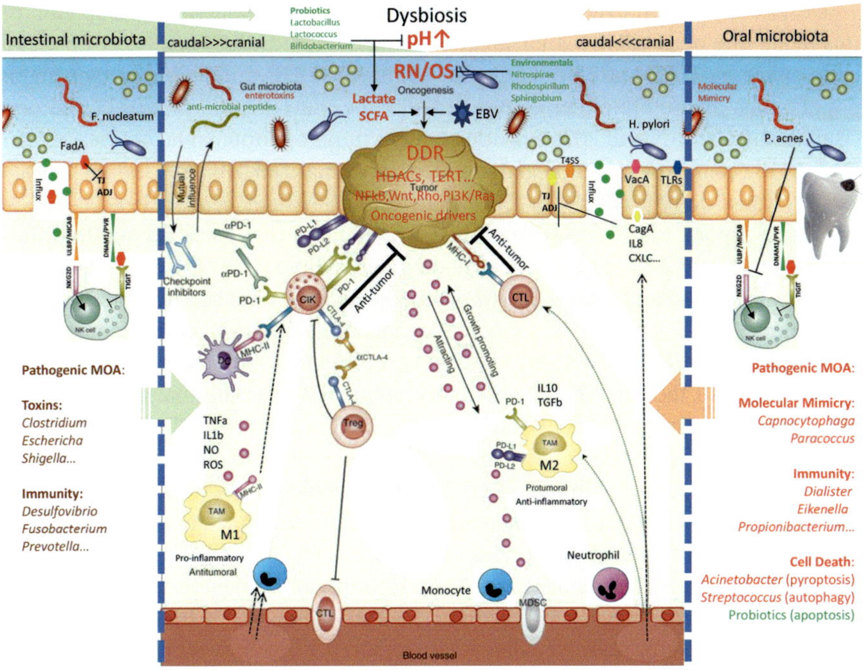

Fig. 4.1 Microbiota in gastric cancer. Overview of pathogenic (red) vs. beneficial (green, probiotics) bacterial strains enriched in the neoplastic human stomach compared with the healthy gastrointestinal tract and the oral cavity including periodontal tissue, saliva, and gastric juice. Bidirectional migration and colonization of intestinal and oral non-HP strains contribute to gastric carcinogenesis beyond H. pylori (HP). The interplay between epithelial barrier disruption by microbiota and submucosal host immune responses is depicted and detailed in the main text. *MOA* mode of action, *ADJ/TJ* adherens/tight junction, *DDR* DNA-damage response, *RN/OS* reactive nitrogen/oxygen species, *TERT* telomerase, *HDAC* histone deacetylase, *SCFA* small-chain fatty acid (e.g., butyrate); Cell types: *MDSC* myeloid-derived suppressor cell, *TAN/M* tumor-associated neutrophil/macrophage, *NK* natural killer cell, *DC* dendritic cell, *T/B* lymphocyte, *CTL* cytotoxic CD8+ T lymphocyte, *CIK* cytokine-induced killer cell (NK or CD4+ helper/CD8+ cytotoxic T cells), *Treg* regulatory (immunosuppressive) T cell

In this context, multiple **pathogenic mode of actions** (MOAs) have been described to be exerted by these species, a fact which may co-trigger and exacerbate carcinogenesis which frequently develops, e.g., by sporadic or inherited mutations, also in absence of HP after its eradication or in non-infected individuals (Li and Yu 2020; Noto and Peek Jr. 2017). Both, increase in abundance and alpha-diversity as well as decrease in the same population parameters have been evinced by a plethora of sequencing approaches for the Correa cascade (Correa 1992) starting from the healthy mucosa to atrophic gastritis, metaplasia, early vs. advanced, metastatic GC (Stewart et al. 2020). The underlying idea of these apparent paradox results is that reduction in the dominant HP species in the stomach upon malignant transformation of the gastric mucosa opens a novel ecological niche to be populated by competing strains from the upper and lower GI tract (Serrano et al. 2021).

Despite lack of an overall consensus, the concept of competitive occupation of this niche of a quasi-sterile stomach after pH rise upon dysfunction/loss of parietal cells either by HP or atrophy allows to stratify non-HP microbiota in two major populations. Those are either commensals of the gut (Chen et al. 2021) and oral (Bakhti and Latifi-Navid 2021) cavities or ubiquitous environmental species (Coker et al. 2018) abundant in natural and polluted, industrialized habitats (Table 4.1) such as soil, water, dairy products, or feces from animals (Elinav et al. 2019).

Scarce reports have recently emerged which claim that there are subtle differences between CMS and histomorphological subtypes of GC. For example, *Fusobacteria, Bacteroidetes, Patescibacteria* seem to be enriched in signet-ring cell carcinoma (SRCC), while *Proteobacteria* and *Acidobacteria* in adenocarcinoma (Ravegnini et al. 2020). Another group, however limited to stool samples, found that diffuse GC had the lowest alpha-diversity compared with the intestinal type and gastrointestinal stromal tumors (GIST). As such, tumor patients had higher abundance of *Enterobacteriaceae* and lower abundance of probiotic *Lactobacillaceae* and *Bifidobacteriaceae* (Sarhadi et al. 2021). Likewise, studies demonstrated contradictory results on decrease or increase of microbiome complexity across early vs. advanced pTNM stages of GC (reviewed in Stewart et al. 2020). No non-HP microbiota have so far been correlated with MALT lymphoma. Taken together, those preliminary studies may in the future allow a stratification of GI tumors by specific microbiota profile for improved diagnosis or therapeutic intervention.

4.5 Pathogenic Mechanisms of Non-HP Microbiota in Gastric Carcinogenesis

Bacteria exert multiple mechanisms to enable efficient adherence, enforce invasion, and achieve persistent colonization of GI epithelia (Levy et al. 2017). This aggressive behavior elicits counter responses by the host which manifest as inflammation and anti-microbial immune responses (e.g., defensins), activation of epithelial signaling, e.g., at adherens/tight junctions and loss of barrier integrity, and direct damage of cells or DNA by microbial toxins or epigenetic changes in the host DNA by bacterial metabolites (Elinav et al. 2019). Overall, the balance between beneficial probiotic microbiota and potentially detrimental strains, which may be selectively targeted by antibiotics, seems to be crucial in maintaining the physiological homeostasis, a delicate network which is disrupted in GC (Stewart et al. 2020). As such, the molecular modes of actions for the following species (Fig. 4.1) have already been deciphered and are not limited to the stomach.

Specific examples for pathogenic mechanisms are highlighted by **Fusobacterium nucleatum** (Brennan and Garrett 2019), originally gut microbiota, enriched (Table 4.1) not only in GC, but also in CRC and pancreatic cancers, which confers poor prognosis in diffuse but not intestinal-type GC (Boehm et al. 2020). In CRC, outer membrane vesicles and the adhesin **FadA** target E-cadherin of epithelial cells, activating β-catenin and Wnt/NFκB signaling, inducing expression of proinflammatory cytokines (IL1/6/8, TNFα) and epithelial-to-mesenchymal transition (EMT).

Adhesin **Fap2** blocks host immunity by binding TIGIT on T/NK cells (Gur et al. 2015). It is unclear if these virulence factors also contribute to GC.

Proteobacteria are abundant in GC, e.g., **Desulfovibrio** (Liu et al. 2021) a sulfate-reducing gut strain was detected in the feces of patients with advanced GC (stage IV) compared to early stages. Mechanistically, H_2S-induced synthesis of inflammatory factors (NO, IL1β, IL18) in CRC cell lines, factors possibly implicated in gastric carcinogenesis as well (Liu et al. 2021). Likewise, **Burkholderia** is abundant in GC, however with unknown etiology, previously known from the environmental saprophyte *B. pseudomallei* causing melioidosis, a frequently lethal tropical systemic or chronic disseminated infection (West et al. 2010). In GC patients, **Stenotrophomonas** and **Selenomonas (Firmicutes)** positively, *Comamonas* and *Gaiella* negatively correlated with BDCA2 + pDC and Foxp3 + Treg cells (Ling et al. 2019), proposing novel targets to attack the immunosuppressive microenvironment in GC. **Paracoccus denitrificans** exploits molecular mimicry to resemble the TIR domain of human TLRs and MyD88 proteins to adopt an identical structure of the host receptor to interfere with proinflammatory signaling and promote immune escape (Chan et al. 2009).

Representative for **Bacteroidetes** enriched in GC is **Acinetobacter baumannii**, a common multidrug-resistant source of nosocomial (hospital-acquired) infections. It induces pyroptosis through activation of caspase-1 and synthesis of IL1β in alveolar macrophage *in vivo* (Dai et al. 2018). (Li et al. 2018) *A. baumannii* triggered type I IFN production, activation of the NLRP3 inflammasome, resulting in mixed pyroptosis and necroptosis, potentially damage triggers also relevant for GC development.

Downward migration toward the stomach and gastric colonization of **oral** bacteria has been previously underrecognized. Dysbiosis of the oral microbiome (Bakhti and Latifi-Navid 2021), with high abundance of **Firmicutes** (e.g., *Pepto/Streptococcus, Dialister*) and **Actinobacteria** (e.g., *Slackia exigua*) in GC, now focused the attention to the association of peri-oral and dental hygiene with upper GI cancer risk (Coker et al. 2018). As above pathogenic mechanisms remain largely elusive or may resemble those exerted by intestinal microbiota. For example, **Peptostreptococcus anaerobius** (Long et al. 2019; Tsoi et al. 2017) adheres to murine and human CRC cells and accelerates tumor development in wt and *Apcmin/+* mice via TLRs or the cell wall protein PCWBR2 and α2/β1 integrin, followed by activation of the PI3K/AKT pathway, leading to increased cell proliferation and NFκB-dependent cytokine expression (IL10, IFNγ), and expansion of myeloid lineages (MDSC, TAMs), promoting cancer progression. **Streptococcus anginosus** is increased in GC and oral squamous cell carcinoma (OSCC) (Xu et al. 2021). In OSCC cell lines, culture supernatants reduced proliferation, migration, and invasion and promoted apoptosis, but increased autophagy, a major driver of cancer progression and resistance. Periodontal strains **Veillonella parvula** and **Streptococcus gordonii** (Hirschfeld et al. 2017) stimulated human peripheral blood neutrophils to release ROS and anti-microbial proteins (elastase, myeloperoxidase, cathepsin G), again exacerbating the inflammatory response.

Similarly, **Bacteroidetes** such as **Prevotella** may play a causal role in GC (Gunathilake et al. 2019), with *P. copri* a predominant strain in the human gut microbiome promoting inflammation and ROS formation. A clinical study in patients with acute dental root abscess (Sousa et al. 2014) showed that Raw264.7 macrophages stimulated with endodontic contents containing **Prevotella nigrescens, Parvimonas micra, Porphyromonas endodontalis,** and **Dialister pneumosintes** endotoxins elicited IL1β and TNFα release promoting inflammation *in vitro*. If this mechanism is valid for bacteria which migrated into the stomach remains to be proven.

Porphyromonas gingivalis secretes cysteine proteases (gingipains), key drivers of chronic periodontitis linked to systemic disease and formation of oral and gastric tract tumors. Mechanistically, it abrogates protection by SPINK6 (Tissue Inhibitor of Human Kallikreins) (Plaza et al. 2016) and evokes formation of periodontitis-related oral tumors in mice (Wu et al. 2018). The oral microbe **Capnocytophaga ochracea** (Martino et al. 2001) exploits a molecular mimicry peptide from its vWFA protein to activate auto-reactive T cells (Szymula et al. 2014). Thus, immune responses to opportunistic pathogens may constitute triggers for autoimmunity or cancer.

Actinobacteria like **Propionibacterium acnes** of the skin were found in GC patients (Gunathilake et al. 2019), suggested to trigger corpus-dominant lymphocytic gastritis via NKG2D, an activatory NK cell receptor system and proinflammatory cytokine production (e.g., IL15) (Montalban-Arques et al. 2016). *P. acnes* overabundance in GC patients' tissues correlated positively with TNM staging, and culture supernatants promoted migration and M2 polarization of macrophages via TLR4/PI3K-AKT signaling *in vitro* (Li et al. 2021), presumably fostering GC progression. The GC-enriched periodontal pathogen **Slackia exigua** (Coker et al. 2018) has been proposed to be causal for rare cases of periprosthetic joint infections (Rieber et al. 2019) and systemic bacteremia (Lee et al. 2016), with mechanisms of action elusive.

Proteobacteria like **Eikenella corrodens** have been isolated from inflammatory CD68+ pseudotumors associated with chronic persistent infection (Lee et al. 2003). *E. corrodens* was also detected in the oral cavity with *Streptococcus constellatus* and *Fusobacterium nucleatum* colonizing the exposed bone of patients with anti-osteoclastic drug-related osteonecrosis of the jaws (Jabbour et al. 2016). Conclusively, future translational and mechanistic studies have to explore and validate the causal role of individual pathogenic strains in GC in view of effective intervention strategies.

4.6 Microbial Metabolites: The Good, the Bad, and the Ugly

4.6.1 Reactive O_2 and N_2 Metabolites

Besides direct attack on host epithelial cells by virulence factors, the metabolism of microbiota generates a plethora of soluble agents which also contribute to the transition of chronic inflammation to carcinogenesis (Tshibangu-Kabamba and Yamaoka

2021). For example, HP produces reactive oxygen and nitrogen species (RO/NS) which evoke DNA-damage including point mutations and double-strand breaks, thus acting as a mutagen (Yamaoka 2010). This direct genotoxic action is exacerbated by HP-induced down-regulation of DNA-repair factors in infected host cells (Koeppel et al. 2015), thereby facilitating genetic instability, a major driver of intestinal-type GC (Fig. 4.1).

Likewise, non-HP bacteria such as **Nitrospirae, Veillonella, Clostridium, Haemophilus, Staphylococcus, Neisseria,** and **Lactobacillus** (Table 4.1) contribute to the generation of pro-carcinogenic N-nitroso compounds (Lundberg et al. 2008). Food-borne nitrite is oxidized to nitrate by oral bacterial in the saliva, which is then further metabolized after entering the stomach. Overall, nitrosating and nitrate-reducing bacteria seem to be enriched in GC patients compared to healthy individuals (Ferreira et al. 2018). Both reactive oxygen and nitrogen compounds trigger lipid peroxidation and DNA-base alterations facilitating carcinogenesis.

4.6.2 Pros and Cons of Lactate

Probiotics are defined by the WHO as "live microorganisms which when administered in adequate amounts confer a health benefit on the host" (Salminen et al. 2021). This broad spectrum includes adverse effect prevention, restoration of eubiosis, and increase of antibiotics efficacies, e.g., during HP eradication. Mechanistically, out-competition within ecological niches (e.g., by biofilm formation) and production of metabolites (e.g., short-chain fatty acids **(SCFAs)** or proteins/peptides "bacteriocins") reduce adhesion and spread of pathogenic bacteria. The most prominent example of organic acids is lactate (Fig. 4.1), which has both pro- and anti-cancer effects (Certo et al. 2021). **Lactobacillus** and **Lactococcus** mitigate gastrointestinal disorders, however, their abundance is increased in GC (Ferreira et al. 2018; Castano-Rodriguez et al. 2017), where they also generate RO/NS compounds. Lactate is a major energy source from anaerobic glycolysis for cancer cells, also known as Warburg effect, fostering angiogenesis, metastasis, and immune tolerance. On the other hand, ample evidence underscores a role for lactate-producing strains in counteracting cancer (Certo et al. 2021). For example, **Lactobacillus gasseri** isolated from the human stomach lowers the synthesis of proinflammatory cytokines (TNFα, IL6) in HP-infected macrophages via inhibition of TNFα-converting enzyme (TACE/ADAM17) (Gebremariam et al. 2019). **Lactococcus lactis** inhibits growth of human GC cells via p53/p21-mediated cell cycle arrest and apoptosis (Kim et al. 2009). **Lactobacillus rhamnosus** homogenates reduced proliferation and metabolism in human GC and CRC cell lines (Orlando et al. 2009) and, as a probiotic supplementation, alleviated HP-associated gastric pathology in humans (Westerik et al. 2018). **Lactobacillus casei** extract induces apoptosis in GC cell lines by inhibiting NFκB and PI3K/AKT/mTOR survival signaling (Hwang et al. 2013), a strain reported to prevent GC. Low abundance of **Bifidobacterium** (e.g., *B. adolescentis, B. longum*) and *Bacteroides* in the gut was associated with

HP-related gastric ulcer and GC in patients (Devi et al. 2021), suggesting a protective role of probiotic supplementation diets, whereas *Dialister* and *Prevotella* were enriched in these disease conditions.

4.6.3 Epigenetic Modulation by SCFAs

An elegant twist in the attack mechanisms exploited by bacteria is their production of metabolites which are actually epigenetic modifiers of the DNA (Fig. 4.1). A landmark study discovered lactate-derived lactylation of histone lysine residues in human and murine macrophages (Zhang et al. 2019). Hypoxia and bacteria (**Escherichia coli, Acinetobacter baumannii,** and **Pseudomonas aeruginosa**) triggered glycolysis-driven lactate production followed by histone lactylation inducing expression of genes responsible for wound healing (e.g., arginase) and tissue homeostasis, thus enforcing repolarization from anti-tumor M1 toward pro-tumor M2 macrophages. Overall, human gut bacteria strains function as inhibitors of class I histone deacetylases (HDACs) through production of butyric acid, a potential antitumor epigenetic drug phenocopied by clinically approved valproic acid (Dai et al. 2020). A screen of phylogenetically diverse gut commensals from healthy human donors identified **Megasphaera massiliensis** (Yuille et al. 2018) as a major butyrate producing strain complemented by valeric and hexanoic acid which inhibited HDAC activity *in vitro*. **Prevotella histicola** (Balakrishnan et al. 2021) was isolated from a human duodenal biopsy and produced acetate and vitamins such as biotin and folate. In a mouse arthritis model, this strain restored eubiosis and via butyrate ameliorated immune and gut homeostasis. In contrast, the activity of HDAC3 was diminished in intestinal epithelial cells of germ-free mice compared with mice harboring physiological microbiomes: Therein, **Escherichia coli** (Wu et al. 2020) stimulated HDAC3 activity through phytate and inositol-1,4,5-trisphosphate (InsP3) to promote epithelial repair and growth of intestinal stem cells, potentiating the risk for neoplastic transformation. All these commensal gut bacteria have been detected in gastric specimens as well, however, no functional data are available so far, to undermine a direct role of these species in shaping the epigenetic profile of DNA-expression during gastric carcinogenesis.

4.7 Microbiota in Prevention and Therapy of GC: From Mice to Patients

Besides the traditional use of probiotics as nutrition additives (e.g., yogurt), novel sophisticated approaches like **fecal microbiota transplantation** (FMT) (Ng et al. 2020) have revolutionized the field by envisioning the therapeutical regain of eubiosis in gastrointestinal diseases. Several reports confirmed this concept for GC in transgenic mice: Colonization of the gut with "altered Schaedler flora" (ASF), containing *Clostridium, Lactobacillus* e.a., promotes GC in HP-infected INS-GAS mice (Lertpiriyapong et al. 2014). Vice versa, depletion of commensal flora delays GC formation under germ-free conditions in the same model (Lofgren et al. 2011). However, no studies were conducted yet for prevention or therapy of GC in humans. Notably, FMT procedures have been recently questioned by an international expert panel, due to variable outcomes and need for standardization and safety (Ng et al. 2020).

4.7.1 Probiotics: Prevention of Gastric Disease

Due to the wide-spread use of **proton pump inhibitors** (PPIs) (Malfertheiner et al. 2017), interest in their association with the gastric microbiome has risen. Long-term intake of PPIs reduces secretion of gastric acid favoring bacterial overgrowth, due to a pH rise as evoked by HP. Consequently, PPIs make profound impact on bacterial diversity and abundance (Duran et al. 2021). For example, high occurrence of oral cavity-derived *Bifidobacteriaceae* (*Bifidobacterium dentium, Scardovia inopinata, Parascardovia denticolens*) in human stomachs with hypochlorhydria was stated in omeprazole-treated gastritis (Mattarelli et al. 2014). *Streptophyta, Clostridiales, Fusobacterium, Veillonella, Oribacterium, Leptotrichia, Prevotella, Porphyromonas, Capnocytophaga, Granulicatella, Campylobacter,* and *Bulleidia* were also increased by PPIs, most of which can colonize the mouth (Parsons et al. 2017; Duran et al. 2021). Meta-analyses already confirmed the association of PPIs and gut colonization with multidrug-resistant strains (Willems et al. 2020) such as *enterobacterales* (β-lactamase+, carbapenemase+), vancomycin-resistant *enterococci*, methicillin/vancomycin-resistant *Staphylococcus aureus,* or multidrug-resistant *Pseudomonas* or *Acinetobacter* species. The oral microbiome is altered by PPIs as well. As such, esomeprazole (Mishiro et al. 2018) raised *Streptococcus* organisms in fecal and oral saliva samples. In GERD patients under PPI use (Shi et al. 2019), higher abundances of "environmentals" (*Planococcaceae, Oxalobacteraceae, Sphingomonadaceae, Methylophilus*) were found in the gastric mucosa. In the gastric refluxate of esophagitis and Barrett's esophagus patients on PPI prescription (Amir et al. 2014) levels of gut commensals (*Enterobacteriaceae, Erysipelotrichaceae, Clostridiales*) were elevated.

Again, the intake of **probiotic** strains together with **NSAIDs** or PPIs prevents some of their damaging adverse effects on gastrointestinal mucosae. For example, *Bifidobacterium* protects against gastric ulcer caused by aspirin in rats (Hsieh et al. 2021), and *Lactobacillus plantarum* from green tea ameliorates alcohol-induced gastric ulcers (Park et al. 2020). Oral supplementation of *Lactobacillus johnsonii* in mice treated with the PPIs rabeprazole or vonoprazan mitigated indomethacin-induced small intestinal damage (Nadatani et al. 2019). In patients (Tsujimoto et al. 2021) who received aspirin and vonoprazan or esomeprazole, increased abundance of *Lactobacillales* positively correlated with gastrin levels. Notably, probiotics in restoring eubiosis could be confirmed in experimental mice, however awaiting the elucidation of the underlying molecular biological mechanisms and validation in large clinical trials.

4.7.2 *Antibiotics: Eradication of* H. pylori

The Maastricht V/Florence (Malfertheiner et al. 2012) and Tapei Consensus Reports (Liou et al. 2020) recommended screening and eradication of HP for GC prevention by PPI-containing triple/quadruple therapy as a first-line treatment. Large clinical trials and field studies confirmed the cancer prevention upon HP eradication (Tshibangu-Kabamba and Yamaoka 2021), however antibiotics resistance is a rising obstacle, as is the perturbation of the gut microbiota and the impact of HP on other disease conditions (e.g., asthma, esophageal cancer). Nonetheless, most agree that HP depletion restores non-HP alpha-diversity in the stomach and the gut by increasing (Table 4.1) the ratio of beneficial to potentially pathogenic strains (Li et al. 2017).

A recent randomized controlled clinical trial evinced diverse microbes associated with gastric disease 1 year after HP eradication (Sung et al. 2020). *Acinetobacter lwoffii, Streptococcus anginosus and Ralstonia* were enriched, probiotic *Faecalibacterium prausnitzii, Roseburia,* and *Sphingomonas* were depleted. Likewise, oral bacteria (*Peptostreptococcus, Streptococcus, Parvimonas, Prevotella, Rothia, Granulicatella*) were associated persistent gastritis. Others confirmed long-term persistence of dysbiosis after HP eradication in patients upon endoscopic ablation of early GC (Watanabe et al. 2021) with loss of probiotic strains (*Blautia, Ralstonia, Faecalibacterium, Methylobacterium, Megamonas*). In young asymptomatic adults, HP eradication restores beneficial GI microbia (*Lactobacillus, Bifidobacterium, Blautia, Lachnoclostridium*), while pathogenic *Alistipes* was depleted (He et al. 2019).

As for **PPI or NSAID** intake, probiotics (*Lactobacillus, Bifidobacterium, Enterococcus, Bacillus*) were demonstrated to augment the efficacy of HP eradication, restore eubiosis, and avert side effects in patients (e.g., vomiting, diarrhea, pain) (Zheng et al. 2019; Wang et al. 2013; McFarland et al. 2016). For example, *Lactobacillus rhamnosus* (Chen et al. 2018b), *johnsonii* (Aiba et al. 2019), and *plantarum* (Pan et al. 2016) prevent or ameliorate HP infection *in vitro* and in mice.

An open clinical trial is assessing the efficacy of *Lactobacillus acidophilus* combined with quadruple therapy and its correlation with gastric pH value (Ji et al. 2018). Randomized controlled trials with quadruple therapy using probiotics supplement *Lactobacillus reuteri* reduced adverse events and improved patients' clinical performance (Poonyam et al. 2019), while triple therapy with *Lactobacillus delbrueckii* and *Streptococcus thermophilus* (Tongtawee et al. 2015) or *Clostridium butyricum* and *Bacillus coagulans* is less effective (Zhang et al. 2020). Meta-analyses (Lau et al. 2016), trial (Bruno et al. 2018), and field study (Westerik et al. 2018) reviews confirmed benefits of *Lactobacillus (acidophilus, reuteri, rhamnosus* e.a.),

Bifidobacterium, Streptococcus faecalis, Bacillus subtilis, yeast (*Saccharomyces*), and mixtures of probiotics in HP-eradicating triple therapy independent of age and ethnicity, and this was true both for the gastric and the gut flora (Oh et al. 2016).

4.7.3 Cancer Therapies

GC patients usually present at advanced stages where effective or even curative treatment options are limited (Wong et al. 2021). Those comprise surgery, radiation, and chemotherapies, the latter often associated with low efficacy and drug resistance. Recent targeted therapies benefit only small subsets of patients, e.g., blocking antibodies against Her2+ overexpressing tumors (Nakamura et al. 2021). Hence, novel approaches are of urgent clinical need. Overwhelmed by the recent success of immunotherapies, microbiota have regained attention in conjunction with boosting the host's tumor immunosurveillance (Elinav et al. 2019; Levy et al. 2017).

4.7.3.1 Surgery

For example, several strains were positively associated with clinical outcomes of **surgery** or endoscopic resection. As such, probiotics lowered post-operative inflammation, enhanced immunity and nutrition indices, improved gut microbiota and general recovery. Randomized controlled trials showed improved post-operative quality of gastric bypass surgery upon supplementation of *Clostridium butyricum* (Chen et al. 2016) and *Bifidobacterium longum*, (Zheng et al. 2019) and reduced severity of disorders upon partial gastrectomy in GC patients after administration of *Bifidobacterium infantis, Lactobacillus acidophilus, Enterococcus faecalis,* and *Bacillus cereus. Lactobacillus (plantarum, rhamnosus, acidophilus) and Bifidobacterium animalis subsp. lactis* improved conditions after gastrectomy in patients and rat models (Zheng et al. 2021). A multicenter retrospective cohort study found that antibiotics and probiotics reduce risk of metachronous GC (Arai et al. 2021) after endoscopic resection.

4.7.3.2 Chemotherapy

Further, **chemotherapy** outcome was reported to be fostered by the presence of certain gut commensal microbiota strains. Chemotherapy reduced the abundance of gut bacteria in GC patients by more than 50% (Zhang et al. 2021), therein *Lactobacillus* and *Megasphaera* were associated with GC. Neoadjuvant chemotherapy (NACT) combined with enteral nutrition improved perioperative immunity, inflammation, and intestinal flora in GC patients (Zong et al. 2019) with a rise in *Bifidobacterium* and *Lactobacillus* and a decline in *Escherichia coli* and *Enterococcus*. Likewise, a higher incidence of post-operative infection in GC patients under NACT occurred, accompanied by intestinal barrier damage, down-regulation of tight junction proteins, and reduced probiotics (*Bifidobacterium, Faecalibacterium, Ruminococcus*) (Wei et al. 2017). *Enterococcus hirae* and *Barnesiella intestinihominis* translocate from the colon to secondary lymphoid organs, increase intratumoral CD8/Treg ratios, infiltration of IFNγ-producing γδT cells and strain-specific memory Th1 cells conferring longer progression-free survival in advanced lung and ovarian cancer patients treated with **cyclophosphamide** chemo-immunotherapy (Daillere et al. 2016). **Oxaliplatin**-induced GI mucositis and damage were mitigated in mice and patients by probiotics (BIO-THREE: *Clostridium butyricum, Enterococcus, Bacillus mesentericus*) (Yuan et al. 2022). *Escherichia coli Nissle* and *Faecalibacterium prausnitzii* supernatants reduced viability and monolayer permeability of intestinal epithelial cell lines and improved preclinical parameters in a rat model of **5-FU**-induced mucositis (Wang et al. 2017). Probiotic *Lactobacillus rhamnosus* augmented the efficacy of **capecitabine** against GC growth in mice (Rahimi et al. 2021). If this holds true for human GC remains to be shown. In contrast to CRC, no reports were recorded on the microbiome and chemo- or targeted therapies in GC patients.

4.7.3.3 Immunotherapy

Similar lack of knowledge pertains for the association of **immunotherapy** with gastric microbiota. The DELIVER (JACCRO GC-08) clinical trial is now recruiting patients to discover novel host-related immune-biomarkers for nivolumab (PD1 Ab) in advanced GC, awaiting results in the future (Sunakawa et al. 2019). Several *in vitro* reports described induction of PD1/PDL1 expression in GC cells by virulence factors (as reviewed in Aydin et al. 2021). A recent landmark paper demonstrated that HP may have a detrimental effect on the survival outcome (OS/PFS) and efficacy of immune checkpoint inhibitors in mouse xenograft models (colon, melanoma) and NSCLC patients, but not for GC (Oster et al. 2022). IRAE and related toxicities seem to correlate to high abundance of gut-associated **Bacteroides intestinalis** in melanoma patients (Andrews et al. 2021). Moreover, defined gut strains in patients or mice under anti-CTLA4/PD1 therapy (**Collinsella, Enterococcus, Bacteroides, Burkholderia, Faecalibacterium, Bifidobacterium, Akkermansia, Ruminococcaceae**) augmented efficacy and prolonged survival while minimizing adverse effects such as colitis (as reviewed by Miller and Carson 2020).

4.7.3.4 Oncomicrobiotics

Besides metabolic or epigenetic mechanisms, bacteria produce active components (e.g., enterotoxins, adjuvants) which directly modulate the infected host to prevent dysbiosis-associated gastrointestinal disorders and potentially prevent or treat cancer. For example, **Enterobacteriaceae** are enriched in GC (Table 4.1). As such, **Shigella Flexneri** whose enterotoxin causes diarrhea, fever, and stomach cramps, induced Bax/Bcl2-dependent apoptosis in pancreatic cancer cell lines (Khodavirdipour et al. 2021), and irinotecan-coupled Shiga toxin via uptake by glycosphingolipid Gb3/CD77 effectively killed GC cell lines *in vitro* (Geyer et al. 2016). Bacillomycin D from **Bacillus subtilis** triggered apoptosis of GC cell lines through PI3K/AKT/FOXO signaling (Lin et al. 2019), and **Clostridium perfringens** enterotoxin exerted cytotoxicity on GC cells and attenuated tumor growth of xenografts in nude mice (Liang et al. 2017). Cholera toxin as a mucosal adjuvant orally administrated to C57BL/6 mice suppressed syngeneic tumor growth by priming cytotoxic CD8+ T cells (Wakabayashi et al. 2008), and super-antigen SEB (Staphylococcal Enterotoxin B) exerted anti-tumor efficacy in co-cultures of GC cells and PBMCs *in vitro* and in rats (Tong et al. 2010).

Specialized environmental bacteria (Table 4.1) degrade harmful compounds (e.g., heterocarbocyclic, aromatic), fix N_2 to ammonia, or reduce N-nitroso-compounds, and thereby may prevent carcinogenesis (Lundberg et al. 2008). For example, asparaginase of **Rhodospirillum rubrum**, an N_2-fixating bacterium identified in GC, prevents tumor growth by down-regulating expression of the catalytic subunit hTERT of the telomerase complex in multiple cancer cell lines and in xenograft models (Zhdanov et al. 2017). **Sphingobium yanoikuyae**, which degrades carcinogenic heterocarbocyclic substances, is depleted in GC patients (Hu et al. 2018), whereas *Neisseria, Alloprevotella, Aggregatibacter, Streptococcus mitis oralis pneumoniae, and Porphyromonas endodontalis* were enriched. It remains to be explored if probiotic supplementation may be exploited to detoxify harmful chemicals in situ.

Alternative approaches repurposing microbiota or its components as active therapeutic agents comprise adoptive cell transfer, e.g., DC-based vaccines (Radojevic et al. 2021) or nano-medicines (Ladaycia et al. 2021): For example, **Lactobacillus kimchicus**-coated gold nano-particles triggered apoptosis in human GC cancer cells (Kim et al. 2019), and purified magnetosomes from **Magnetospirillum gryphiswaldense** combined with agonistic TNF-receptor Ab (CD137/4-11BB) prevented tumor formation in mice (Tang et al. 2019). Decades ago, it was already evident that "biological response modifiers" [**Streptococcus pyogenes, Bacillus Calmette-Guerin (BCG), Corynebacterium parvum**] mount anti-tumor responses in GC patients (Nakayama et al. 1998). Nonetheless, translational validation of defined immunotherapeutic "**oncomicrobiota**" against GC is hitherto lacking.

4.7.3.5 Perspectives

With pathogenic and therapeutic modes of actions (MOAs) of defined bacteria still to be unraveled, the knowledge of other kingdoms (virome, phagome, mycobiota) and "macrobiota" (helminths, nematodes) is even scarcer. Meta-analyses proposed non-EBV viruses (HBV, CMV, HPV e.a.) as GC risk factors (Wang et al. 2020b), and dysbiosis of intestinal fungi impacts on anti-tumor immune responses upon radiation in mice (breast cancer, melanoma) (Shiao et al. 2021). As such, *Candida albicans* infection was associated with gastric carcinogenesis (Zhong et al. 2021), while probiotic *Saccharomyces cerevisiae var. boulardii* supernatant inhibited survivin gene expression and induced apoptosis in human GC cells (Pakbin et al. 2021). Single case reports associated parasitic worm infections with regression of MALT lymphoma after co-eradication with HP (Singh et al. 2018). Conclusively, a holistic, individualized and mechanistic understanding of the heterogeneity of inter-kingdom ecosystems around, on, and in our body is needed to develop novel patient-tailored strategies to diagnose, prevent, or treat GC.

Author Contributions All the authors contributed to the writing and editing of the review. All the authors approved the final version.

Funding EB received funding from Deutsche Forschungsgemeinschaft (DFG, BU2285). EB and ME were supported by GRK 2727 [DFG Graduate School: Innate Immune Checkpoints in Cancer and Tissue Damage (InCheck)].

Compliance with Ethical Standards

Conflict of interest: All authors declare no conflict of **interest.**

Ethical approval and ethical standards: Not applicable. This is a review of published literature review and contains no original data.

References

Aiba Y, et al. Synergistic effect of anti-Helicobacter pylori urease immunoglobulin Y from egg yolk of immunized hens and Lactobacillus johnsonii No.1088 to inhibit the growth of Helicobacter pylori in vitro and in vivo. Vaccine. 2019;37(23):3106–12.

Amir I, et al. Gastric microbiota is altered in oesophagitis and Barrett's oesophagus and further modified by proton pump inhibitors. Environ Microbiol. 2014;16(9):2905–14.

Andrews MC, et al. Gut microbiota signatures are associated with toxicity to combined CTLA-4 and PD-1 blockade. Nat Med. 2021;27(8):1432–41.

Arai J, et al. Use of antibiotics and probiotics reduces the risk of metachronous gastric cancer after endoscopic resection. Biology (Basel). 2021;10(6):455.

Aydin EM, et al. The crosstalk between H. pylori virulence factors and the PD1:PD-L1 immune checkpoint inhibitors in progression to gastric cancer. Immunol Lett. 2021;239:1–11.

Bakhti SZ, Latifi-Navid S. Oral microbiota and Helicobacter pylori in gastric carcinogenesis: what do we know and where next? BMC Microbiol. 2021;21(1):71.

Balakrishnan B, et al. Prevotella histicola protects from arthritis by expansion of Allobaculum and augmenting butyrate production in humanized mice. Front Immunol. 2021;12:609644.

Boehm ET, et al. Fusobacterium nucleatum is associated with worse prognosis in Lauren's diffuse type gastric cancer patients. Sci Rep. 2020;10(1):16240.

Brennan CA, Garrett WS. Fusobacterium nucleatum—symbiont, opportunist and oncobacterium. Nat Rev Microbiol. 2019;17(3):156–66.

Bruno G, et al. Helicobacter pylori infection and gastric dysbiosis: can probiotics administration be useful to treat this condition? Can J Infect Dis Med Microbiol. 2018;2018:6237239.

Cancer Genome Atlas Research Network. Comprehensive molecular characterization of gastric adenocarcinoma. Nature. 2014;513(7517):202–9.

Castano-Rodriguez N, et al. Dysbiosis of the microbiome in gastric carcinogenesis. Sci Rep. 2017;7(1):15957.

Certo M, et al. Lactate modulation of immune responses in inflammatory versus tumour microenvironments. Nat Rev Immunol. 2021;21(3):151–61.

Chan SL, et al. Molecular mimicry in innate immunity: crystal structure of a bacterial TIR domain. J Biol Chem. 2009;284(32):21386–92.

Chen JC, et al. Effect of probiotics on postoperative quality of gastric bypass surgeries: a prospective randomized trial. Surg Obes Relat Dis. 2016;12(1):57–61.

Chen X, et al. Comparisons between bacterial communities in mucosa in patients with gastric antrum ulcer and a duodenal ulcer. Front Cell Infect Microbiol. 2018a;8:126.

Chen ME, et al. Baicalin, Baicalein, and Lactobacillus Rhamnosus JB3 alleviated Helicobacter pylori infections in vitro and in vivo. J Food Sci. 2018b;83(12):3118–25.

Chen CC, et al. The interplay between Helicobacter pylori and gastrointestinal microbiota. Gut Microbes. 2021;13(1):1–22.

Coker OO, et al. Mucosal microbiome dysbiosis in gastric carcinogenesis. Gut. 2018;67(6):1024–32.

Correa P. Human gastric carcinogenesis: a multistep and multifactorial process—First American Cancer Society Award Lecture on Cancer Epidemiology and Prevention. Cancer Res. 1992;52(24):6735–40.

Dai M, et al. The antimicrobial cathelicidin peptide hlF(1-11) attenuates alveolar macrophage pyroptosis induced by Acinetobacter baumannii in vivo. Exp Cell Res. 2018;364(1):95–103.

Dai Z, Ramesh V, Locasale JW. The evolving metabolic landscape of chromatin biology and epigenetics. Nat Rev Genet. 2020;21(12):737–53.

Daillere R, et al. Enterococcus hirae and Barnesiella intestinihominis facilitate cyclophosphamide-induced therapeutic immunomodulatory effects. Immunity. 2016;45(4):931–43.

Devi TB, et al. Low Bifidobacterium abundance in the lower gut microbiota is associated with Helicobacter pylori-related gastric ulcer and gastric cancer. Front Microbiol. 2021;12:631140.

Duran C, et al. Nonlinear machine learning pattern recognition and bacteria-metabolite multilayer network analysis of perturbed gastric microbiome. Nat Commun. 2021;12(1):1926.

Elinav E, et al. The cancer microbiome. Nat Rev Cancer. 2019;19(7):371–6.

Ferreira RM, et al. Gastric microbial community profiling reveals a dysbiotic cancer-associated microbiota. Gut. 2018;67(2):226–36.

Gebremariam HG, et al. Lactobacillus gasseri suppresses the production of proinflammatory cytokines in Helicobacter pylori-infected macrophages by inhibiting the expression of ADAM17. Front Immunol. 2019;10:2326.

Geyer PE, et al. Gastric adenocarcinomas express the glycosphingolipid Gb3/CD77: targeting of gastric cancer cells with Shiga toxin B-subunit. Mol Cancer Ther. 2016;15(5):1008–17.

Gunathilake MN, et al. Association between the relative abundance of gastric microbiota and the risk of gastric cancer: a case-control study. Sci Rep. 2019;9(1):13589.

Gur C, et al. Binding of the Fap2 protein of Fusobacterium nucleatum to human inhibitory receptor TIGIT protects tumors from immune cell attack. Immunity. 2015;42(2):344–55.

He C, et al. The eradication of Helicobacter pylori restores rather than disturbs the gastrointestinal microbiota in asymptomatic young adults. Helicobacter. 2019;24(4):e12590.

Hirschfeld J, et al. Modulation of neutrophil extracellular trap and reactive oxygen species release by periodontal bacteria. Infect Immun. 2017;85(12):e00297–17.

Hsieh SY, et al. Combined Lycium barbarum polysaccharides and C-phycocyanin increase gastric Bifidobacterium relative abundance and protect against gastric ulcer caused by aspirin in rats. Nutr Metab (Lond). 2021;18(1):4.

Hu YL, et al. The gastric microbiome is perturbed in advanced gastric adenocarcinoma identified through shotgun metagenomics. Front Cell Infect Microbiol. 2018;8:433.

Huang JQ, et al. Meta-analysis of the relationship between cagA seropositivity and gastric cancer. Gastroenterology. 2003;125(6):1636–44.

Human Microbiome Project Consortium. Structure, function and diversity of the healthy human microbiome. Nature. 2012;486(7402):207–14.

Hwang JW, et al. Lactobacillus casei extract induces apoptosis in gastric cancer by inhibiting NF-kappaB and mTOR-mediated signaling. Integr Cancer Ther. 2013;12(2):165–73.

Jabbour Z, et al. Profile of bacteria colonizing the exposed bone of patients with anti-osteoclastic drug-related osteonecrosis of the jaws. Can J Microbiol. 2016;62(9):772–80.
Ji W, Chen WQ, Tian X. Efficacy of compound Lactobacillus acidophilus tablets combined with quadruple therapy for Helicobacter pylori eradication and its correlation with pH value in the stomach: a study protocol of a randomised, assessor-blinded, single-centre study. BMJ Open. 2018;8(10):e023131.
Khodavirdipour A, et al. To study the anti-cancer effects of shigella Flexneri in AspC-1 pancreatic cancer cell line in approach to Bax and bcl-2 genes. J Gastrointest Cancer. 2021;52(2):593–9.
Kim SY, et al. Lactococcus lactis ssp. lactis inhibits the proliferation of SNU-1 human stomach cancer cells through induction of G0/G1 cell cycle arrest and apoptosis via p53 and p21 expression. Ann N Y Acad Sci. 2009;1171:270–5.
Kim YJ, et al. Development of Lactobacillus kimchicus DCY51(T)-mediated gold nanoparticles for delivery of ginsenoside compound K: in vitro photothermal effects and apoptosis detection in cancer cells. Artif Cells Nanomed Biotechnol. 2019;47(1):30–44.
Koeppel M, et al. Helicobacter pylori infection causes characteristic DNA damage patterns in human cells. Cell Rep. 2015;11(11):1703–13.
Ladaycia A, et al. Microbiota and cancer: in vitro and in vivo models to evaluate nanomedicines. Adv Drug Deliv Rev. 2021;170:44–70.
Lau CS, Ward A, Chamberlain RS. Probiotics improve the efficacy of standard triple therapy in the eradication of Helicobacter pylori: a meta-analysis. Infect Drug Resist. 2016;9:275–89.
Lee SH, et al. Inflammatory pseudotumour associated with chronic persistent Eikenella corrodens infection: a case report and brief review. J Clin Pathol. 2003;56(11):868–70.
Lee MY, et al. A case of bacteremia caused by Dialister pneumosintes and Slackia exigua in a patient with periapical abscess. Anaerobe. 2016;38:36–8.
Lertpiriyapong K, et al. Gastric colonisation with a restricted commensal microbiota replicates the promotion of neoplastic lesions by diverse intestinal microbiota in the Helicobacter pylori INS-GAS mouse model of gastric carcinogenesis. Gut. 2014;63(1):54–63.
Levy M, et al. Dysbiosis and the immune system. Nat Rev Immunol. 2017;17(4):219–32.
Li Q, Yu H. The role of non-H. pylori bacteria in the development of gastric cancer. Am J Cancer Res. 2020;10(8):2271–81.
Li TH, et al. Alterations in gastric microbiota after H. pylori eradication and in different histological stages of gastric carcinogenesis. Sci Rep. 2017;7:44935.
Li Y, et al. Type I IFN operates pyroptosis and necroptosis during multidrug-resistant A. baumannii infection. Cell Death Differ. 2018;25(7):1304–18.
Li Q, et al. Propionibacterium acnes overabundance in gastric cancer promote M2 polarization of macrophages via a TLR4/PI3K/Akt signaling. Gastric Cancer. 2021;24(6):1242–53.
Liang ZY, et al. Effect of Clostridium perfringens enterotoxin on gastric cancer cells SGC7901 which highly expressed claudin-4 protein. World J Gastrointest Oncol. 2017;9(4):153–9.
Lin F, et al. Bacillomycin D-C16 triggers apoptosis of gastric cancer cells through the PI3K/Akt and FoxO3a signaling pathways. Anticancer Drugs. 2019;30(1):46–55.
Ling Z, et al. Regulatory T cells and plasmacytoid dendritic cells within the tumor microenvironment in gastric cancer are correlated with gastric microbiota dysbiosis: a preliminary study. Front Immunol. 2019;10:533.
Liou JM, et al. Screening and eradication of Helicobacter pylori for gastric cancer prevention: the Taipei global consensus. Gut. 2020;69(12):2093–112.
Liu S, et al. Intestinal bacteria are potential biomarkers and therapeutic targets for gastric cancer. Microb Pathog. 2021;151:104747.
Lofgren JL, et al. Lack of commensal flora in Helicobacter pylori-infected INS-GAS mice reduces gastritis and delays intraepithelial neoplasia. Gastroenterology. 2011;140(1):210–20.
Long X, et al. Peptostreptococcus anaerobius promotes colorectal carcinogenesis and modulates tumour immunity. Nat Microbiol. 2019;4(12):2319–30.
Lundberg JO, Weitzberg E, Gladwin MT. The nitrate-nitrite-nitric oxide pathway in physiology and therapeutics. Nat Rev Drug Discov. 2008;7(2):156–67.

Malfertheiner P, et al. Management of Helicobacter pylori infection—the Maastricht IV/Florence Consensus Report. Gut. 2012;61(5):646–64.
Malfertheiner P, Kandulski A, Venerito M. Proton-pump inhibitors: understanding the complications and risks. Nat Rev Gastroenterol Hepatol. 2017;14(12):697–710.
Martino R, et al. Bacteremia caused by Capnocytophaga species in patients with neutropenia and cancer: results of a multicenter study. Clin Infect Dis. 2001;33(4):E20–2.
Matson V, et al. The commensal microbiome is associated with anti-PD-1 efficacy in metastatic melanoma patients. Science. 2018;359(6371):104–8.
Mattarelli P. et al. Occurrence of Bifidobacteriaceae in human hypochlorhydria stomach. Microb Ecol Health Dis. 2014:25.
McFarland LV, et al. Systematic review and meta-analysis: multi-strain probiotics as adjunct therapy for Helicobacter pylori eradication and prevention of adverse events. United European Gastroenterol J. 2016;4(4):546–61.
Miller PL, Carson TL. Mechanisms and microbial influences on CTLA-4 and PD-1-based immunotherapy in the treatment of cancer: a narrative review. Gut Pathog. 2020;12:43.
Mishiro T, et al. Oral microbiome alterations of healthy volunteers with proton pump inhibitor. J Gastroenterol Hepatol. 2018;33(5):1059–66.
Montalban-Arques A, et al. Propionibacterium acnes overabundance and natural killer group 2 member D system activation in corpus-dominant lymphocytic gastritis. J Pathol. 2016;240(4):425–36.
Nadatani Y, et al. Gastric acid inhibitor aggravates indomethacin-induced small intestinal injury via reducing Lactobacillus johnsonii. Sci Rep. 2019;9(1):17490.
Nakamura Y, et al. Biomarker-targeted therapies for advanced-stage gastric and gastro-oesophageal junction cancers: an emerging paradigm. Nat Rev Clin Oncol. 2021;18(8):473–87.
Nakayama F, et al. Effect of streptococcal lyzate OK-432 on peripheral blood mononuclear cells in gastric cancer patients. J Med. 1998;29(3–4):199–215.
Ng SC, et al. Scientific frontiers in faecal microbiota transplantation: joint document of Asia-Pacific Association of Gastroenterology (APAGE) and Asia-Pacific Society for Digestive Endoscopy (APSDE). Gut. 2020;69(1):83–91.
Noto JM, Peek RM Jr. The gastric microbiome, its interaction with Helicobacter pylori, and its potential role in the progression to stomach cancer. PLoS Pathog. 2017;13(10):e1006573.
Oh B, et al. The effect of probiotics on gut microbiota during the Helicobacter pylori eradication: randomized controlled trial. Helicobacter. 2016;21(3):165–74.
Orlando A, et al. Effects of Lactobacillus rhamnosus GG on proliferation and polyamine metabolism in HGC-27 human gastric and DLD-1 colonic cancer cell lines. Immunopharmacol Immunotoxicol. 2009;31(1):108–16.
Oster P, et al. Helicobacter pylori infection has a detrimental impact on the efficacy of cancer immunotherapies. Gut. 2022;71(3):457–66.
Pakbin B, et al. Probiotic Saccharomyces cerevisiae var. boulardii supernatant inhibits survivin gene expression and induces apoptosis in human gastric cancer cells. Food Sci Nutr. 2021;9(2):692–700.
Pan M, et al. Changes in gastric microbiota induced by Helicobacter pylori infection and preventive effects of Lactobacillus plantarum ZDY 2013 against such infection. J Dairy Sci. 2016;99(2):970–81.
Park CH, et al. Network construction of gastric microbiome and organization of microbial modules associated with gastric carcinogenesis. Sci Rep. 2019a;9(1):12444.
Park CH, et al. Evaluation of gastric microbiome and metagenomic function in patients with intestinal metaplasia using 16S rRNA gene sequencing. Helicobacter. 2019b;24(1):e12547.
Park H, et al. Amelioration of alcohol induced gastric ulcers through the administration of Lactobacillus plantarum APSulloc 331261 isolated from green tea. Front Microbiol. 2020;11:420.
Parsons BN, et al. Comparison of the human gastric microbiota in hypochlorhydric states arising as a result of Helicobacter pylori-induced atrophic gastritis, autoimmune atrophic gastritis and proton pump inhibitor use. PLoS Pathog. 2017;13(11):e1006653.

Plaza K, et al. Gingipains of Porphyromonas gingivalis affect the stability and function of serine protease inhibitor of Kazal-type 6 (SPINK6), a tissue inhibitor of human kallikreins. J Biol Chem. 2016;291(36):18753–64.

Poonyam P, Chotivitayatarakorn P, Vilaichone RK. High effective of 14-day high-dose PPI-bismuth-containing quadruple therapy with probiotics supplement for Helicobacter pylori eradication: a double blinded-randomized placebo-controlled study. Asian Pac J Cancer Prev. 2019;20(9):2859–64.

Radojevic D, et al. Fecal microbiota composition associates with the capacity of human peripheral blood monocytes to differentiate into immunogenic dendritic cells in vitro. Gut Microbes. 2021;13(1):1–20.

Rahimi AM, et al. Probiotic Lactobacillus rhamnosus supplementation improved capecitabine protective effect against gastric cancer growth in male BALB/c mice. Nutr Cancer. 2021;73(10):2089–99.

Ravegnini G, et al. Gastric adenocarcinomas and signet-ring cell carcinoma: unraveling gastric cancer complexity through microbiome analysis-deepening heterogeneity for a personalized therapy. Int J Mol Sci. 2020;21(24):9735.

Rieber H, Frontzek A, Schmitt H. Slackia exigua, an anaerobic Gram-positive rod and part of human oral microbiota associated with periprosthetic joint infection of the hip. First case and review of the literature. Anaerobe. 2019;56:130–2.

Salama NR, Hartung ML, Muller A. Life in the human stomach: persistence strategies of the bacterial pathogen Helicobacter pylori. Nat Rev Microbiol. 2013;11(6):385–99.

Salminen S, et al. The International Scientific Association of Probiotics and Prebiotics (ISAPP) consensus statement on the definition and scope of postbiotics. Nat Rev Gastroenterol Hepatol. 2021;18(9):649–67.

Sarhadi V, et al. Gut microbiota of patients with different subtypes of gastric cancer and gastrointestinal stromal tumors. Gut Pathog. 2021;13(1):11.

Serrano C, et al. Interactions between H. pylori and the gastric microbiome: impact on gastric homeostasis and disease. Curr Opin Physiol. 2021;21:57–64.

Shi YC, et al. Effects of proton pump inhibitors on the gastrointestinal microbiota in gastroesophageal reflux disease. Genomics Proteomics Bioinformatics. 2019;17(1):52–63.

Shiao SL, et al. Commensal bacteria and fungi differentially regulate tumor responses to radiation therapy. Cancer Cell. 2021;39(9):1202–1213.e6.

Singh K, Gandhi S, Doratotaj B. Synchronous MALT lymphoma of the colon and stomach and regression after eradication of Strongyloides stercoralis and Helicobacter pylori. BMJ Case Rep. 2018;2018:bcr2018224795.

Sousa EL, et al. Macrophage cell activation with acute apical abscess contents determined by interleukin-1 Beta and tumor necrosis factor alpha production. J Endod. 2014;40(11):1752–7.

Stewart OA, Wu F, Chen Y. The role of gastric microbiota in gastric cancer. Gut Microbes. 2020;11(5):1220–30.

Sunakawa Y, et al. DELIVER (JACCRO GC-08) trial: discover novel host-related immune-biomarkers for nivolumab in advanced gastric cancer. Future Oncol. 2019;15(21):2441–7.

Sung JJY, et al. Gastric microbes associated with gastric inflammation, atrophy and intestinal metaplasia 1 year after Helicobacter pylori eradication. Gut. 2020;69(9):1572–80.

Szymula A, et al. T cell epitope mimicry between Sjogren's syndrome antigen A (SSA)/Ro60 and oral, gut, skin and vaginal bacteria. Clin Immunol. 2014;152(1–2):1–9.

Tang YS, et al. Preparation and anti-tumor efficiency evaluation of bacterial magnetosome-anti-4-1BB antibody complex: bacterial magnetosome as antibody carriers isolated from Magnetospirillum gryphiswaldense. Biotechnol Appl Biochem. 2019;66(3):290–7.

Tong Q, et al. Construction and characterization of a novel fusion protein MG7-scFv/SEB against gastric cancer. J Biomed Biotechnol. 2010;2010:121094.

Tongtawee T, et al. Effect of pretreatment with Lactobacillus delbrueckii and Streptococcus thermophillus on tailored triple therapy for Helicobacter pylori eradication: a prospective randomized controlled clinical trial. Asian Pac J Cancer Prev. 2015;16(12):4885–90.

Tshibangu-Kabamba E, Yamaoka Y. Helicobacter pylori infection and antibiotic resistance—from biology to clinical implications. Nat Rev Gastroenterol Hepatol. 2021;18(9):613–29.

Tsoi H, et al. Peptostreptococcus anaerobius induces intracellular cholesterol biosynthesis in colon cells to induce proliferation and causes dysplasia in mice. Gastroenterology. 2017;152(6):1419–1433 e5.

Tsujimoto H, et al. Effect of a proton-pump inhibitor on intestinal microbiota in patients taking low-dose aspirin. Eur J Clin Pharmacol. 2021;

Wakabayashi A, et al. Suppression of an already established tumor growing through activated mucosal CTLs induced by oral administration of tumor antigen with cholera toxin. J Immunol. 2008;180(6):4000–10.

Wang ZH, Gao QY, Fang JY. Meta-analysis of the efficacy and safety of Lactobacillus-containing and Bifidobacterium-containing probiotic compound preparation in Helicobacter pylori eradication therapy. J Clin Gastroenterol. 2013;47(1):25–32.

Wang H, et al. Effects of supernatants from Escherichia coli Nissle 1917 and Faecalibacterium prausnitzii on intestinal epithelial cells and a rat model of 5-fluorouracil-induced mucositis. Nutr Cancer. 2017;69(2):307–18.

Wang Z, et al. Changes of the gastric mucosal microbiome associated with histological stages of gastric carcinogenesis. Front Microbiol. 2020a;11:997.

Wang H, et al. Associations between gastric cancer risk and virus infection other than Epstein-Barr virus: a systematic review and meta-analysis based on epidemiological studies. Clin Transl Gastroenterol. 2020b;11(7):e00201.

Watanabe T, et al. Long-term persistence of gastric dysbiosis after eradication of Helicobacter pylori in patients who underwent endoscopic submucosal dissection for early gastric cancer. Gastric Cancer. 2021;24(3):710–20.

Wei Z, et al. The influence of neoadjuvant chemotherapy on gastric cancer patients' postoperative infectious complications: what is the negative role played by the intestinal barrier dysfunction? Oncotarget. 2017;8(26):43376–88.

West TE, et al. Pathogenicity of high-dose enteral inoculation of Burkholderia pseudomallei to mice. Am J Trop Med Hyg. 2010;83(5):1066–9.

Westerik N, et al. The probiotic Lactobacillus rhamnosus for alleviation of Helicobacter pylori-associated gastric pathology in East Africa. Front Microbiol. 2018;9:1873.

Willems RPJ, et al. Evaluation of the association between gastric acid suppression and risk of intestinal colonization with multidrug-resistant microorganisms: a systematic review and meta-analysis. JAMA Intern Med. 2020;180(4):561–71.

Wong MCS, et al. Global incidence and mortality of gastric cancer, 1980-2018. JAMA Netw Open. 2021;4(7):e2118457.

Wu JS, et al. Porphyromonas gingivalis promotes 4-nitroquinoline-1-oxide-induced oral carcinogenesis with an alteration of fatty acid metabolism. Front Microbiol. 2018;9:2081.

Wu SE, et al. Microbiota-derived metabolite promotes HDAC3 activity in the gut. Nature. 2020;586(7827):108–12.

Xu Y, et al. Effect of Streptococcus anginosus on biological response of tongue squamous cell carcinoma cells. BMC Oral Health. 2021;21(1):141.

Yamaoka Y. Mechanisms of disease: Helicobacter pylori virulence factors. Nat Rev Gastroenterol Hepatol. 2010;7(11):629–41.

Yuan, W., et al., Probiotic therapy (BIO-THREE) mitigates intestinal microbial imbalance and intestinal damage caused by oxaliplatin. Probiotics Antimicrob Proteins, 2022;14(1):60-71.

Yuille S, et al. Human gut bacteria as potent class I histone deacetylase inhibitors in vitro through production of butyric acid and valeric acid. PLoS One. 2018;13(7):e0201073.

Zhang D, et al. Metabolic regulation of gene expression by histone lactylation. Nature. 2019;574(7779):575–80.

Zhang J, et al. The efficacy and safety of Clostridium butyricum and Bacillus coagulans in Helicobacter pylori eradication treatment: an open-label, single-arm pilot study. Medicine (Baltimore). 2020;99(45):e22976.

Zhang Y, et al. Gut microbiome analysis as a predictive marker for the gastric cancer patients. Appl Microbiol Biotechnol. 2021;105(2):803–14.

Zhdanov DD, et al. Rhodospirillum rubrum l-asparaginase targets tumor growth by a dual mechanism involving telomerase inhibition. Biochem Biophys Res Commun. 2017;492(2):282–8.

Zheng C, et al. A randomised trial of probiotics to reduce severity of physiological and microbial disorders induced by partial gastrectomy for patients with gastric cancer. J Cancer. 2019;10(3):568–76.

Zheng C, et al. Adjuvant treatment and molecular mechanism of probiotic compounds in patients with gastric cancer after gastrectomy. Food Funct. 2021;12(14):6294–308.

Zhong M, et al. Candida albicans disorder is associated with gastric carcinogenesis. Theranostics. 2021;11(10):4945–56.

Zong L, Li H, Li S. Effects of neoadjuvant chemotherapy combined with enteral nutrition on perioperative immunity, inflammation and intestinal flora in gastric cancer patients. J BUON. 2019;24(3):1113–9.

Chapter 5
Microbiota and Liver Cancer

Chun-Ying Wu and Ching-Hung Tseng

Abstract Hepatocellular carcinoma (HCC) is the most prevalent cancer and a leading cause of cancer-related deaths worldwide. Chronic hepatitis B, hepatitis C, alcoholism, and non-alcohol fatty liver disease are the most common etiologies of HCC. Most etiologies lead to the oncogenesis pathways via chronic inflammation, which has been shown to be closely related to dysbiosis, the unbalanced status of symbionts and pathobionts. Trillions of microbes live in the human gastrointestinal tract, renowned as the gut microbiome, and perform a variety of functions that support human physiology. As they become more understood, these gut symbiotic microorganisms also cause diseases when they go wrong, including cancer. Given the tremendous abundance and physical proximity to our digestive tract, the gut microbiome has been widely studied for its association, mechanism, and even causality to liver cancer. In principle, the gut microbiome not only alters in composition along with liver disease progression, but also demonstrates the critical role in carcinogenesis by disrupting host immune response, abolishing liver metabolism, and inducing chronic inflammation. This chapter is organized to first introduce the relationships between cancer and the gut microbiome, and then to review the studies (from association to mechanism) looking at microbial roles in the gut–liver axis, HCC-inducing liver diseases, and HCC. Finally, according to the recently prominent advances in cancer immunotherapy, the last section will discuss the role and application of gut microbes in cancer treatment and the progress achieved in HCC immunotherapy. This compilation aims to provide a comprehensive review and up-to-date

C.-Y. Wu (✉)
College of Medicine, National Yang Ming Chiao Tung University, Taipei, Taiwan

Institute of Biomedical Informatics, National Yang Ming Chiao Tung University, Taipei, Taiwan

Division of Translational Research, Taipei Veterans General Hospital, Taipei, Taiwan

Taiwan Microbiota Consortium, Taipei, Taiwan

C.-H. Tseng
Taiwan Microbiota Consortium, Taipei, Taiwan

Germark Biotechnology, Co., Ltd., Taichung, Taiwan

J. Yu (ed.), *Microbiome in Gastrointestinal Cancer*,
https://doi.org/10.1007/978-981-19-4492-5_5

understanding of the gut microbiome in HCC and hopefully to inspire new ideas translating these pieces of knowledge into therapeutic strategies for patients.

Keywords Microbiome · Hepatocellular carcinoma · Immune response · Immunotherapy

5.1 Cancer and Gut Microbiome

Cancer is a type of disease resulting from uncontrolled cell growth and division, often caused by accumulated mutations (or damages) in chromosome DNA. In comparison with benign tumors, cancer (i.e., malignant tumors) causes harm more likely to the host, including death, as it is with the potential to metastasize to distant sites of the body.

In general, cancer progression begins with a genetic defect to accelerate cell division, leading to a cellular condition called hyperplasia. At this stage, the cells look normal under a microscope. As the cells continue to divide, further mutations are likely to worsen the cellular condition with abnormal appearance, called dysplasia. Following that, the dysplastic cells may become in situ cancer, characterized by abnormal structure, loss of differentiation, and loss of contact with surrounding cells, but are still confined to the epithelial layer from which they grew. Finally, cancer forms with the ability to invade tissue and penetrate blood vessels or lymph nodes, shedding cancerous cells into blood or lymph and metastasizing to remote sites.

For a long time, microbial infection has been listed as one of the risk factors for carcinogenesis, and infection-induced chronic inflammation is acknowledged as a pivotal cause. The most well-known microbial carcinogen is *Helicobacter pylori*, of which the infection in stomach increases the risk of developing peptic ulcer disease and gastric cancer (O'Connor et al. 2017). Other carcinogenic microorganisms include hepatitis B and C viruses for liver cancer (El-Serag 2012) and Epstein–Barr viruses for nasopharyngeal cancer (Wong et al. 2021). Recently, mounting evidence has blamed the carcinogenic effects of these microbial challenges to the induced gut dysbiosis (i.e., the disequilibrium state of gut microbial composition associated with disease) (Zitvogel et al. 2015), which in turn gives rise to chronic inflammation and, finally, carcinogenesis (Fig. 5.1). However, not all microorganisms are detrimental. Several commensal bacteria have been found essential in the development of the host immune system (Zhao and Elson 2018). For example, indigenous *Clostridium* species promote the expansion and differentiation of regulatory T (T_{reg}) cells by providing bacterial antigens and creating an environment rich in transforming growth factor-β (TGF-β) in the colon (Atarashi et al. 2011, 2013).

In summary, gut microbiome is an indispensable part of the human body, and the composed member types (pathogenic or commensal) and abundance configuration

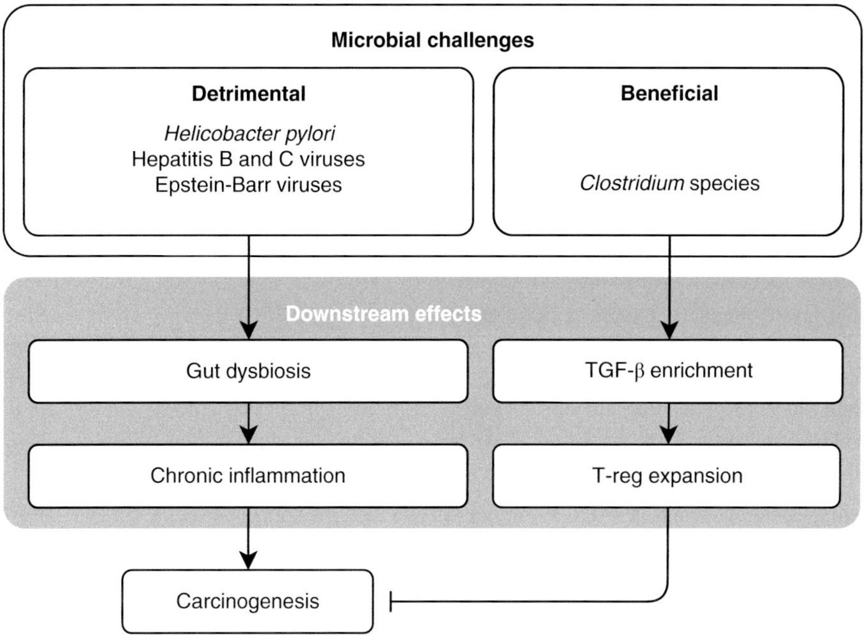

Fig. 5.1 Known microbial challenges and downstream effects associated with carcinogenesis

(dysbiotic or eubiotic) determine the health status of host. Concerning the carcinogenesis of HCC, a plethora of studies has successfully revealed the pivotal roles played by gut microbes, and how these microbial roles involve and participate in the gut–liver axis and carcinogenic liver diseases such as hepatitis viral infection, alcoholic liver disease (ALD), and non-alcoholic fatty liver disease (NAFLD) will be sequentially discussed in the following sections.

5.2 Liver Diseases and Gut Microbiome

According to the GLOBOCAN 2020, primary liver cancer is the sixth most common cancer and the third leading cause of cancer death worldwide, and most of cases (about 75–85%) are HCC (Sung et al. 2021). In Taiwan, HCC also represents a prominent cause of cancer-related death and ranks second among all cancer types by a mortality rate of 18% in 2020 (The Ministry of Health and Welfare of Taiwan ROC 2021). HCC is the cancerous outcome of chronic liver inflammation and cirrhosis, which can be induced by various factors such as hepatitis viral infection, ALD, and NAFLD. The growing pandemic of obesity and type 2 diabetes, the major risk factors for NAFLD and related cirrhosis, forecasts NAFLD being the major cause of HCC by 2030 (Huang et al. 2021).

5.2.1 The Gut–Liver Axis

Although without anatomical connection, the liver communicates with the gut via the portal vein, systemic circulation, and biliary tract, forming the gut–liver axis (Tremaroli and Backhed 2012). The portal vein supplies the major portion of blood to the liver, and provides the opportunity for gut microbe-derived metabolites and products (also known as microbe-associated molecular patterns, MAMPs) to reach the liver when the gut barrier function is aberrant (Wiest et al. 2017). MAMPs are mostly structural components of bacteria. In particular, lipopolysaccharides (LPS), the Gram-negative bacterial outer-membrane component triggering inflammation via toll-like receptor (TLR) 4 (Seki et al. 2007), represent a typical messenger of MAMPs in the gut–liver axis. In the liver, TLR4-activated Kupffer cells (i.e., stellate macrophages), hepatic stellate cells, and hepatocytes can be activated by LPS to release inflammatory cytokines in response (Schwabe and Greten 2020), resulting in hepatic inflammation and chronic liver diseases (Fig. 5.2).

In addition to being a passive recipient of MAMPs from the gut, the liver regulates gut microbiota by one class of its metabolites, bile acids (Wahlstrom et al.

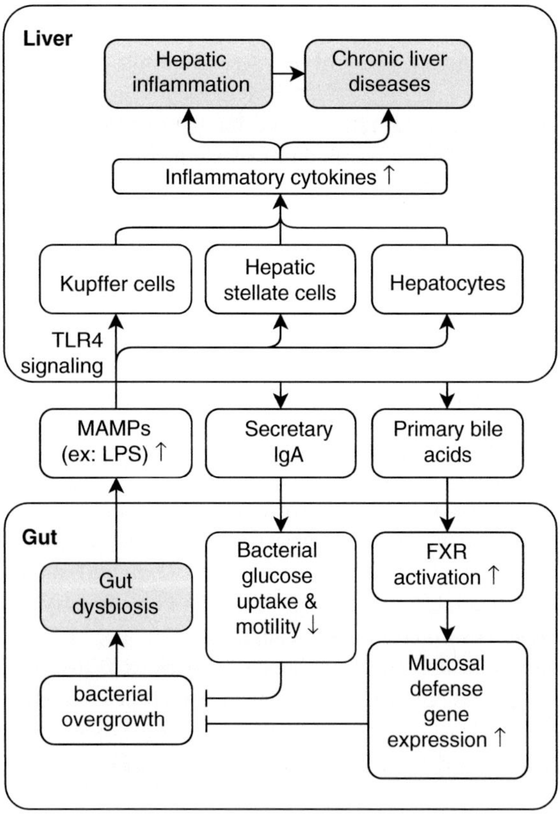

Fig. 5.2 The gut–liver axis and associated molecular communications regulating gut microbial homeostasis and liver health. The gray background represents the disease state. *FXR* farnesoid X receptor, *IgA* immunoglobulin A, *LPS* lipopolysaccharides, *MAMPs* microbe-associated molecular patterns, *TLR* toll-like receptor

2016). Bile acids activate the farnesoid X receptor (FXR), a nuclear receptor majorly expressed in ileum, and protect the intestine from bacterial overgrowth by up-regulating genes involved in mucosal defense like angiogenin, inducible NO synthase, and pro-inflammatory cytokine IL18 (Fig. 5.2) (Inagaki et al. 2006). Plus, by the activation of intestinal FXR, the altered gut microbiota was found to improve hepatic glucose and insulin sensitivity (Pathak et al. 2018), which was in part due to the reduced abundance of gut bacteria carrying bile salt hydrolase (Sun et al. 2018). Considering that FXR is required for diet-induced obesity by gut microbiota (Parseus et al. 2017), different bile acids (or other FXR agonists) are supposed to be responsible for different downstream metabolic response.

The liver also produces IgA, an immunoglobulin isotype dominated in the intestinal lumen and lately discovered central in regulating gut microbiota (Macpherson et al. 2015). The intrahepatic IgA-producing plasma cells originate from the Peyer's patches (Moro-Sibilot et al. 2016) and secrete IgA across biliary epithelium into the bile. In the intestine, secretory IgA, the IgA found in secretions, coats differentially among gut microbes such as *Enterobacteriaceae* (Tsuruta et al. 2010) and colitogenic intestinal bacteria (Palm et al. 2014), and regulates microbial functional fitness such as glucose uptake and cell motility (Rollenske et al. 2021). Furthermore, the recognition of IgA to gut microbes prevents bacterial overgrowth (Fig. 5.2) (Fagarasan et al. 2002), maintains a homeostatic gut flora more tolerant to intestinal injury (Reikvam et al. 2012), and promotes neonatal microbiota maturation (Mirpuri et al. 2014), all of which demonstrates the indispensable function of IgA in host-microbiota homeostasis.

Taken together, the gut–liver axis is established on the communication between the gut microbes and liver via hepatic portal system. Dysregulated intestinal barrier function increases the chance of MAMPs flowing through the liver, elevating the risk of hepatic inflammation. However, the liver-produced bile acids and IgA regulate the gut microbial configuration, and thus affects the composition of MAMPs. These intricate interactions demonstrate the critical role of the gut microbiota in the liver health.

5.2.2 *Hepatitis Viral Infection and Gut Microbiome*

Chronic infection with hepatitis B virus (HBV) or hepatitis C virus (HCV) is the most common risk factor for HCC, and HBV is more common compared with HCV in Asia and developing countries. Both viruses infect hepatocytes and trigger host immune response for clearance. Failure in viral clearance results in the persistent viral infection and causes microbial metabolite translocation and chronic inflammation, leading to the progressive development of fibrosis, liver cirrhosis, and ultimately HCC (Guicciardi and Gores 2005; Sandler et al. 2011). The treatment of viral hepatitis is commonly achieved by using nucleoside (or nucleotide) analogues (NAs) to block viral replication. In Taiwan, a nationwide investigation comparing two groups of hepatitis patients, receiving antiviral therapy or not, identified NAs also possessing the anti-HCC effects, as demonstrated by the lower HCC occurrence (Wu et al. 2014) and recurrence (Wu et al. 2012) in patients using NAs. Besides that, the matured gut microbiota is required for rapid HBV clearance via effective stimulation on host immunity (Chou et al. 2015).

By tapping into next-generation sequencing technology, the patients of HBV-related cirrhosis harbored a distinct gut microbiota compared with healthy controls (e.g., increased *Veillonella*, *Streptococcus*, *Clostridium*, and *Prevotella,* and decreased *Eubacterium* and *Alistipes*), and the enrichment of oral species suggests the mouth-to-gut microbial translocation being common in cirrhosis patients (Fig. 5.3) (Qin et al. 2014). The later investigation also correspondingly discovered *Veillonella* and *Streptococcus* positively correlated with hepatitis B severity (Wang et al. 2017). In comparison with healthy controls, the gut microbial diversity, as evaluated by Shannon and Simpson indices, reduced in cirrhosis (Ren et al. 2019) and rebounded in par in HBV-related HCC patients (Liu et al. 2019). Meanwhile, the diversity also reduced more, though not significantly, in patients of early than moderate hepatitis B and both were lower than healthy controls (Fig. 5.3) (Wang et al. 2017).

Collectively, the gut microbial diversity seems to reduce at the early HBV infection and rebound to the level parallel to healthy controls along with the liver disease progresses. The expansion of oral bacteria in gut, particularly *Veillonella* and *Streptococcus* species, represents a compositional signature associated with late-stage HBV infection. These gut microbial alterations associated with HBV

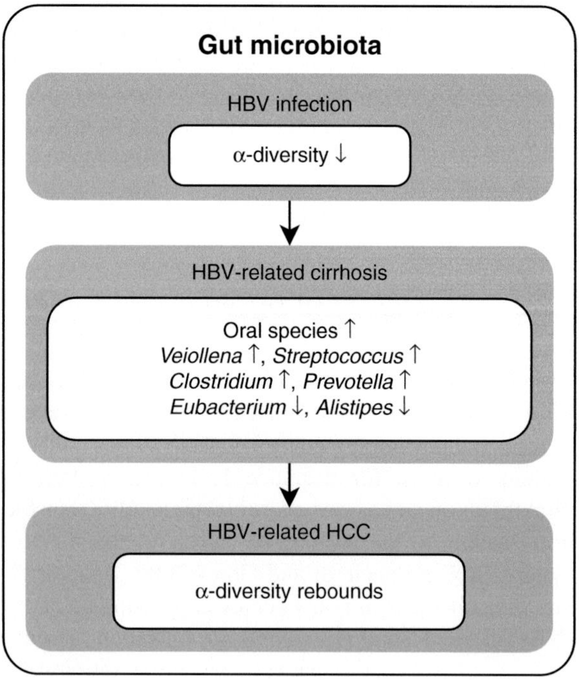

Fig. 5.3 Gut microbiota alterations associated with the progression of HBV-related liver diseases. The gray background represents the disease state. *HBV* hepatitis B virus, *HCC* hepatocellular carcinoma

infection are speculated to in part arise from the abnormal bile acids secretion and composition, which in turn disrupts the antimicrobial protection of bile acids and permits the translocation of oral species.

5.2.3 Alcoholic Liver Disease and Gut Microbiome

Alcohol overconsumption is one of risk factors causing a wide range of liver diseases such as alcoholic fatty liver disease, alcoholic hepatitis, and alcoholic cirrhosis, collectively termed as alcohol liver disease (ALD) (Seitz et al. 2018). The harmful effect of alcohol misuse is blamed on the by-products of its metabolism. In the hepatocyte, alcohol is oxidized to mainly acetaldehyde (by alcohol dehydrogenase) and marginally reactive oxygen species (ROS, by cytochrome P450 2E1), both of which are toxic and carcinogenic to the liver under a long-term exposure (Fig. 5.4) (Seitz and Becker 2007). However, among heavy drinkers up to 90% would develop fatty liver, 20–40% fibrosis, and 20% or even fewer cirrhosis (Mathurin and Bataller 2015), indicating that the risk of ALD progression not only depends on alcohol consumption but also other personalized traits, including the modifiable organ, gut microbiota (Szabo 2015).

Although alcohol is majorly metabolized in the liver, it can also be metabolized by intestinal enzymes (Cederbaum 2012) and microbes (Bishehsari et al. 2017). Therefore, the excessive intake of alcohol elevates luminal acetaldehyde and ROS, and consequently disrupts the gut ecology by impairing gut barrier function (Dunagan et al. 2012; Wang et al. 2014) and promoting gut dysbiosis (Fig. 5.4) (Mutlu et al. 2012), which change the gut microbial composition. As proof, alcoholic hepatitis reduced *Akkermansia* compared with healthy controls (Grander et al. 2018) and reduced more in severe patients (Lang et al. 2020). *Bacteroides*, *Bilophila*, *Alistipes*, *Butyricimonas*, and *Clostridium* XIVa exhibited higher abundance in mice receiving fecal transplant from the alcoholics of severe hepatitis than no hepatitis (Llopis et al. 2016). Furthermore, alcoholic hepatitis increased bacterial DNA in the circulating blood than non-alcohol-drinking controls, with decreased DNA from *Bacteroidetes* but increased from *Fusobacteria* in abundance (Puri et al. 2018). As for alcoholic cirrhosis, decreased *Bacteroidetes* and increased *Proteobacteria* and *Fusobacteria* were discovered in patients compared with healthy controls (Chen et al. 2011). Likewise, less *Bacteroidetes* and more *Proteobacteria* (especially *Gammaproteobacteria*) characterized the alcoholics with gut dysbiosis (Mutlu et al. 2012). A larger cohort involved 219 patients with cirrhosis demonstrated decreases in *Firmicutes* (including *Clostridiales* XIV, *Lachnospiraceae*, and *Ruminococcaceae*) and increases in *Proteobacteria* (including *Enterobacteriaceae* and *Halomonadaceae*) compared with healthy controls (Bajaj et al. 2014). The repetitive observation of increased *Proteobacteria* corresponds to the reported elevation in serum endotoxin in cirrhosis (Mutlu et al. 2012; Bajaj et al. 2014).

The functional profile of gut microbiota is changed with community structure, which is affected by ALD. By the shotgun metagenomic sequencing, the look at genome-level rather than 16S information provides views on metabolic capability for the gut microbiota (Quince et al. 2017). Comparing alcoholic hepatitis patients with healthy controls showed that genes in the urea cycle pathway were increased (Gao et al. 2020), which was consistent with the impaired liver function of urea synthesis in patients with liver injury. The predicted functional profile based on 16S sequencing discovered the enrichment of genes for aromatic amino acids metabolism in alcoholic hepatitis compared with alcoholics without hepatitis (Smirnova et al. 2020). Among alcoholic cirrhotics, functional preference significantly occurred in genes for alcohol metabolism (e.g., alcohol, aldehyde, and acetaldehyde dehydrogenases), while those for bile metabolism and microbial virulence had undetectable changes from healthy controls (Dubinkina et al. 2017). Glutathione metabolism in gut microbiome was predicted to increase in cirrhosis patients with severe hepatitis, which plausibly reflects the elevated intestinal oxidative stress as a result of liver abnormality (Fig. 5.4) (Ciocan et al. 2018). Apparently, these functional

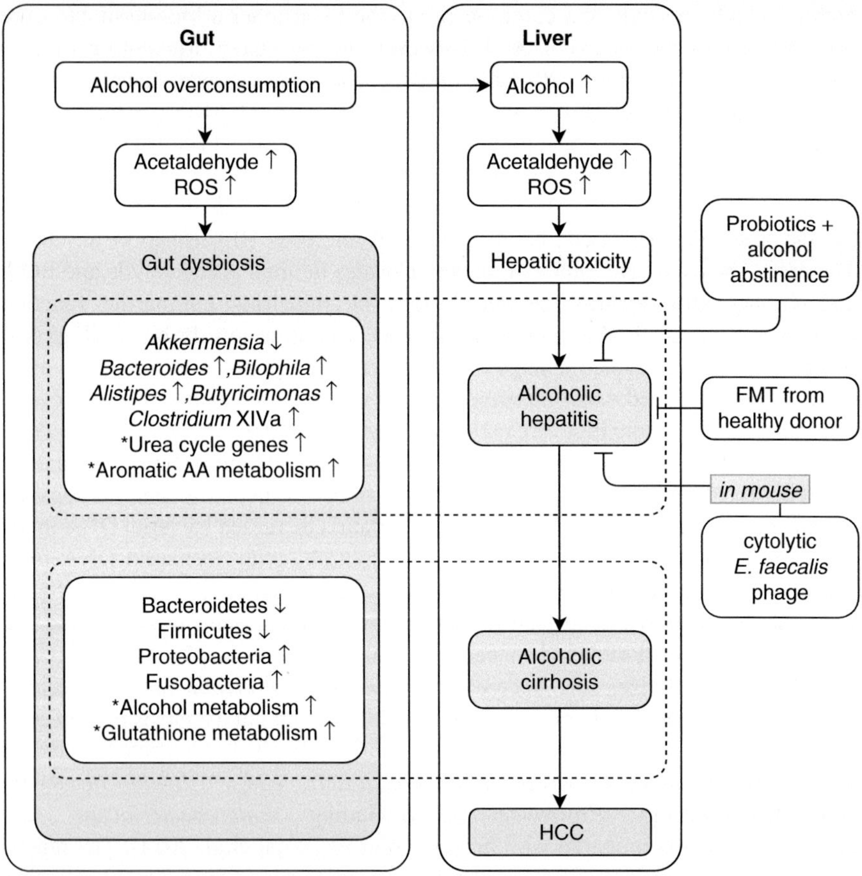

Fig. 5.4 ALD associated gut microbiome (compositional and functional) alterations and potential mitigations. Asterisk indicates functional changes. The gray background represents the disease state. *AA* amino acid, *ALD* alcoholic liver disease, *E. faecalis Enterococcus faecalis*, *FMT* fecal microbiota transplant, *HCC* hepatocellular carcinoma, *ROS* reactive oxygen species

alterations in gut microbiota are related to liver dysfunction, thereby forcibly shifting the metabolic demands on to the intestinal bacteria and exacerbating disease progression through the gut–liver axis.

Microbial interventions for ameliorating ALD have been trialed in various studies (Fig. 5.4). The oral supplementation of probiotics *Lactobacillus subtilis* and *Enterococcus faecium* (formally classified as *Streptococcus* genus) coupled with alcohol abstinence restored gut microbiota, improved liver function, and reduced inflammation in patients of alcoholic hepatitis (Han et al. 2015). However, the increases in *Bifidobacterium* and *Lactobacillus* in liver cirrhosis remind the need for caution regarding probiotics intervention in patients with ALD (Dubinkina et al. 2017). Patients with severe alcoholic hepatitis receiving fecal microbiota transplant (FMT) from healthy donors improved survival compared with patients receiving standard cares (Philips et al. 2017) or conventional medications (Philips et al. 2018). Lastly, the bacteriophage targeting cytolytic *Enterococcus faecalis*, a gut bacterium correlating with the severity and mortality in patients with alcoholic hepatitis, has been successfully applied in mice for attenuating liver disease (Duan et al. 2019), showing the potential of strain-level manipulation in gut microbiota.

5.2.4 Non-alcoholic Fatty Liver Disease and Gut Microbiome

In addition to alcohol, metabolic syndrome (e.g., obesity, insulin resistance, and hyperlipidemia) and other health complications damage the liver and cause non-alcoholic fatty liver disease (NAFLD), of which the main stages include simple steatosis, non-alcoholic steatohepatitis (NASH), fibrosis, and cirrhosis. Metabolic syndromes induce chronic inflammation and alter lipid metabolisms, deteriorating the liver disease progression and ending up with HCC (Park et al. 2010). NAFLD has been demonstrated to dysregulate lipid metabolism, leading to the depletion of $CD4^+$ T cells and successively promoting hepatocarcinogenesis (Fig. 5.5) (Ma et al. 2016). Similarly, the liver-accumulated IgA^+ cells in NASH patients with fibrosis promote hepatocarcinogenesis by limiting the activation of $CD8^+$ T cells (Fig.5.5) (Shalapour et al. 2017). Although the incidence of HCC by NAFLD is lower than other liver diseases (Huang et al. 2021), the growing prevalence of metabolic syndrome makes NAFLD an unneglectable cause to HCC.

The etiological association of gut bacteria to NAFLD was firstly verified in mice by replicating NAFLD-associated hepatic alterations through co-housing (Henao-Mejia et al. 2012) and FMT (Le Roy et al. 2013) experiments. The subsequent induction of NALFD in mice using FMT from patients with NASH (Chiu et al. 2017) and non-diabetic, obese women with simple steatosis (Hoyles et al. 2018) emphasized the participation of gut microbiota in the pathogenesis of NAFLD. The gut microbiota contributes to NAFLD when disrupted by metabolic syndromes (Leung et al. 2016). In brief, gut dysbiosis alters the bile acid pool and thus impairs bile acid and lipid homeostasis via FXR dysregulation (Sinal et al. 2000; Ridlon et al. 2014), stimulating hepatic triglyceride accumulation and inflammation (Li et al. 2013).

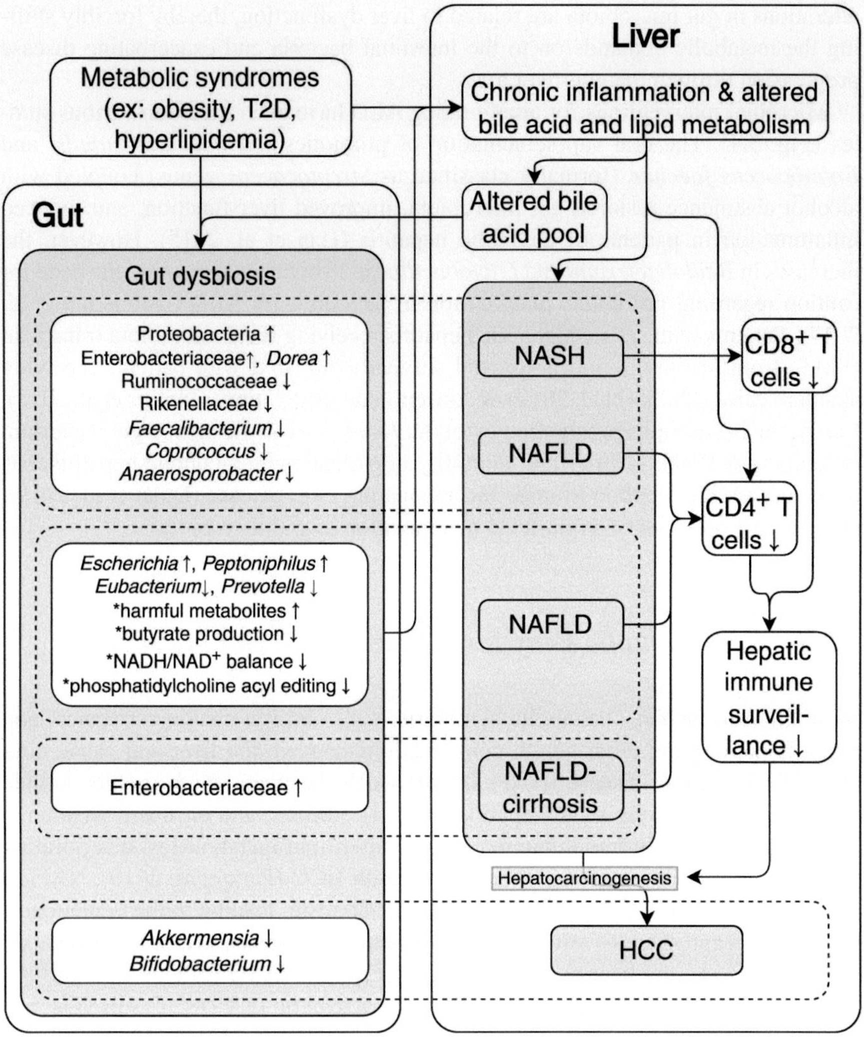

Fig. 5.5 NAFLD-associated gut microbiome (compositional and functional) alterations and downstream modifications in the liver metabolism caused by metabolic syndromes. The gray background represents the disease state. Asterisk indicates functional changes. *NAFLD* non-alcoholic fatty liver disease, *NASH* non-alcoholic steatohepatitis, *T2D* type 2 diabetes, *HCC* hepatocellular carcinoma

The gut microbial signature contrasting NAFLD with healthy controls has been adequately summarized (Aron-Wisnewsky et al. 2020). The increases in Proteobacteria, Enterobacteriaceae, *Dorea*, and decreases in Ruminococcaceae, Rikenellaceae, *Faecalibacterium*, *Coprococcus*, and *Anaerosporobacter* represent concordant signatures in the gut of NAFLD and NASH patients, while increases in *Escherichia* and *Peptoniphilus* and decreases in *Eubacterium* and *Prevotella* favorably observed in patients with NAFLD (Fig. 5.5). The significant overlap among signatures for NAFLD and NASH is probably because NASH is also a type of NAFLD. Among features predicting NAFLD-cirrhosis, the detection of increased Enterobacteriaceae reflected its haunting role in the progression of NAFLD (Caussy et al. 2019). Coincidentally, two Enterobacteriaceae strains belonging to *Klebsiella pneumonia* were discovered to produce ethanol endogenously in Chinese patients with NAFLD, explaining in part the origin of NAFLD among non-drinkers (Yuan et al. 2019). The re-analysis of multiple published shotgun metagenomes from NAFLD cohorts extended the microbial association to species and functional level (Wang et al. 2021); in addition to identifying pathogenic species enriched in patients with NAFLD, these gut microbes seemed to worsen the disease progression by producing harmful products, breaking NADH/NAD$^+$ balance, weakening butyrate production and phosphatidylcholine acyl editing (Fig. 5.5). The diminished *Akkermansia* and *Bifidobacterium* species in patients with NAFLD-related HCC compared with NASH cirrhosis manifested that gut dysbiosis may deteriorate NAFLD progression to hepatocarcinogenesis (Ponziani et al. 2019).

5.2.5 Hepatocellular Carcinoma and Gut Microbiome

HCC develops most frequently in patients with chronic liver diseases, among which liver cirrhosis represents the primary cause. However, because liver cirrhosis is the common end before HCC of various liver diseases (e.g., viral hepatitis, ALD, and NAFLD), in a broad sense, these diseases are all potential cues triggering HCC. Concerning the microbial cause for HCC, the gut–liver axis is responsible for almost all communications between the gut microbiota and the liver (Yu and Schwabe 2017). Although the liver produces bile acids and IgA to regulate gut microbial homeostasis, the gut dysbiosis caused by other complications would indirectly harm the liver by immersing hepatocytes in MAMPs, which initiates a vicious cycle that compromises normal liver function and exacerbates gut dysbiosis. As exemplified in rats, either exposure with penicillin (to disrupt microbial homeostasis) or dextran sulfate sodium (to damage gut barrier) elevated endotoxin and inflammatory cytokines in the systemic circulation and in turn promoted hepatic tumor formation (Zhang et al. 2012). In addition to the pro-inflammatory effect, further research also demonstrated the gut bacterial LPS being carcinogenic to the liver, mainly through the activation of TLR4 on hepatic stellate cells and hepatocytes (Dapito et al. 2012).

Primary bile acids are produced by the liver and transformed into various secondary forms by gut bacteria to expand their functional roles for lipid digestion, cell signaling, microbiota modulation, and even pathogen resistance (Jia et al. 2018; Buffie et al. 2015). However, the elevated level of deoxycholic acid, a secondary bile acid known to damage DNA, in obesity was found to promote HCC (Yoshimoto et al. 2013), suggesting the disrupted bile acid pool by obesity-induced gut dysbiosis also affecting the liver health. Recently, primary bile acids were found to have a role in HCC suppression by inducing the accumulation of CXCR6$^+$ natural killer T (NKT) cells in the liver, which perform immune surveillance and in turn downregulate the tumor growth (Fig. 5.6) (Ma et al. 2018). Furthermore, the colonization of a bile acid converting species, *Clostridium scindens*, in mice reduced hepatic NKT levels and increased liver tumors compared with counterparts fed with antibiotics or a species not converting bile acid, suggesting the regulatory role of gut bacteria catalyzing bile acid transformation in HCC development.

Dietary fibers are essential to gut health because they can be fermented by gut bacteria to short-chain fatty acids (SCFAs), which fuel colonocytes and participate in numerous signaling pathways (Koh et al. 2016). An experimental attempt treating colitis model mice with inulin, one type of soluble fibers, to alleviate metabolic syndromes unexpectedly resulted in elevated bilirubin levels and liver dysfunction, and prolonged consumption of inulin together with gut dysbiosis induced cholestasis, hepatocyte death, neutrophilic inflammation, and finally HCC in mice (Fig. 5.6) (Singh et al. 2018). This results were reproduced by incorporating the other soluble fibers pectin and fructooligosaccharides but not the insoluble fiber cellulose. Therefore, the effects of soluble fibers are highly dependent on the gut microbiota, and subjects suffering from dysbiosis should be cautious to a long-term supplementation enriched with soluble fibers.

Among 30 patients with cirrhosis, those with HCC demonstrated only *Escherichia coli* overabundant relative to non-HCC counterparts (Grat et al. 2016). Compared with healthy controls, NAFLD-cirrhotics with and without HCC identified decreased *Akkermansia* but *Bifidobacterium* only in those with HCC; these two genera also

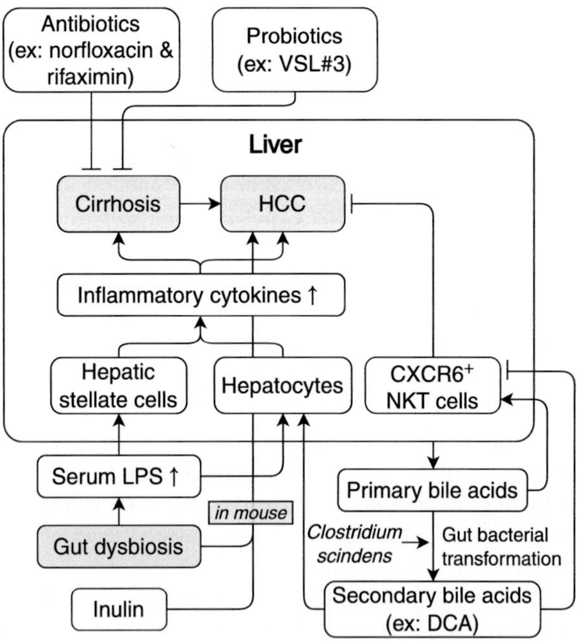

Fig. 5.6 Gut microbiome associations and molecular mechanisms in the liver correlating with HCC development. The gray background represents the disease state. *DCA* deoxycholic acid, *HCC* hepatocellular carcinoma, *LPS* lipopolysaccharide, *NKT cells* natural killer T cells

inversely correlated with fecal calprotectin and inflammation cytokine levels, implying that lacking certain bacteria in patients with NAFLD-associated cirrhosis enhances hepatocarcinogenesis by promoting systemic inflammation (Ponziani et al. 2019). A sizeable Chinese cohort including healthy controls, patients with cirrhosis, and early HCC reported more *Actinobacteria* phylum and 13 genera in early HCC than cirrhosis; 12 genera (e.g., *Alistipes*, *Phascolarctobacterium*, and butyrate-producing genera) reduced and 6 genera (e.g., *Klebsiella* and *Haemophilus*) increased in early HCC compared to controls (Ren et al. 2019). Non-viral HCC patients harbored more *Escherichia-Shigella*, *Enterococcus* and less Faecalibacterium, *Ruminococcus*, and *Ruminoclostridium* than healthy controls and HBV-related HCC (Liu et al. 2019). These data suggest that HCC is associated with increases in pro-inflammatory and decreases in SCFA-producing and probiotic genera. Nonetheless, the gut microbiota showed only slight differences but the bile acids concentration ratio in plasma over feces seemed discriminative for HCC and intrahepatic cholangiocarcinoma patients (Jia et al. 2020). HCC of different etiologies lead to different gut microbiota configurations, and therefore the microbes of potential therapeutic benefits plausibly depend on the causes of HCC.

While discovering the mechanisms behind the scenes, small-scale clinical trials have successively documented gut microbial interventions (e.g., antibiotics and probiotics) as ameliorative options for liver diseases (Fig. 5.6). Norfloxacin and rifaximin improve survival and reduce the risk of developing spontaneous bacterial peritonitis and hepatorenal syndrome in patients with cirrhosis (Fernandez et al. 2007; Vlachogiannakos et al. 2013). Probiotics modulation with VSL#3 also demonstrates beneficial effects in cirrhosis (Dhiman et al. 2014) and obese children with non-alcoholic steatohepatitis (Alisi et al. 2014). As being the essential regulator in hepatic lipid and glucose homeostasis, FXR agonists have been proposed as therapeutic agents for NAFLD (Carr and Reid 2015; Jiao et al. 2015). Moreover, probiotics seem to inhibit the growth of HCC in rodents (Zhang et al. 2012; Li et al. 2016).

5.3 Microbiota and Immunotherapy

Advances in cancer immunotherapy such as immune checkpoint inhibitors (ICI) in the past 5 years have revolutionized the way we treat cancer. Based on the close interaction of intestinal bacteria with human physiology, gut dysbiosis has been etiologically associated with human diseases, including cancer, by various dysbiosis-induced responses (Zitvogel et al. 2015). Preclinical experiments in mice have successively confirmed that the gut microbiota affects the responsiveness of cancer treatments (Cheng et al. 2020), such as chemotherapy (Viaud et al. 2013), CpG-oligonucleotide (Iida et al. 2013), and anti-programmed death ligand 1 (anti-PD-L1) immunotherapy (Sivan et al. 2015). As for mechanisms, studies in mice revealed that gut commensals were required for the cancer drug cyclophosphamide (CTX) to induce its antitumor immune response (Viaud et al. 2013), and especially *Enterococcus hirae* and *Barnesiella intestinihominis* represented the species beneficial to CTX treatment by enhancing tumor immunosurveillance in secondary lymphoid organs and the colon, respectively (Daillere et al. 2016). In addition, *Bacteroides* species improved the efficacy of cytotoxic T-lymphocyte-associated protein 4 (CTLA-4) blockade treatment for melanoma by inducing T helper 1 immune responses in the lymph nodes and promoting the maturation of intratumoral dendritic cells (Vetizou et al. 2015).

These promising data encouraged following trials in cancer patients. In non-small cell lung cancer (NSCLC) and renal cell cancer patients, antibiotics treatment significantly compromised the antitumor effects of anti-PD-1/PD-L1 immunotherapy, and the abundance and detection frequency of fecal *A. muciniphila* were both higher in responders than non-responders (Routy et al. 2018). Recently, *H. pylori* seropositivity was reported to be associated with a decreased survival in NSCLC patients on anti-PD-1 immunotherapy (Oster et al. 2022). Among melanoma patients receiving anti-PD-1 treatment, the responders exhibited significantly higher fecal alpha diversity, more *Ruminococcaceae* family members, and enhanced systemic and antitumor immunity compared with non-responders (Gopalakrishnan et al. 2018). At the beginning of 2021, two clinical trials reported the outcome of treating melanoma with FMT derived from immunotherapy responders. The Israel study reported 3 out of 10 patients showing improved response to anti-PD-1 immunotherapy and favorable changes in immune cell infiltration and gene expression profile in both the gut lamina propria and the tumor microenvironment (Baruch et al. 2021); the USA study demonstrated clinical benefits in 6 out of 15 patients and found alterations in microbiota and immune profiles associated with response to anti-PD-1 in responders (Davar et al. 2021). These results suggest responder-derived FMT as a potential alternative for overcoming immunotherapy resistance in patients. Lastly, the tumor microenvironment was found reprogrammable by microbiota-derived stimulator of interferon genes (STING), which improves responsiveness in patients with melanoma (Lam et al. 2021).

Studies on immunotherapy for HCC are still at the early stage with vibrant activities. Regarding the molecular mechanisms, NASH-induced hepatic accumulation of IgA-producing cells suppressed $CD8^+$ T cells, thereby reducing immune surveillance and promoting hepatocarcinogenesis (Fig. 5.5) (Shalapour et al. 2017). Liver metastases, in mouse and patients, reduced immunotherapy efficacy by depleting systemic $CD8^+$ T cells, and the antitumor immunity was proposed to be rescued by liver-directed radiotherapy in combination with immunotherapy (Yu et al. 2021). Several clinical trials deploying ICIs for HCC treatment are underway, for example, either by using alone the antibody targeting CTLA-4 (Agdashian et al. 2019), anti-PD-1 antibody (Finn et al. 2020a), CD133-directed chimeric antigen receptor T cells (Dai et al. 2020), or in combination (Finn et al. 2020b). The molecular effects of beneficial drug combinations have been revealed in regorafenib, an anti-angiogenic kinase inhibitor, plus anti-PD-1 (by controlling tumor vasculature and increasing intra-tumor $CXCR3^+$ $CD8^+$ T-cell infiltration) (Shigeta et al. 2020) and in lenvatinib plus anti-PD-1 (by reducing T_{reg} cell infiltration and inhibiting TGF-β signaling) (Torrens et al. 2021). The combination using anti-PD-L1 and synthetic double-strand RNA was newly discovered to overcome the immune-suppressive liver environment in metastasized liver cancer by boosting hepatic innate immunity (Xin et al. 2022). Lastly, gut microbiota was reportedly associated with HCC promotion (Shalapour et al. 2017) and affected the response of anti-PD-1 therapy in HCC patients, among whom the responders possessed a higher taxa richness and gene count, more *Akkermansia muciniphila* and *Ruminococcaceae* spp., and enriched carbohydrate metabolism and methanogenesis compared with non-responders (Zheng et al. 2019). However, the mechanistic role played by gut microbes associated with the immunotherapy response for HCC remained underexplored.

5.4 Conclusion

The gut microbiome is a conceptual organ with dynamic nature, and whether it is a friend or foe heavily depends on the composed members. When the imbalance of gut microbiome occurs, the compromised gut barrier function increases the translocation of MAMPs from gut to liver through the portal circulation. As being the important immune organ consistently processing the antigen-rich blood, the elevated MAMPs activate the innate and adaptive immune response in the liver and cause chronic liver damage under long-term exposure, which may increase the risk of HCC. Chronic liver disease is the prevailed cause of HCC, and each affects the gut microbiome in its own way. In viral hepatitis, the diversity of gut microbiome decreases at the beginning and rebounds along with the disease progresses. The increased diversity of late-stage viral hepatitis is partly contributed by the appearance of oral species in the gut, which could be ascribed to the abnormal bile acid secretion that protects them from being killed and promotes colonization. ALD and NAFLD are similar in terms of disease progression stages, and gut dysbiosis emerges as the paramount factor initiating and regulating the development of both diseases. The enrichment of Enterobacteriaceae shared by ALD and NAFLD emphasizes the detrimental influence of dysbiosis-induced inflammation on liver health. However, in addition to ALD-induced cirrhosis, the carcinogenicity of ALD also derives from the increased acetaldehyde and oxidative stress accompanied by alcohol metabolism in the liver and intestines, which successively disturb bile acid secretion, sabotage antimicrobial protection, and increase gene mutation. The carcinogenicity of NAFLD is enhanced by the continuous inflammation from metabolic syndromes, which cause gut dysbiosis and then overexpose the liver to MAMPs, and by abolishing immune surveillance performed by $CD4^+$ and $CD8^+$ T cells. The HCC-associated gut microbes exert detrimental effects *indirectly* by modulating the metabolites and molecules in circulation, such as secondary bile acids and LPS. Consumption of inulin and other soluble fibers might unexpectedly increase the risk of HCC when combined with gut dysbiosis. The diverse cause for HCC reminds us to categorize HCC by its primitive etiology (e.g., cirrhosis, NAFLD) and stages before studying the associated microbiome, to reduce the interference from unseen variables and better resolve the microbial alterations corresponding to patient conditions in downstream analysis. Based on the observed synergism with chemo drugs and immunotherapy, modulating the gut microbiome has called attention to improving tailored treatment for patients suffering from refractory cancers, although the case for HCC is still in scarcity. The differential efficacy reported in clinical trials using responder-derived FMT encourages more investigations in recipients, of which the gut microbial configuration prior to inoculation ought to be as well important. Fulfilling these knowledge gaps will certainly transform the clinical practice for patients with HCC and other cancers.

Acknowledgments This work was supported in part by the Ministry of Science and Technology, Taiwan, under the grant number MOST 108-2321-B-075-002, MOST 109-2327-B-010-003, MOST 110-2327-B-A49A-001, and MOST 111-2327-B-A49-005.

Conflicts of Interest The authors declare no competing interests.

References

Agdashian D, ElGindi M, Xie C, Sandhu M, Pratt D, Kleiner DE, Figg WD, Rytlewski JA, Sanders C, Yusko EC, Wood B, Venzon D, Brar G, Duffy AG, Greten TF, Korangy F. The effect of anti-CTLA4 treatment on peripheral and intra-tumoral T cells in patients with hepatocellular carcinoma. Cancer Immunol Immunother. 2019;68(4):599–608. https://doi.org/10.1007/s00262-019-02299-8.

Alisi A, Bedogni G, Baviera G, Giorgio V, Porro E, Paris C, Giammaria P, Reali L, Anania F, Nobili V. Randomised clinical trial: the beneficial effects of VSL#3 in obese children with non-alcoholic steatohepatitis. Aliment Pharmacol Ther. 2014;39(11):1276–85. https://doi.org/10.1111/apt.12758.

Aron-Wisnewsky J, Vigliotti C, Witjes J, Le P, Holleboom AG, Verheij J, Nieuwdorp M, Clement K. Gut microbiota and human NAFLD: disentangling microbial signatures from metabolic disorders. Nat Rev Gastroenterol Hepatol. 2020;17(5):279–97. https://doi.org/10.1038/s41575-020-0269-9.

Atarashi K, Tanoue T, Shima T, Imaoka A, Kuwahara T, Momose Y, Cheng G, Yamasaki S, Saito T, Ohba Y, Taniguchi T, Takeda K, Hori S, Ivanov II, Umesaki Y, Itoh K, Honda K. Induction of colonic regulatory T cells by indigenous Clostridium species. Science. 2011;331(6015):337–41. https://doi.org/10.1126/science.1198469.

Atarashi K, Tanoue T, Oshima K, Suda W, Nagano Y, Nishikawa H, Fukuda S, Saito T, Narushima S, Hase K, Kim S, Fritz JV, Wilmes P, Ueha S, Matsushima K, Ohno H, Olle B, Sakaguchi S, Taniguchi T, Morita H, Hattori M, Honda K. Treg induction by a rationally selected mixture of Clostridia strains from the human microbiota. Nature. 2013;500(7461):232–6. https://doi.org/10.1038/nature12331.

Bajaj JS, Heuman DM, Hylemon PB, Sanyal AJ, White MB, Monteith P, Noble NA, Unser AB, Daita K, Fisher AR, Sikaroodi M, Gillevet PM. Altered profile of human gut microbiome is associated with cirrhosis and its complications. J Hepatol. 2014;60(5):940–7. https://doi.org/10.1016/j.jhep.2013.12.019.

Baruch EN, Youngster I, Ben-Betzalel G, Ortenberg R, Lahat A, Katz L, Adler K, Dick-Necula D, Raskin S, Bloch N, Rotin D, Anafi L, Avivi C, Melnichenko J, Steinberg-Silman Y, Mamtani R, Harati H, Asher N, Shapira-Frommer R, Brosh-Nissimov T, Eshet Y, Ben-Simon S, Ziv O, Khan MAW, Amit M, Ajami NJ, Barshack I, Schachter J, Wargo JA, Koren O, Markel G,

Boursi B. Fecal microbiota transplant promotes response in immunotherapy-refractory melanoma patients. Science. 2021;371(6529):602–9. https://doi.org/10.1126/science.abb5920.

Bishehsari F, Magno E, Swanson G, Desai V, Voigt RM, Forsyth CB, Keshavarzian A. Alcohol and gut-derived inflammation. Alcohol Res. 2017;38(2):163–71.

Buffie CG, Bucci V, Stein RR, McKenney PT, Ling L, Gobourne A, No D, Liu H, Kinnebrew M, Viale A, Littmann E, van den Brink MR, Jenq RR, Taur Y, Sander C, Cross JR, Toussaint NC, Xavier JB, Pamer EG. Precision microbiome reconstitution restores bile acid mediated resistance to Clostridium difficile. Nature. 2015;517(7533):205–8. https://doi.org/10.1038/nature13828.

Carr RM, Reid AE. FXR agonists as therapeutic agents for non-alcoholic fatty liver disease. Curr Atheroscler Rep. 2015;17(4):500. https://doi.org/10.1007/s11883-015-0500-2.

Caussy C, Tripathi A, Humphrey G, Bassirian S, Singh S, Faulkner C, Bettencourt R, Rizo E, Richards L, Xu ZZ, Downes MR, Evans RM, Brenner DA, Sirlin CB, Knight R, Loomba R. A gut microbiome signature for cirrhosis due to nonalcoholic fatty liver disease. Nat Commun. 2019;10(1):1406. https://doi.org/10.1038/s41467-019-09455-9.

Cederbaum AI. Alcohol metabolism. Clin Liver Dis. 2012;16(4):667–85. https://doi.org/10.1016/j.cld.2012.08.002.

Chen Y, Yang F, Lu H, Wang B, Chen Y, Lei D, Wang Y, Zhu B, Li L. Characterization of fecal microbial communities in patients with liver cirrhosis. Hepatology. 2011;54(2):562–72. https://doi.org/10.1002/hep.24423.

Cheng WY, Wu CY, Yu J. The role of gut microbiota in cancer treatment: friend or foe? Gut. 2020;69(10):1867–76. https://doi.org/10.1136/gutjnl-2020-321153.

Chiu CC, Ching YH, Li YP, Liu JY, Huang YT, Huang YW, Yang SS, Huang WC, Chuang HL. Nonalcoholic fatty liver disease is exacerbated in high-fat diet-fed gnotobiotic mice by colonization with the gut microbiota from patients with nonalcoholic steatohepatitis. Nutrients. 2017;9(11):1220. https://doi.org/10.3390/nu9111220.

Chou HH, Chien WH, Wu LL, Cheng CH, Chung CH, Horng JH, Ni YH, Tseng HT, Wu D, Lu X, Wang HY, Chen PJ, Chen DS. Age-related immune clearance of hepatitis B virus infection requires the establishment of gut microbiota. Proc Natl Acad Sci U S A. 2015;112(7):2175–80. https://doi.org/10.1073/pnas.1424775112.

Ciocan D, Voican CS, Wrzosek L, Hugot C, Rainteau D, Humbert L, Cassard AM, Perlemuter G. Bile acid homeostasis and intestinal dysbiosis in alcoholic hepatitis. Aliment Pharmacol Ther. 2018;48(9):961–74. https://doi.org/10.1111/apt.14949.

Dai H, Tong C, Shi D, Chen M, Guo Y, Chen D, Han X, Wang H, Wang Y, Shen P. Efficacy and biomarker analysis of CD133-directed CAR T cells in advanced hepatocellular carcinoma: a single-arm, open-label, phase II trial. Oncoimmunology. 2020;9(1):1846926. https://doi.org/10.1080/2162402X.2020.1846926.

Daillere R, Vetizou M, Waldschmitt N, Yamazaki T, Isnard C, Poirier-Colame V, Duong CPM, Flament C, Lepage P, Roberti MP, Routy B, Jacquelot N, Apetoh L, Becharef S, Rusakiewicz S, Langella P, Sokol H, Kroemer G, Enot D, Roux A, Eggermont A, Tartour E, Johannes L, Woerther PL, Chachaty E, Soria JC, Golden E, Formenti S, Plebanski M, Madondo M, Rosenstiel P, Raoult D, Cattoir V, Boneca IG, Chamaillard M, Zitvogel L. Enterococcus hirae and Barnesiella intestinihominis facilitate cyclophosphamide-induced therapeutic immunomodulatory effects. Immunity. 2016;45(4):931–43. https://doi.org/10.1016/j.immuni.2016.09.009.

Dapito DH, Mencin A, Gwak GY, Pradere JP, Jang MK, Mederacke I, Caviglia JM, Khiabanian H, Adeyemi A, Bataller R, Lefkowitch JH, Bower M, Friedman R, Sartor RB, Rabadan R, Schwabe RF. Promotion of hepatocellular carcinoma by the intestinal microbiota and TLR4. Cancer Cell. 2012;21(4):504–16. https://doi.org/10.1016/j.ccr.2012.02.007.

Davar D, Dzutsev AK, McCulloch JA, Rodrigues RR, Chauvin JM, Morrison RM, Deblasio RN, Menna C, Ding Q, Pagliano O, Zidi B, Zhang S, Badger JH, Vetizou M, Cole AM, Fernandes MR, Prescott S, Costa RGF, Balaji AK, Morgun A, Vujkovic-Cvijin I, Wang H, Borhani AA, Schwartz MB, Dubner HM, Ernst SJ, Rose A, Najjar YG, Belkaid Y, Kirkwood JM, Trinchieri

G, Zarour HM. Fecal microbiota transplant overcomes resistance to anti-PD-1 therapy in melanoma patients. Science. 2021;371(6529):595–602. https://doi.org/10.1126/science.abf3363.

Dhiman RK, Rana B, Agrawal S, Garg A, Chopra M, Thumburu KK, Khattri A, Malhotra S, Duseja A, Chawla YK. Probiotic VSL#3 reduces liver disease severity and hospitalization in patients with cirrhosis: a randomized, controlled trial. Gastroenterology. 2014;147(6):1327–1337.e1323. https://doi.org/10.1053/j.gastro.2014.08.031.

Duan Y, Llorente C, Lang S, Brandl K, Chu H, Jiang L, White RC, Clarke TH, Nguyen K, Torralba M, Shao Y, Liu J, Hernandez-Morales A, Lessor L, Rahman IR, Miyamoto Y, Ly M, Gao B, Sun W, Kiesel R, Hutmacher F, Lee S, Ventura-Cots M, Bosques-Padilla F, Verna EC, Abraldes JG, Brown RS Jr, Vargas V, Altamirano J, Caballeria J, Shawcross DL, Ho SB, Louvet A, Lucey MR, Mathurin P, Garcia-Tsao G, Bataller R, Tu XM, Eckmann L, van der Donk WA, Young R, Lawley TD, Starkel P, Pride D, Fouts DE, Schnabl B. Bacteriophage targeting of gut bacterium attenuates alcoholic liver disease. Nature. 2019;575(7783):505–11. https://doi.org/10.1038/s41586-019-1742-x.

Dubinkina VB, Tyakht AV, Odintsova VY, Yarygin KS, Kovarsky BA, Pavlenko AV, Ischenko DS, Popenko AS, Alexeev DG, Taraskina AY, Nasyrova RF, Krupitsky EM, Shalikiani NV, Bakulin IG, Shcherbakov PL, Skorodumova LO, Larin AK, Kostryukova ES, Abdulkhakov RA, Abdulkhakov SR, Malanin SY, Ismagilova RK, Grigoryeva TV, Ilina EN, Govorun VM. Links of gut microbiota composition with alcohol dependence syndrome and alcoholic liver disease. Microbiome. 2017;5(1):141. https://doi.org/10.1186/s40168-017-0359-2.

Dunagan M, Chaudhry K, Samak G, Rao RK. Acetaldehyde disrupts tight junctions in Caco-2 cell monolayers by a protein phosphatase 2A-dependent mechanism. Am J Physiol Gastrointest Liver Physiol. 2012;303(12):G1356–64. https://doi.org/10.1152/ajpgi.00526.2011.

El-Serag HB. Epidemiology of viral hepatitis and hepatocellular carcinoma. Gastroenterology. 2012;142(6):1264–1273.e1261. https://doi.org/10.1053/j.gastro.2011.12.061.

Fagarasan S, Muramatsu M, Suzuki K, Nagaoka H, Hiai H, Honjo T. Critical roles of activation-induced cytidine deaminase in the homeostasis of gut flora. Science. 2002;298(5597):1424–7. https://doi.org/10.1126/science.1077336.

Fernandez J, Navasa M, Planas R, Montoliu S, Monfort D, Soriano G, Vila C, Pardo A, Quintero E, Vargas V, Such J, Gines P, Arroyo V. Primary prophylaxis of spontaneous bacterial peritonitis delays hepatorenal syndrome and improves survival in cirrhosis. Gastroenterology. 2007;133(3):818–24. https://doi.org/10.1053/j.gastro.2007.06.065.

Finn RS, Ryoo BY, Merle P, Kudo M, Bouattour M, Lim HY, Breder V, Edeline J, Chao Y, Ogasawara S, Yau T, Garrido M, Chan SL, Knox J, Daniele B, Ebbinghaus SW, Chen E, Siegel AB, Zhu AX, Cheng AL, KEYNOTE-240 Investigators. Pembrolizumab as second-line therapy in patients with advanced hepatocellular carcinoma in KEYNOTE-240: a randomized, double-blind, phase III trial. J Clin Oncol. 2020a;38(3):193–202. https://doi.org/10.1200/JCO.19.01307.

Finn RS, Qin S, Ikeda M, Galle PR, Ducreux M, Kim TY, Kudo M, Breder V, Merle P, Kaseb AO, Li D, Verret W, Xu DZ, Hernandez S, Liu J, Huang C, Mulla S, Wang Y, Lim HY, Zhu AX, Cheng AL, IMbrave150 Investigators. Atezolizumab plus bevacizumab in unresectable hepatocellular carcinoma. N Engl J Med. 2020b;382(20):1894–905. https://doi.org/10.1056/NEJMoa1915745.

Gao B, Duan Y, Lang S, Barupal D, Wu TC, Valdiviez L, Roberts B, Choy YY, Shen T, Byram G, Zhang Y, Fan S, Wancewicz B, Shao Y, Vervier K, Wang Y, Zhou R, Jiang L, Nath S, Loomba R, Abraldes JG, Bataller R, Tu XM, Starkel P, Lawley TD, Fiehn O, Schnabl B. Functional microbiomics reveals alterations of the gut microbiome and host co-metabolism in patients with alcoholic hepatitis. Hepatology Commun. 2020;4(8):1168–82. https://doi.org/10.1002/hep4.1537.

Gopalakrishnan V, Spencer CN, Nezi L, Reuben A, Andrews MC, Karpinets TV, Prieto PA, Vicente D, Hoffman K, Wei SC, Cogdill AP, Zhao L, Hudgens CW, Hutchinson DS, Manzo T, Petaccia de Macedo M, Cotechini T, Kumar T, Chen WS, Reddy SM, Szczepaniak Sloane R, Galloway-Pena J, Jiang H, Chen PL, Shpall EJ, Rezvani K, Alousi AM, Chemaly RF, Shelburne S, Vence

LM, Okhuysen PC, Jensen VB, Swennes AG, McAllister F, Marcelo Riquelme Sanchez E, Zhang Y, Le Chatelier E, Zitvogel L, Pons N, Austin-Breneman JL, Haydu LE, Burton EM, Gardner JM, Sirmans E, Hu J, Lazar AJ, Tsujikawa T, Diab A, Tawbi H, Glitza IC, Hwu WJ, Patel SP, Woodman SE, Amaria RN, Davies MA, Gershenwald JE, Hwu P, Lee JE, Zhang J, Coussens LM, Cooper ZA, Futreal PA, Daniel CR, Ajami NJ, Petrosino JF, Tetzlaff MT, Sharma P, Allison JP, Jenq RR, Wargo JA. Gut microbiome modulates response to anti-PD-1 immunotherapy in melanoma patients. Science. 2018;359(6371):97–103. https://doi.org/10.1126/science.aan4236.

Grander C, Adolph TE, Wieser V, Lowe P, Wrzosek L, Gyongyosi B, Ward DV, Grabherr F, Gerner RR, Pfister A, Enrich B, Ciocan D, Macheiner S, Mayr L, Drach M, Moser P, Moschen AR, Perlemuter G, Szabo G, Cassard AM, Tilg H. Recovery of ethanol-induced Akkermansia muciniphila depletion ameliorates alcoholic liver disease. Gut. 2018;67(5):891–901. https://doi.org/10.1136/gutjnl-2016-313432.

Grat M, Wronka KM, Krasnodebski M, Masior L, Lewandowski Z, Kosinska I, Grat K, Stypulkowski J, Rejowski S, Wasilewicz M, Galecka M, Szachta P, Krawczyk M. Profile of gut microbiota associated with the presence of hepatocellular cancer in patients with liver cirrhosis. Transplant Proc. 2016;48(5):1687–91. https://doi.org/10.1016/j.transproceed.2016.01.077.

Guicciardi ME, Gores GJ. Apoptosis: a mechanism of acute and chronic liver injury. Gut. 2005;54(7):1024–33. https://doi.org/10.1136/gut.2004.053850.

Han SH, Suk KT, Kim DJ, Kim MY, Baik SK, Kim YD, Cheon GJ, Choi DH, Ham YL, Shin DH, Kim EJ. Effects of probiotics (cultured Lactobacillus subtilis/Streptococcus faecium) in the treatment of alcoholic hepatitis: randomized-controlled multicenter study. Eur J Gastroenterol Hepatol. 2015;27(11):1300–6. https://doi.org/10.1097/MEG.0000000000000458.

Henao-Mejia J, Elinav E, Jin C, Hao L, Mehal WZ, Strowig T, Thaiss CA, Kau AL, Eisenbarth SC, Jurczak MJ, Camporez JP, Shulman GI, Gordon JI, Hoffman HM, Flavell RA. Inflammasome-mediated dysbiosis regulates progression of NAFLD and obesity. Nature. 2012;482(7384):179–85. https://doi.org/10.1038/nature10809.

Hoyles L, Fernandez-Real JM, Federici M, Serino M, Abbott J, Charpentier J, Heymes C, Luque JL, Anthony E, Barton RH, Chilloux J, Myridakis A, Martinez-Gili L, Moreno-Navarrete JM, Benhamed F, Azalbert V, Blasco-Baque V, Puig J, Xifra G, Ricart W, Tomlinson C, Woodbridge M, Cardellini M, Davato F, Cardolini I, Porzio O, Gentileschi P, Lopez F, Foufelle F, Butcher SA, Holmes E, Nicholson JK, Postic C, Burcelin R, Dumas ME. Molecular phenomics and metagenomics of hepatic steatosis in non-diabetic obese women. Nat Med. 2018;24(7):1070–80. https://doi.org/10.1038/s41591-018-0061-3.

Huang DQ, El-Serag HB, Loomba R. Global epidemiology of NAFLD-related HCC: trends, predictions, risk factors and prevention. Nat Rev Gastroenterol Hepatol. 2021;18(4):223–38. https://doi.org/10.1038/s41575-020-00381-6.

Iida N, Dzutsev A, Stewart CA, Smith L, Bouladoux N, Weingarten RA, Molina DA, Salcedo R, Back T, Cramer S, Dai RM, Kiu H, Cardone M, Naik S, Patri AK, Wang E, Marincola FM, Frank KM, Belkaid Y, Trinchieri G, Goldszmid RS. Commensal bacteria control cancer response to therapy by modulating the tumor microenvironment. Science. 2013;342(6161):967–70. https://doi.org/10.1126/science.1240527.

Inagaki T, Moschetta A, Lee YK, Peng L, Zhao G, Downes M, Yu RT, Shelton JM, Richardson JA, Repa JJ, Mangelsdorf DJ, Kliewer SA. Regulation of antibacterial defense in the small intestine by the nuclear bile acid receptor. Proc Natl Acad Sci U S A. 2006;103(10):3920–5. https://doi.org/10.1073/pnas.0509592103.

Jia W, Xie G, Jia W. Bile acid-microbiota crosstalk in gastrointestinal inflammation and carcinogenesis. Nat Rev Gastroenterol Hepatol. 2018;15(2):111–28. https://doi.org/10.1038/nrgastro.2017.119.

Jia X, Lu S, Zeng Z, Liu Q, Dong Z, Chen Y, Zhu Z, Hong Z, Zhang T, Du G, Xiang J, Wu D, Bai W, Yang B, Li Y, Huang J, Li H, Safadi R, Lu Y. Characterization of gut microbiota, bile acid metabolism, and cytokines in intrahepatic cholangiocarcinoma. Hepatology. 2020;71(3):893–906. https://doi.org/10.1002/hep.30852.

Jiao Y, Lu Y, Li XY. Farnesoid X receptor: a master regulator of hepatic triglyceride and glucose homeostasis. Acta Pharmacol Sin. 2015;36(1):44–50. https://doi.org/10.1038/aps.2014.116.

Koh A, De Vadder F, Kovatcheva-Datchary P, Backhed F. From dietary fiber to host physiology: short-chain fatty acids as key bacterial metabolites. Cell. 2016;165(6):1332–45. https://doi.org/10.1016/j.cell.2016.05.041.

Lam KC, Araya RE, Huang A, Chen Q, Di Modica M, Rodrigues RR, Lopes A, Johnson SB, Schwarz B, Bohrnsen E, Cogdill AP, Bosio CM, Wargo JA, Lee MP, Goldszmid RS. Microbiota triggers STING-type I IFN-dependent monocyte reprogramming of the tumor microenvironment. Cell. 2021;184(21):5338–5356.e5321. https://doi.org/10.1016/j.cell.2021.09.019.

Lang S, Fairfied B, Gao B, Duan Y, Zhang X, Fouts DE, Schnabl B. Changes in the fecal bacterial microbiota associated with disease severity in alcoholic hepatitis patients. Gut Microbes. 2020;12(1):1785251. https://doi.org/10.1080/19490976.2020.1785251.

Le Roy T, Llopis M, Lepage P, Bruneau A, Rabot S, Bevilacqua C, Martin P, Philippe C, Walker F, Bado A, Perlemuter G, Cassard-Doulcier AM, Gerard P. Intestinal microbiota determines development of non-alcoholic fatty liver disease in mice. Gut. 2013;62(12):1787–94. https://doi.org/10.1136/gutjnl-2012-303816.

Leung C, Rivera L, Furness JB, Angus PW. The role of the gut microbiota in NAFLD. Nat Rev Gastroenterol Hepatol. 2016;13(7):412–25. https://doi.org/10.1038/nrgastro.2016.85.

Li Y, Jadhav K, Zhang Y. Bile acid receptors in non-alcoholic fatty liver disease. Biochem Pharmacol. 2013;86(11):1517–24. https://doi.org/10.1016/j.bcp.2013.08.015.

Li J, Sung CY, Lee N, Ni Y, Pihlajamaki J, Panagiotou G, El-Nezami H. Probiotics modulated gut microbiota suppresses hepatocellular carcinoma growth in mice. Proc Natl Acad Sci U S A. 2016;113(9):E1306–15. https://doi.org/10.1073/pnas.1518189113.

Liu Q, Li F, Zhuang Y, Xu J, Wang J, Mao X, Zhang Y, Liu X. Alteration in gut microbiota associated with hepatitis B and non-hepatitis virus related hepatocellular carcinoma. Gut Pathog. 2019;11:1. https://doi.org/10.1186/s13099-018-0281-6.

Llopis M, Cassard AM, Wrzosek L, Boschat L, Bruneau A, Ferrere G, Puchois V, Martin JC, Lepage P, Le Roy T, Lefevre L, Langelier B, Cailleux F, Gonzalez-Castro AM, Rabot S, Gaudin F, Agostini H, Prevot S, Berrebi D, Ciocan D, Jousse C, Naveau S, Gerard P, Perlemuter G. Intestinal microbiota contributes to individual susceptibility to alcoholic liver disease. Gut. 2016;65(5):830–9. https://doi.org/10.1136/gutjnl-2015-310585.

Ma C, Kesarwala AH, Eggert T, Medina-Echeverz J, Kleiner DE, Jin P, Stroncek DF, Terabe M, Kapoor V, ElGindi M, Han M, Thornton AM, Zhang H, Egger M, Luo J, Felsher DW, McVicar DW, Weber A, Heikenwalder M, Greten TF. NAFLD causes selective CD4(+) T lymphocyte loss and promotes hepatocarcinogenesis. Nature. 2016;531(7593):253–7. https://doi.org/10.1038/nature16969.

Ma C, Han M, Heinrich B, Fu Q, Zhang Q, Sandhu M, Agdashian D, Terabe M, Berzofsky JA, Fako V, Ritz T, Longerich T, Theriot CM, McCulloch JA, Roy S, Yuan W, Thovarai V, Sen SK, Ruchirawat M, Korangy F, Wang XW, Trinchieri G, Greten TF. Gut microbiome-mediated bile acid metabolism regulates liver cancer via NKT cells. Science. 2018;360(6391):eaan5931. https://doi.org/10.1126/science.aan5931.

Macpherson AJ, Koller Y, McCoy KD. The bilateral responsiveness between intestinal microbes and IgA. Trends Immunol. 2015;36(8):460–70. https://doi.org/10.1016/j.it.2015.06.006.

Mathurin P, Bataller R. Trends in the management and burden of alcoholic liver disease. J Hepatol. 2015;62(1 Suppl):S38–46. https://doi.org/10.1016/j.jhep.2015.03.006.

Mirpuri J, Raetz M, Sturge CR, Wilhelm CL, Benson A, Savani RC, Hooper LV, Yarovinsky F. Proteobacteria-specific IgA regulates maturation of the intestinal microbiota. Gut Microbes. 2014;5(1):28–39. https://doi.org/10.4161/gmic.26489.

Moro-Sibilot L, Blanc P, Taillardet M, Bardel E, Couillault C, Boschetti G, Traverse-Glehen A, Defrance T, Kaiserlian D, Dubois B. Mouse and human liver contain immunoglobulin A-secreting cells originating from Peyer's patches and directed against intestinal antigens. Gastroenterology. 2016;151(2):311–23. https://doi.org/10.1053/j.gastro.2016.04.014.

Mutlu EA, Gillevet PM, Rangwala H, Sikaroodi M, Naqvi A, Engen PA, Kwasny M, Lau CK, Keshavarzian A. Colonic microbiome is altered in alcoholism. Am J Physiol Gastrointest Liver Physiol. 2012;302(9):G966–78. https://doi.org/10.1152/ajpgi.00380.2011.

O'Connor A, O'Morain CA, Ford AC. Population screening and treatment of Helicobacter pylori infection. Nat Rev Gastroenterol Hepatol. 2017;14(4):230–40. https://doi.org/10.1038/nrgastro.2016.195.

Oster P, Vaillant L, Riva E, McMillan B, Begka C, Truntzer C, Richard C, Leblond MM, Messaoudene M, Machremi E, Limagne E, Ghiringhelli F, Routy B, Verdeil G, Velin D. Helicobacter pylori infection has a detrimental impact on the efficacy of cancer immunotherapies. Gut. 2022;71(3):457–66. https://doi.org/10.1136/gutjnl-2020-323392.

Palm NW, de Zoete MR, Cullen TW, Barry NA, Stefanowski J, Hao L, Degnan PH, Hu J, Peter I, Zhang W, Ruggiero E, Cho JH, Goodman AL, Flavell RA. Immunoglobulin A coating identifies colitogenic bacteria in inflammatory bowel disease. Cell. 2014;158(5):1000–10. https://doi.org/10.1016/j.cell.2014.08.006.

Park EJ, Lee JH, Yu GY, He G, Ali SR, Holzer RG, Osterreicher CH, Takahashi H, Karin M. Dietary and genetic obesity promote liver inflammation and tumorigenesis by enhancing IL-6 and TNF expression. Cell. 2010;140(2):197–208. https://doi.org/10.1016/j.cell.2009.12.052.

Parseus A, Sommer N, Sommer F, Caesar R, Molinaro A, Stahlman M, Greiner TU, Perkins R, Backhed F. Microbiota-induced obesity requires farnesoid X receptor. Gut. 2017;66(3):429–37. https://doi.org/10.1136/gutjnl-2015-310283.

Pathak P, Xie C, Nichols RG, Ferrell JM, Boehme S, Krausz KW, Patterson AD, Gonzalez FJ, Chiang JYL. Intestine farnesoid X receptor agonist and the gut microbiota activate G-protein bile acid receptor-1 signaling to improve metabolism. Hepatology. 2018;68(4):1574–88. https://doi.org/10.1002/hep.29857.

Philips CA, Pande A, Shasthry SM, Jamwal KD, Khillan V, Chandel SS, Kumar G, Sharma MK, Maiwall R, Jindal A, Choudhary A, Hussain MS, Sharma S, Sarin SK. Healthy donor fecal microbiota transplantation in steroid-ineligible severe alcoholic hepatitis: a pilot study. Clin Gastroenterol Hepatol. 2017;15(4):600–2. https://doi.org/10.1016/j.cgh.2016.10.029.

Philips CA, Phadke N, Ganesan K, Ranade S, Augustine P. Corticosteroids, nutrition, pentoxifylline, or fecal microbiota transplantation for severe alcoholic hepatitis. Indian J Gastroenterol. 2018;37(3):215–25. https://doi.org/10.1007/s12664-018-0859-4.

Ponziani FR, Bhoori S, Castelli C, Putignani L, Rivoltini L, Del Chierico F, Sanguinetti M, Morelli D, Paroni Sterbini F, Petito V, Reddel S, Calvani R, Camisaschi C, Picca A, Tuccitto A, Gasbarrini A, Pompili M, Mazzaferro V. Hepatocellular carcinoma is associated with gut microbiota profile and inflammation in nonalcoholic fatty liver disease. Hepatology. 2019;69(1):107–20. https://doi.org/10.1002/hep.30036.

Puri P, Liangpunsakul S, Christensen JE, Shah VH, Kamath PS, Gores GJ, Walker S, Comerford M, Katz B, Borst A, Yu Q, Kumar DP, Mirshahi F, Radaeva S, Chalasani NP, Crabb DW, Sanyal AJ, TREAT Consortium. The circulating microbiome signature and inferred functional metagenomics in alcoholic hepatitis. Hepatology. 2018;67(4):1284–302. https://doi.org/10.1002/hep.29623.

Qin N, Yang F, Li A, Prifti E, Chen Y, Shao L, Guo J, Le Chatelier E, Yao J, Wu L, Zhou J, Ni S, Liu L, Pons N, Batto JM, Kennedy SP, Leonard P, Yuan C, Ding W, Chen Y, Hu X, Zheng B, Qian G, Xu W, Ehrlich SD, Zheng S, Li L. Alterations of the human gut microbiome in liver cirrhosis. Nature. 2014;513(7516):59–64. https://doi.org/10.1038/nature13568.

Quince C, Walker AW, Simpson JT, Loman NJ, Segata N. Shotgun metagenomics, from sampling to analysis. Nat Biotechnol. 2017;35(9):833–44. https://doi.org/10.1038/nbt.3935.

Reikvam DH, Derrien M, Islam R, Erofeev A, Grcic V, Sandvik A, Gaustad P, Meza-Zepeda LA, Jahnsen FL, Smidt H, Johansen FE. Epithelial-microbial crosstalk in polymeric Ig receptor deficient mice. Eur J Immunol. 2012;42(11):2959–70. https://doi.org/10.1002/eji.201242543.

Ren Z, Li A, Jiang J, Zhou L, Yu Z, Lu H, Xie H, Chen X, Shao L, Zhang R, Xu S, Zhang H, Cui G, Chen X, Sun R, Wen H, Lerut JP, Kan Q, Li L, Zheng S. Gut microbiome analysis as a tool towards targeted non-invasive biomarkers for early hepatocellular carcinoma. Gut. 2019;68(6):1014–23. https://doi.org/10.1136/gutjnl-2017-315084.

Ridlon JM, Kang DJ, Hylemon PB, Bajaj JS. Bile acids and the gut microbiome. Curr Opin Gastroenterol. 2014;30(3):332–8. https://doi.org/10.1097/MOG.0000000000000057.

Rollenske T, Burkhalter S, Muerner L, von Gunten S, Lukasiewicz J, Wardemann H, Macpherson AJ. Parallelism of intestinal secretory IgA shapes functional microbial fitness. Nature. 2021;598(7882):657–61. https://doi.org/10.1038/s41586-021-03973-7.

Routy B, Le Chatelier E, Derosa L, Duong CPM, Alou MT, Daillere R, Fluckiger A, Messaoudene M, Rauber C, Roberti MP, Fidelle M, Flament C, Poirier-Colame V, Opolon P, Klein C, Iribarren K, Mondragon L, Jacquelot N, Qu B, Ferrere G, Clemenson C, Mezquita L, Masip JR, Naltet C, Brosseau S, Kaderbhai C, Richard C, Rizvi H, Levenez F, Galleron N, Quinquis B, Pons N, Ryffel B, Minard-Colin V, Gonin P, Soria JC, Deutsch E, Loriot Y, Ghiringhelli F, Zalcman G, Goldwasser F, Escudier B, Hellmann MD, Eggermont A, Raoult D, Albiges L, Kroemer G, Zitvogel L. Gut microbiome influences efficacy of PD-1-based immunotherapy against epithelial tumors. Science. 2018;359(6371):91–7. https://doi.org/10.1126/science.aan3706.

Sandler NG, Koh C, Roque A, Eccleston JL, Siegel RB, Demino M, Kleiner DE, Deeks SG, Liang TJ, Heller T, Douek DC. Host response to translocated microbial products predicts outcomes of patients with HBV or HCV infection. Gastroenterology. 2011;141(4):1220–30, 1230 e1221-1223. https://doi.org/10.1053/j.gastro.2011.06.063.

Schwabe RF, Greten TF. Gut microbiome in HCC—mechanisms, diagnosis and therapy. J Hepatol. 2020;72(2):230–8. https://doi.org/10.1016/j.jhep.2019.08.016.

Seitz HK, Becker P. Alcohol metabolism and cancer risk. Alcohol Res Health. 2007;30(1):38–41, 44–37.

Seitz HK, Bataller R, Cortez-Pinto H, Gao B, Gual A, Lackner C, Mathurin P, Mueller S, Szabo G, Tsukamoto H. Alcoholic liver disease. Nat Rev Dis Primers. 2018;4(1):16. https://doi.org/10.1038/s41572-018-0014-7.

Seki E, De Minicis S, Osterreicher CH, Kluwe J, Osawa Y, Brenner DA, Schwabe RF. TLR4 enhances TGF-beta signaling and hepatic fibrosis. Nat Med. 2007;13(11):1324–32. https://doi.org/10.1038/nm1663.

Shalapour S, Lin XJ, Bastian IN, Brain J, Burt AD, Aksenov AA, Vrbanac AF, Li W, Perkins A, Matsutani T, Zhong Z, Dhar D, Navas-Molina JA, Xu J, Loomba R, Downes M, Yu RT, Evans RM, Dorrestein PC, Knight R, Benner C, Anstee QM, Karin M. Inflammation-induced IgA+ cells dismantle anti-liver cancer immunity. Nature. 2017;551(7680):340–5. https://doi.org/10.1038/nature24302.

Shigeta K, Matsui A, Kikuchi H, Klein S, Mamessier E, Chen IX, Aoki S, Kitahara S, Inoue K, Shigeta A, Hato T, Ramjiawan RR, Staiculescu D, Zopf D, Fiebig L, Hobbs GS, Quaas A, Dima S, Popescu I, Huang P, Munn LL, Cobbold M, Goyal L, Zhu AX, Jain RK, Duda DG. Regorafenib combined with PD1 blockade increases CD8 T-cell infiltration by inducing CXCL10 expression in hepatocellular carcinoma. J Immunother Cancer. 2020;8(2):e001435. https://doi.org/10.1136/jitc-2020-001435.

Sinal CJ, Tohkin M, Miyata M, Ward JM, Lambert G, Gonzalez FJ. Targeted disruption of the nuclear receptor FXR/BAR impairs bile acid and lipid homeostasis. Cell. 2000;102(6):731–44. https://doi.org/10.1016/s0092-8674(00)00062-3.

Singh V, Yeoh BS, Chassaing B, Xiao X, Saha P, Aguilera Olvera R, Lapek JD Jr, Zhang L, Wang WB, Hao S, Flythe MD, Gonzalez DJ, Cani PD, Conejo-Garcia JR, Xiong N, Kennett MJ, Joe B, Patterson AD, Gewirtz AT, Vijay-Kumar M. Dysregulated microbial fermentation of soluble fiber induces cholestatic liver cancer. Cell. 2018;175(3):679–694.e622. https://doi.org/10.1016/j.cell.2018.09.004.

Sivan A, Corrales L, Hubert N, Williams JB, Aquino-Michaels K, Earley ZM, Benyamin FW, Lei YM, Jabri B, Alegre ML, Chang EB, Gajewski TF. Commensal Bifidobacterium promotes antitumor immunity and facilitates anti-PD-L1 efficacy. Science. 2015;350(6264):1084–9. https://doi.org/10.1126/science.aac4255.

Smirnova E, Puri P, Muthiah MD, Daitya K, Brown R, Chalasani N, Liangpunsakul S, Shah VH, Gelow K, Siddiqui MS, Boyett S, Mirshahi F, Sikaroodi M, Gillevet P, Sanyal AJ. Fecal microbiome distinguishes alcohol consumption from alcoholic hepatitis but does not discriminate disease severity. Hepatology. 2020;72(1):271–86. https://doi.org/10.1002/hep.31178.

Sun L, Xie C, Wang G, Wu Y, Wu Q, Wang X, Liu J, Deng Y, Xia J, Chen B, Zhang S, Yun C, Lian G, Zhang X, Zhang H, Bisson WH, Shi J, Gao X, Ge P, Liu C, Krausz KW, Nichols RG, Cai J, Rimal B, Patterson AD, Wang X, Gonzalez FJ, Jiang C. Gut microbiota and intestinal FXR mediate the clinical benefits of metformin. Nat Med. 2018;24(12):1919–29. https://doi.org/10.1038/s41591-018-0222-4.

Sung H, Ferlay J, Siegel RL, Laversanne M, Soerjomataram I, Jemal A, Bray F. Global cancer statistics 2020: GLOBOCAN estimates of incidence and mortality worldwide for 36 cancers in 185 countries. CA Cancer J Clin. 2021;71(3):209–49. https://doi.org/10.3322/caac.21660.

Szabo G. Gut-liver axis in alcoholic liver disease. Gastroenterology. 2015;148(1):30–6. https://doi.org/10.1053/j.gastro.2014.10.042.

The Ministry of Health and Welfare of Taiwan ROC. Statistics on the causes of death of Taiwanese people in 2020. 2021. https://www.mohw.gov.tw/cp-5017-61533-1.html. Accessed 23 Sept 2021.

Torrens L, Montironi C, Puigvehi M, Mesropian A, Leslie J, Haber PK, Maeda M, Balaseviciute U, Willoughby CE, Abril-Fornaguera J, Pique-Gili M, Torres-Martin M, Peix J, Geh D, Ramon-Gil E, Saberi B, Friedman SL, Mann DA, Sia D, Llovet JM. Immunomodulatory effects of lenvatinib plus anti-programmed cell death protein 1 in mice and rationale for patient enrichment in hepatocellular carcinoma. Hepatology. 2021;74(5):2652–69. https://doi.org/10.1002/hep.32023.

Tremaroli V, Backhed F. Functional interactions between the gut microbiota and host metabolism. Nature. 2012;489(7415):242–9. https://doi.org/10.1038/nature11552.

Tsuruta T, Inoue R, Iwanaga T, Hara H, Yajima T. Development of a method for the identification of S-IgA-coated bacterial composition in mouse and human feces. Biosci Biotechnol Biochem. 2010;74(5):968–73. https://doi.org/10.1271/bbb.90801.

Vetizou M, Pitt JM, Daillere R, Lepage P, Waldschmitt N, Flament C, Rusakiewicz S, Routy B, Roberti MP, Duong CP, Poirier-Colame V, Roux A, Becharef S, Formenti S, Golden E, Cording S, Eberl G, Schlitzer A, Ginhoux F, Mani S, Yamazaki T, Jacquelot N, Enot DP, Berard M, Nigou J, Opolon P, Eggermont A, Woerther PL, Chachaty E, Chaput N, Robert C, Mateus C, Kroemer G, Raoult D, Boneca IG, Carbonnel F, Chamaillard M, Zitvogel L. Anticancer immunotherapy by CTLA-4 blockade relies on the gut microbiota. Science. 2015;350(6264):1079–84. https://doi.org/10.1126/science.aad1329.

Viaud S, Saccheri F, Mignot G, Yamazaki T, Daillere R, Hannani D, Enot DP, Pfirschke C, Engblom C, Pittet MJ, Schlitzer A, Ginhoux F, Apetoh L, Chachaty E, Woerther PL, Eberl G, Berard M, Ecobichon C, Clermont D, Bizet C, Gaboriau-Routhiau V, Cerf-Bensussan N, Opolon P, Yessaad N, Vivier E, Ryffel B, Elson CO, Dore J, Kroemer G, Lepage P, Boneca IG, Ghiringhelli F, Zitvogel L. The intestinal microbiota modulates the anticancer immune effects of cyclophosphamide. Science. 2013;342(6161):971–6. https://doi.org/10.1126/science.1240537.

Vlachogiannakos J, Viazis N, Vasianopoulou P, Vafiadis I, Karamanolis DG, Ladas SD. Long-term administration of rifaximin improves the prognosis of patients with decompensated alcoholic cirrhosis. J Gastroenterol Hepatol. 2013;28(3):450–5. https://doi.org/10.1111/jgh.12070.

Wahlstrom A, Sayin SI, Marschall HU, Backhed F. Intestinal crosstalk between bile acids and microbiota and its impact on host metabolism. Cell Metab. 2016;24(1):41–50. https://doi.org/10.1016/j.cmet.2016.05.005.

Wang Y, Tong J, Chang B, Wang B, Zhang D, Wang B. Effects of alcohol on intestinal epithelial barrier permeability and expression of tight junction-associated proteins. Mol Med Rep. 2014;9(6):2352–6. https://doi.org/10.3892/mmr.2014.2126.

Wang J, Wang Y, Zhang X, Liu J, Zhang Q, Zhao Y, Peng J, Feng Q, Dai J, Sun S, Zhao Y, Zhao L, Zhang Y, Hu Y, Zhang M. Gut microbial dysbiosis is associated with altered hepatic functions and serum metabolites in chronic hepatitis B patients. Front Microbiol. 2017;8:2222. https://doi.org/10.3389/fmicb.2017.02222.

Wang T, Guo XK, Xu H. Disentangling the progression of non-alcoholic fatty liver disease in the human gut microbiota. Front Microbiol. 2021;12:728823. https://doi.org/10.3389/fmicb.2021.728823.

Wiest R, Albillos A, Trauner M, Bajaj JS, Jalan R. Targeting the gut-liver axis in liver disease. J Hepatol. 2017;67(5):1084–103. https://doi.org/10.1016/j.jhep.2017.05.007.

Wong KCW, Hui EP, Lo KW, Lam WKJ, Johnson D, Li L, Tao Q, Chan KCA, To KF, King AD, Ma BBY, Chan ATC. Nasopharyngeal carcinoma: an evolving paradigm. Nat Rev Clin Oncol. 2021;18(11):679–95. https://doi.org/10.1038/s41571-021-00524-x.

Wu CY, Chen YJ, Ho HJ, Hsu YC, Kuo KN, Wu MS, Lin JT. Association between nucleoside analogues and risk of hepatitis B virus-related hepatocellular carcinoma recurrence following liver resection. JAMA. 2012;308(18):1906–14. https://doi.org/10.1001/2012.jama.11975.

Wu CY, Lin JT, Ho HJ, Su CW, Lee TY, Wang SY, Wu C, Wu JC. Association of nucleos(t)ide analogue therapy with reduced risk of hepatocellular carcinoma in patients with chronic hepatitis B: a nationwide cohort study. Gastroenterology. 2014;147(1):143–151.e145. https://doi.org/10.1053/j.gastro.2014.03.048.

Xin B, Yang M, Wu P, Du L, Deng X, Hui E, Feng GS. Enhancing the therapeutic efficacy of PD-L1 antibody for metastasized liver cancer by overcoming hepatic immunotolerance. Hepatology. 2022;76(3):630–45. https://doi.org/10.1002/hep.32266.

Yoshimoto S, Loo TM, Atarashi K, Kanda H, Sato S, Oyadomari S, Iwakura Y, Oshima K, Morita H, Hattori M, Honda K, Ishikawa Y, Hara E, Ohtani N. Obesity-induced gut microbial metabolite promotes liver cancer through senescence secretome. Nature. 2013;499(7456):97–101. https://doi.org/10.1038/nature12347.

Yu LX, Schwabe RF. The gut microbiome and liver cancer: mechanisms and clinical translation. Nat Rev Gastroenterol Hepatol. 2017;14(9):527–39. https://doi.org/10.1038/nrgastro.2017.72.

Yu J, Green MD, Li S, Sun Y, Journey SN, Choi JE, Rizvi SM, Qin A, Waninger JJ, Lang X, Chopra Z, El Naqa I, Zhou J, Bian Y, Jiang L, Tezel A, Skvarce J, Achar RK, Sitto M, Rosen BS, Su F, Narayanan SP, Cao X, Wei S, Szeliga W, Vatan L, Mayo C, Morgan MA, Schonewolf CA, Cuneo K, Kryczek I, Ma VT, Lao CD, Lawrence TS, Ramnath N, Wen F, Chinnaiyan AM, Cieslik M, Alva A, Zou W. Liver metastasis restrains immunotherapy efficacy via macrophage-mediated T cell elimination. Nat Med. 2021;27(1):152–64. https://doi.org/10.1038/s41591-020-1131-x.

Yuan J, Chen C, Cui J, Lu J, Yan C, Wei X, Zhao X, Li N, Li S, Xue G, Cheng W, Li B, Li H, Lin W, Tian C, Zhao J, Han J, An D, Zhang Q, Wei H, Zheng M, Ma X, Li W, Chen X, Zhang Z, Zeng H, Ying S, Wu J, Yang R, Liu D. Fatty liver disease caused by high-alcohol-producing Klebsiella pneumoniae. Cell Metab. 2019;30(6):1172. https://doi.org/10.1016/j.cmet.2019.11.006.

Zhang HL, Yu LX, Yang W, Tang L, Lin Y, Wu H, Zhai B, Tan YX, Shan L, Liu Q, Chen HY, Dai RY, Qiu BJ, He YQ, Wang C, Zheng LY, Li YQ, Wu FQ, Li Z, Yan HX, Wang HY. Profound impact of gut homeostasis on chemically-induced pro-tumorigenic inflammation and hepatocarcinogenesis in rats. J Hepatol. 2012;57(4):803–12. https://doi.org/10.1016/j.jhep.2012.06.011.

Zhao Q, Elson CO. Adaptive immune education by gut microbiota antigens. Immunology. 2018;154(1):28–37. https://doi.org/10.1111/imm.12896.

Zheng Y, Wang T, Tu X, Huang Y, Zhang H, Tan D, Jiang W, Cai S, Zhao P, Song R, Li P, Qin N, Fang W. Gut microbiome affects the response to anti-PD-1 immunotherapy in patients with hepatocellular carcinoma. J Immunother Cancer. 2019;7(1):193. https://doi.org/10.1186/s40425-019-0650-9.

Zitvogel L, Galluzzi L, Viaud S, Vetizou M, Daillere R, Merad M, Kroemer G. Cancer and the gut microbiota: an unexpected link. Sci Transl Med. 2015;7(271):271ps271. https://doi.org/10.1126/scitranslmed.3010473.

Chapter 6
Non-bacteria Microbiome (Virus, Fungi, and Archaea) in Gastrointestinal Cancer

Olabisi Oluwabukola Coker

Abstract Gastrointestinal cancers account for about a third of cancer incidences and deaths in the world and remain a global health burden. Compared to bacteria, much less is known about the roles of viruses, fungi, and archaea in gastrointestinal cancers including colorectal, esophageal, gastric pancreatic, and liver cancers. Advancements in sequencing and taxonomy profiling methods have allowed insights into the possibilities of the non-bacteria microbiome's role in the transformation of normal epithelial cells into cancerous ones. This chapter describes the known associations between non-bacteria gut microbes and gastrointestinal cancers, and the potential mechanisms through which they influence carcinogenesis in the gut including distortion of entire microbe, production of carcinogens, and infection of host cells.

Keywords Virus · Fungi and archaea · Gastric cancer · Colorectal cancer

6.1 Introduction

Cancers in the gastrointestinal tract continue to pose major challenges to public health globally as they account for about a third of cancer incidences and deaths (Sung et al. 2021). Genetics and environmental factors are the two major triggers of this burden. At the center of the environmental factors is the gut microbiome which has been described to be altered by diet, exercise, smoking, and antibiotic use, among other lifestyles. The gut microbiome benefits the host through gut permeability maintenance, metabolisms of nutrients, modulation of the immune system, and prevention of infection, among others. Because of the alteration to the homeostatic state of the gut microbiome, the beneficial roles it plays are perturbed, shifting

O. O. Coker (✉)
Cumming School of Medicine, University of calgary, Calgary, Canada
e-mail: olabisi.coker1@ucalgary.ca

J. Yu (ed.), *Microbiome in Gastrointestinal Cancer*,
https://doi.org/10.1007/978-981-19-4492-5_6

the balance toward pathogenicity, which has been linked to the incidence and progression of gastrointestinal carcinogenesis. Physiologic and metabolic changes in gastrointestinal cancer patients may lead to the alteration of the gut microbes. However, direct and indirect roles of the gut microbiome in the initiation and progression of gastrointestinal cancers have been reported in several studies (Xavier et al. 2020; Aleman and Valenzano 2019). Gut microbiome-linked cancers have been demonstrated in the human colon, pancreas, stomach, esophagus, and liver (Coker 2022).

Bacteria involvement in gastrointestinal cancers is the most studied. This is because, compared to viruses, fungi, and archaea, commensal bacteria residing along the gastrointestinal tract are the most abundant, and as such, easily detected by sequencing technologies (Weng et al. 2019). Alterations in gut bacteriome in association with colon, gastric, esophageal, pancreatic, and liver cancers have been documented. Recent advancements in sequencing technologies and taxonomy profiling bioinformatics software have opened up the possibilities of describing the changes in the less abundant viruses, fungi, and archaea in association with human diseases including gastrointestinal cancers. This chapter describes the links between non-bacteria gut microbes and gastrointestinal cancers, and the potential mechanisms through which they influence carcinogenesis in the gut.

6.2 Functions of Non-bacteria Microbes in the Gut

6.2.1 Viruses in the Gut

Viruses are proportionately lower than bacteria in the gut, but they have been characterized as members of the stable commensal microbial community along the gastrointestinal tract (Beller and Matthijnssens 2019; Shkoporov et al. 2019; Deshpande et al. 2018; Coker et al. 2018; Santiago-Rodriguez and Hollister 2019). The most abundant enteric viruses are bacteriophages and are involved in several functions in the gut. Through their lytic and lysogenic stages of life cycles, bacteriophages can control the population of enteric bacteria. It was shown that the bacterial community of the gut microbiome is associated with human health and with the proportion of bacteriophages (Shkoporov et al. 2019; Santiago-Rodriguez and Hollister 2019). The fitness of host bacteria and their colonization of specific niches are reportedly influenced by lysogenic phages along the gastrointestinal tract (Santiago-Rodriguez and Hollister 2019). Modulation of enteric bacteria population by viruses was demonstrated by the finding that PreforPro, a phage that targets *E. coli* and was administered to humans reduced the abundance of pathogenic *Clostridium perfringens* while expanding the abundance of gut beneficial *Eubacterium*, a butyrate-producing bacterial genus (Febvre et al. 2019). In addition, phages that adhere to the mucosal surface of the gut can proffer defence against colonization of pathogenic bacteria, supporting host immunity (Barr et al. 2015). Viruses also support immune balance in the gut. Persistent stimulation of the immune system demonstrated by protection against pathogenic infection by *Listeria monocytogenes* was shown by latent gammaherpesvirus 68 infection in a mouse model (Barton et al. 2007). Similarly, murine norovirus facilitated IFNγ and IgA production resulting in crypt-villi production in another mouse model (Kernbauer et al. 2014).

6.2.2 Fungi in the Gut

Fungi are established as residents of the gastrointestinal tract of healthy humans but the composition is largely influenced by lifestyle especially diet (Hallen-Adams and Suhr 2017). They have been described in the gastric compartment, colon, pancreas, and esophagus albeit in a much lower proportion compared to bacteria (Coker 2022). Recent studies are beginning to reveal the importance of fungi in the gut. Fungi including *Candida, Saccharomyces, Cryptococcus, Malassezia, Cladosporium, Debaryomyces, Trichosporon,* and *Galactomyces* have been described in the healthy human gastrointestinal tract (Hallen-Adams and Suhr 2017). Fungi are involved in the maintenance of gut homeostasis. They have also been shown to play roles such as in systemic immunity, control of inflammatory responses and defence against infection (Perez 2021). Fungi reportedly induced T helper 17 cells, which are pivotal to host defence against infection (Fiers et al. 2019) and participate in the maturation of secondary lymphoid organs and calibration of host immunological and inflammatory responses. Moreover, enteric fungi modulate the function of host tissues such as the repair of the gut epithelial layer (Jiang et al. 2017; Zhang et al. 2016; Gaitanis et al. 2008; Mexia et al. 2015). Interactions among fungi and bacteria in the gut are associated with the maintenance of microbial ecology in the gut (Coker et al. 2019). The use of antibiotics usually leads to the overgrowth of fungi in the gut (Samonis et al. 1993), indicating a yet-to-be fully understood but important role for fungi in gut microbial homeostasis.

6.2.3 Archaea in the Gut

The advancement in sequencing and bioinformatic analysis has enabled the study of archaea, which is less studied compared to bacteria, viruses, and fungi in the gut. Based on 16S ribosomal RNA sequences, the archaea domain was identified as a unique group of prokaryotic organisms (Gribaldo and Brochier-Armanet 2006), characterized by lack of fatty acids, peptidoglycan, esters, and D-glycerol in their cell wall (Kandler and Konig 1998). Archaea were generally believed to be found in habitats with extreme environmental conditions, however recent studies have identified them in mesophilic conditions including human skin, nose, oral cavity, vagina, and the gut (Lurie-Weinberger and Gophna 2015). In the gut, both methanogenic archaea and haloarchaea have been described (Kim et al. 2020), the relative abundances of which vary according to individual (Kim et al. 2020). Archaea participate in host processes such as in nutrient fermentation involving gut bacteria (Nakamura et al. 2010). During nutrient digestion, the methanogenic archaea reduce carbon dioxide to generate methane, thereby contributing to the disposal of hydrogen, a process which helps in maintaining gut health (Roccarina et al. 2010). Moreover, archaea in the gut also help in the disposal of trimethylamine, produced by gut bacteria from the digestion of choline. The removal of trimethylamine by archaea including *Methanobrevibacter smithii* was reportedly associated with a lower risk of atherosclerosis (Ramezani et al. 2018; Blais Lecours et al. 2014; Brugere et al. 2014). As with fungi and viruses, archaea can play role in the maintenance of gut homeostasis by activating the adaptive immune responses in an antigen-specific fashion (Bang and Schmitz 2015). *Halobacterium salinarum,* a halophilic archaeon reportedly acted as an adjuvant in $CD8^+$ T-cell immunity induction, a means of modulating the immune system (Bang and Schmitz 2015).

6.3 Non-bacteria Gut Microbes and Gastrointestinal Cancers

6.3.1 Colorectal Cancer

Colorectal cancer (CRC) is the third most common cancer globally with 3.4 million cases projected in 2040 (Xi and Xu 2021). Several environmental and lifestyle factors are known to contribute to the initiation and progression of CRC. The colon and rectum house the highest proportion of gastrointestinal microbiome. Direct and indirect links showing the function of differentially abundant bacteria and ecological networks along the stages of colorectal cancer have been reported (Wong and Yu 2019). Similar studies focusing on enteric viruses revealed that the abundances of some enteric viruses are altered in CRC patients when compared to healthy subjects (Nakatsu et al. 2018). Virus families *Circoviridae* and *Anelloviridae* are commonly found in healthy human gut (Kernbauer et al. 2014). Bacteria infecting phages including Mulikevirus, Epsilon15likevirus, *Betabaculus* virus, *Inovirus,* and *Orthobunyavirus* were more abundant in CRC patients and determined to be associated with CRC morbidity and mortality in a shotgun metagenomic analysis of fecal samples (Nakatsu et al. 2018). Human eukaryotic viruses reportedly induce DNA alterations in the colon and a number of them were identified as either present or comparatively more abundant in CRC tissues (Massimino et al. 2021). Human cytomegalovirus (CMV) was observed to preferentially infect neoplastic colon tissues in a Taiwanese population and was associated with worse outcome (Chen et al. 2012). Also, infection with human polyomavirus 2 was identified in the colonic mucosa of CRC patients, suggesting a role in colon carcinogenesis (Laghi et al. 1999). The risk of developing CRC was found to be increased with hepatitis B virus (HBV) infection, suggesting a link between liver infection and CRC (Su et al. 2020). Studies have also shown the enrichment of human papillomavirus (HPV) in CRC tissues compared with colon tissues of healthy controls (Kirgan et al. 1990; Mahmoudvand et al. 2015) as well as worse prognosis for HPV-infected CRC patients (Li et al.

2015). Moreover, differential gene expression analysis revealed that CRC-associated genes including WNT-5A, c-Myc, matrix metalloproteinase 7 (MMP-7), and AXIN2 were upregulated in HPV-positive CRC tissues (Qiu et al. 2020). HPV coinfection with Epstein–Barr virus (EBV) was also found in CRC tissues and associated with invasiveness (Malki et al. 2020). In a dextran sulfate sodium-induced colitis mouse model, the severity of colitis was heightened in mice pretreated with antiviral drugs (Yang et al. 2016), giving more evidence to the association of viruses in CRC.

As found with enteric viruses, the association of gut fungi with CRC has been reported in several studies, which consistently identify that enteric fungi in CRC patients are compositionally different from those from healthy humans. Change to the ratio of the two most abundant fungi genera Ascomycota and Basidiomycota which is an index of dysbiosis was observed in CRC patients (Coker et al. 2019; Gao et al. 2017). Enrichment of pathogenic fungi including some species of *Aspergillus, Acremonium,* and *Malassezia*, and depletion of host beneficial fungi, including *Saccharomyces cerevisiae* were observed in CRC patients compared to healthy control subjects (Coker et al. 2019; Elaskandrany et al. 2021). Host factors also play a role in susceptibility to fungi infection and CRC. Infections with *Candida* species are prevalent in human with mutation in genes of the immune system. Mutations in Th17 and Th1 predispose the host to *Candida* overgrowth (Patel and Kuchroo 2015). Moreover, the SKY-CARD9 signaling pathway had been linked with the maintenance of enteric fungal balance. Abnormalities in the SKY-CARD9 signaling accentuated colitis and its associated development of CRC by increased abundance of *Candida tropicalis*, through interleukin 18 cytokines and inflammasomes (Malik et al. 2018). As with antivirals, aggravation of colitis and CRC were observed in mice treated with an antifungal drug. The aggravation was observed to be mediated through enhanced inflammasome activation (Malik et al. 2018).

The gut microbiome of CRC patients, colorectal adenoma patients, and healthy subjects were shown to present distinguishing archaeal profiles, suggesting an association with carcinogenesis. Enrichment of halophiles and depletion of methanogens characterized the archaeome of CRC and precancerous adenoma patients. Natrinema *sp. J7–2* sequentially increased along the stages of colorectal carcinogenesis (Coker et al. 2020). Moreover, observed associations of enteric archaeal and bacteria in healthy humans were lost in CRC patients (Coker et al. 2020). Archaea have also been shown to be associated with other human diseases to which links were established with the microbiome. These include obesity, inflammatory bowel diseases, and periodontitis (Lepp et al. 2004; Basseri et al. 2012). Diseases in the esophagus were reportedly linked to the archaeal component of the esophageal microbiome (Deshpande et al. 2018). It is most likely that their role in cancers exists but uncovered. Indeed, a large-scale study of archaeal metabolites showed that cancer-associated metabolites such as short chain fatty acids and polyamines are most common in the oral cavity and the gut which houses higher diversities of human archaeome. Euryarchaeota and Methanobacteria reportedly encode the genes expressing the cancer-associated metabolites (Cai et al. 2022).

6.3.2 Gastric Cancer

Malignant growth of cells in the stomach lining is gastric cancer (GC). It is the fourth leading cause of global cancer-related deaths (Sung et al. 2021). As with CRC, the DNA(s) of viruses have been detected in GC tissues. The association of EBV with GC is well documented. Moreover, characteristic clinicopathological features are associated with GC tissues that are EBV-positive (Sun et al. 2020; Bocian and Januszkiewicz-Lewandowska 2011). Chronic HBV infection is also reportedly linked with GC with an odd ratio (OR) of 1.56 in a meta-analysis, which was also true in *Helicobacter pylori-infected* GC patients. A positive association between GC and Hepatitis C virus (HCV) was reported in a meta-analysis with a pooled hazard ratio of 1.8 (Yang et al. 2021). Increased risk of GC development was found in with greater than 2.09, 1.53, 2.28 OR in CMV, HPV, and human polyomavirus infected GC patients, respectively (Wang et al. 2020). Using molecular methods, another study reported CMV with a higher copy number in cancer tissues than in adjacent non-cancerous tissues of GC patients. The presence of CMV in the GC tissues was further associated with tendencies for metastasis (Zhang et al. 2017a).

Dysbiotic fungal composition had also been described in GC. With ITS rDNA gene sequencing, a low abundance of fungi and distinct mycobiome signature was found in tissues of GC patients compared to healthy controls (Zhong et al. 2021; Yang et al. 2022). The abundances of fungi genera *Thermomyces* and *Saitozyma* were reduced in GC patients, while *Alternaria* and *Candida* were more abundant. At the species level, *C. albicans* was enriched in GC patients and was identified as a potential GC biomarker (Zhong et al. 2021). In another study, Basidiomycota to Ascomycota ratio was found to increase in GC with higher abundances of *Malassezia* and *Cutaneotrichosporon*, and lower abundances of *Rhodotorula, Lecanactis, Cystobasidium,* and *Rhizopus*. Pro-inflammatory and anti-inflammatory chemokines and cytokines were found to be correlated with the fungi signature of GC tissues. Anti-inflammatory cytokines YM-1 IL-6, IL-8, IL-4, and CCL17 correlated with GC-depleted fungi *Rhodotorula* and *Rhizopus* positively. On the other hand, pro-inflammatory TNF-α, CXCL10, CXCL9, and CXCL11 correlated positively with *Cutaneotrichosporon, Sarocladium, Apiotrichum,* and *Simplicillium* which were enriched in GC. These together suggest a potential for fungi in influencing gastric carcinogenesis (Yang et al. 2022).

6.3.3 Esophageal Cancer

Esophageal cancer (EC) is the cancer of the esophagus, a muscular tube that conveys food from the mouth to the gastric compartment. EC ranks seventh in global cancer with most incidences reported in men (Arnold et al. 2020). The presence of viral DNA that belongs to Gammapapillomavirus, Betaherpesvirus, and Gammaherpesvirus in the microbiome of the esophagus has been documented. The composition of the esophageal microbiome varies with factors such as age and genetics and has been linked with the development of adenocarcinoma. The risk of developing esophageal squamous cell carcinoma (ESCC) was heightened with the presence of HPV and EBV infections (Xu et al. 2015), with HPV DNA discovered from esophageal neoplasia (Syrjanen et al. 1982). In another study, a higher prevalence of HPV was indicated for EC and HPV16 infection was identified as a prognostic marker of ESCC. HPV was also suggested to act in combination with genetic susceptibility to heighten the risk of EC development (Yang et al. 2014). Interestingly, telomeres were found to be longer in EC tissues of HPV-infected patients compared to non-infected patients. Also, chemoradiation response was increased in EC patients infected with HPV (Zhang et al. 2017b), a yet-to-be-understood observation.

EC patients usually experience a high rate of fungi infections with inflammation, which may indicate a probable association with the esophageal carcinogenesis (Stoner and Gupta 2001). This may be due to the general knowledge that frequent and chronic fungi infections occur in immunocompromised individuals. Increased risk of EC was found with chronic *Candida* infections (Domingues-Ferreira et al. 2009). Infections with *C. albicans* were detected in ESCC patients (Rautemaa et al. 2007). Other fungi were also implicated in ESCC. For example, in a mouse model, the severity of ESCC was found to increase by *Cladosporium cladosporioides* infection. This severity was reversed with antifungal treatment (Zhu et al. 2017) underscoring the role of fungi in the development of esophageal cancer.

6.3.4 Pancreatic Cancer

Pancreatic cancer (PC) is the abnormal development of pancreatic cells. One outstanding feature of this cancer is the high mortality rate. This is because it is often diagnosed at stages III and IV as there is no established procedure for screening and early diagnosis (Meng et al. 2018). PC is the twelfth most common cancer and the seventh in terms of cancer-related deaths (Arnold et al. 2020). Association of HBV with carcinogenesis of the pancreas has been suggested (Iloeje et al. 2010). Also, HCV infection was linked to a higher risk of PC development (Huang et al. 2013). A metanalysis however did not find statistical significance in the association between PC risk and infections with HBV or HCV, although a positive association was almost always suggested (Abe et al. 2016; Maronek et al. 2020). It was observed that enteric fungi can migrate to the pancreas, alter the pancreatic microbiome, and contribute to carcinogenesis. This was demonstrated in a mouse model and humans by an increased pancreatic abundance of *Malassezia* in pancreatic ductal adenocarcinoma PDA (Aykut et al. 2019).

6.3.5 Liver Cancer

Liver cancer is the sixth most diagnosed cancer globally and the fourth leading cause of death, with higher incidences and mortality in men (Arnold et al. 2020). Associations between liver cancer and viral infections especially HBV and HCV are

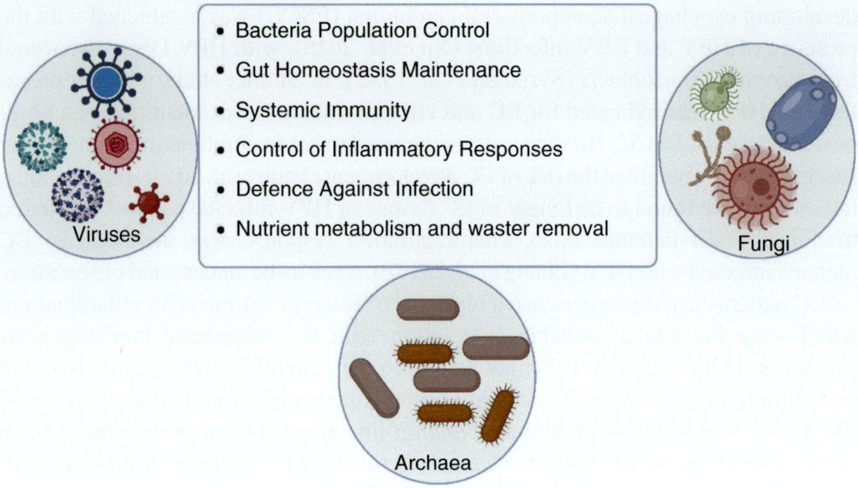

Fig. 6.1 Functions of viruses, fungi, and archaea in the gastrointestinal tract

well documented, with the latter mostly found in the western world and the former occurring more frequently in the developing world (Maucort-Boulch et al. 2018). In addition to HBV and HCV, other viruses have been linked with the incidences of liver cancer development. For example, EBV was detected in about 28% of liver cancer patients. In addition, EBV-positive tumor-infiltrating leukocytes were associated with a worse prognosis (Kang et al. 2019; Li et al. 2004). Downregulation of EBV gene, EBI3 was found to be linked to poor prognosis after surgery in liver cancer patients (Song et al. 2018). Moreover, synergistic relationships between viruses could reportedly promote liver cancer. HPV coinfection with HBV was also found to promote liver cancer development (Scinicariello et al. 1992). The functions of non-bacteria gastrointestinal microbes are summarized in Fig. 6.1.

6.4 Mechanisms of Non-bacteria Microbiome Involvement in Gastrointestinal Cancers

6.4.1 Alteration of the Microbiome

Bacteria, fungi, viruses, and archaea co-exist in a homeostatic state in healthy humans. This balanced state can be affected when there is a change in the abundance of potentially pathogenic microbes due to environmental or host factors, making the microbiome shift toward an oncogenic state. For example, bacteriophages can infect, overwhelm, and reduce the abundance of certain bacteria species thereby distorting the entire gut microbiome, resulting in a dysbiosis state in the gut. Indeed, a shift in enteric bacteriophages and their interactions with bacteria were observed in CRC patients compared with control subjects. This phenomenon was described to be associated with CRC severity and mortality (Nakatsu et al. 2018). Moreover, the gut microbiome of HBV-infected liver cancer patients clustered distinctly from those without HBV infection, which may represent a mechanism in liver carcinogenesis (Liu et al. 2019). Enteric fungi have been suggested to modulate the microbiome. Co-exclusive associations were observed between bacteria and fungi in CRC patients, contributed by *Proteobacteria* and *Ascomycota* (Coker et al. 2019), suggesting that fungi may play a role in gastrointestinal cancer by microbiome dysbiosis. A similar potential mechanism reported for viruses and fungi was also documented for archaea in gastrointestinal cancer. A homeostatic co-occurrence relationship between enteric bacteria and archaea which was identified in healthy subjects was absent in CRC patients, suggesting that modulation of the microbiome is a means through which archaea may impact carcinogenesis (Coker et al. 2020), suggesting a trans-kingdom modulation as means of by which archaea impact carcinogenesis in the gastrointestinal tract. Indeed, fecal samples from CRC patients which harbored altered bacteria, viruses, fungi, and archaea (Coker et al. 2018, 2019, 2020; Nakatsu et al. 2018) promoted colon carcinogenesis in both conventional and germ-free mice (Wong et al. 2017). The altered non-bacterial microbes in the fecal samples likely contributed to the carcinogenesis observed in the recipient mice.

6.4.2 Production of Carcinogenic Products

The production of carcinogens by enteric bacteria to induce gastrointestinal cancer has been studied. Enterotoxigenic *Bacteroide fragilis and colibactin-producing E. coli produce Bacteroides fragilis* toxin (BFT) and colibactin, respectively, leading to inflammation, tissue injury, and DNA damage in CRC (Brennan and Garrett 2016). Similarly, non-bacteria microbes can produce carcinogens that contribute to carcinogenesis in the gut. Although *C. albicans* is a normal commensal, its abundance is increasingly identified to be expanded in gastrointestinal cancers as described above. During its metabolism, *C. albicans* can produce carcinogenic nitrosamines which can activate oncogenes in cancer development (Ramirez-Garcia et al. 2016). Nitrosamine intake had been characterized to increase the risk of GC development (La Vecchia et al. 1995). Nitrosamine production may contribute to carcinogenesis in *C. albicans* enriched GC. Moreover, *C. albicans* expresses alcohol dehydrogenase involved in metabolizing ethanol into acetaldehyde which in turn produces DNA adducts, distorts cytosine methylation, and alters DNA replication, leading to mutations and chromosomal abnormalities (Ramirez-Garcia et al. 2016; Seitz and Stickel 2007). Acetaldehyde also increases reactive oxygen species and induces mitochondria damage in cancer (Ramirez-Garcia et al. 2016; Manzo-Avalos and Saavedra-Molina 2010). Species of *Malassezia* were found enriched in CRC, PDA, and inflammatory bowel disease. It was demonstrated that *Malassezia* can produce extracellular nanovesicles containing proteins that could stimulate the production of IL-6 and activate the nuclear factor- kappa B (NF-KB) pathway in the immune microenvironment of keratinocytes (Zhang et al. 2019). IL-6 and NF-KB signaling pathways are important in carcinogenesis (Hibi et al. 1990; Xia et al. 2018). The production of toxins as a means of promoting diseases can also be attributed to viruses. Some bacteriophages encode toxins and polypeptides which get expressed after infecting bacteria. Some of these polypeptides have been described in human diseases such as botulism, diarrhea, and gastroenteritis. Pseudomonas aeruginosa is the bacteria host for Phage ΦCTX. Phage ΦCTX encodes a cytotoxin (Ctx) which play a role in cytotoxicity of leucocytes (Boyd 2012). Phage Φ 13 infects *Staphylococcus aureus* and expresses enterotoxin (Etx) (Boyd 2012) implicated in the development of gastroenteritis. Further investigation is warranted to delineate the contribution of virus-encoded toxins in the development of gastrointestinal cancers. Although the association between the archaeome and gastrointestinal cancer has been suggested, little is known about the mechanism through which such might occur. Archaeal metabolites which may explain the linkage had been explored. Acetate, lactic acid, trimethylamine, hydrogen sulfide, inorganic acid, and acetaldehyde are some of the metabolites produced by archaea and associated with DNA damage, inflammation, production of reactive oxygen species, genotoxicity, and impairment of intestinal barrier (Cai et al. 2022). Investigation of the direct or indirect role of these metabolites in the initiation and progression of gastrointestinal cancer will increase our understanding of their mode of involvement in promoting aberrant growth in the gastrointestinal tract.

6.4.3 Infection of Epithelial Cells

Human oncogenic viruses such as EBV, HBV, HPV, and HCV can infect cells of the epithelial lining, where they promote tumorigenesis by inserting their genomes into host cells. The insertion into the host genome disrupts normal DNA replication and repair through distortion of critical signaling pathways. Tumor suppressor pathway (TSP) is one of the targets of infecting viruses because tumor suppressor pathways are a critical defence against cancerous transformation of cells. With the disruption of TSP, processes such as apoptosis, DNA damage repair, senescence, and cell cycle arrest are distorted paving way for cancer development (Sherr and McCormick 2002). Oncoproteins from infecting viruses can repress the functions of important tumor suppressive genes like p53 and pRB, which in turn favor virus propagation (Sherr and McCormick 2002; McLaughlin-Drubin and Munger 2008). Gastrointestinal cancer-associated EBV and HPV were found able to drive the cell cycle into the S phase by inactivating p53 and pRB. These were reported in HBV-infected liver cancer patients in which a complex was formed between p53 and HBV-X protein resulting in p53 not being able to perform its function in transcription control (Ringelhan et al. 2015).

Infecting oncoviruses can also target host signaling pathways controlling the proliferation of cells. HPV and EBV could activate the PI3K–AKT–mTOR pathway which plays an important role in cell proliferation and progression of the cell cycle. LMP2A, an EBV-encoded protein induced the PI3K-AKT pathway resulting in an epithelial cell differentiation (Scholle et al. 2000). HPV oncoproteins E5, E6, and E7 also targeted the PI3K–AKT–mTOR pathway promoting uncontrolled cell division and tumor progression (Zhang et al. 2015). Other signaling pathways such as NF-κB WNT/B-catenin, Notch, and MAPK signaling have been reportedly distorted by gastrointestinal cancer-associated oncogenic viruses including EBV, and HBV. EBV oncoprotein LMP1 promoted cell proliferation by activating NF-κB and downstream tumor necrosis factor receptor (TNFR), interleukin-1 receptor-associated kinase 1 (IRAK1), and TNF receptor-associated factor 6 (TRAF6) (Wang et al. 2017). Persistent infection is another way through which viruses can manipulate the host immune system in promoting cancer. Viruses can evade detection by the host, avoid inflammatory responses, and protect their host cells from being killed, a mechanism that promotes the cancerous transformation of cells (Hopcraft and Damania 2017).

6.5 Conclusion and Future Perspective

Advancements in sequencing, bioinformatics, and molecular technologies have advanced knowledge about the associations of non-bacterial members of the gut microbiome in gastrointestinal cancers. The potentials of viruses, fungi, and archaea in colon, liver, gastric, esophageal, and pancreatic cancers are increasingly being uncovered. As with gut bacteria, more research is needed to decipher their direct role and exact mechanisms through which they exert their impact in promoting carcinogenesis in the gut. This will enable their inclusion and consideration in microbiome-targeted gastrointestinal cancer prevention strategies.

References

Abe SK, Inoue M, Sawada N, Iwasaki M, Shimazu T, Yamaji T, Sasazuki S, Saito E, Tanaka Y, Mizokami M, et al. Hepatitis B and C virus infection and risk of pancreatic cancer: a population-based cohort study (JPHC study cohort II). Cancer Epidemiol Biomarkers Prev. 2016;25(3):555–7.

Aleman FDD, Valenzano DR. Microbiome evolution during host aging. PLoS Pathog. 2019;15(7):e1007727.

Arnold M, Abnet CC, Neale RE, Vignat J, Giovannucci EL, McGlynn KA, Bray F. Global burden of 5 Major types of gastrointestinal cancer. Gastroenterology. 2020;159(1):335–349.e15.

Aykut B, Pushalkar S, Chen RN, Li QH, Abengozar R, Kim JI, Shadaloey SA, Wu DL, Preiss P, Verma N, et al. The fungal mycobiome promotes pancreatic oncogenesis via activation of MBL. Nature. 2019;574(7777):264–7.

Bang C, Schmitz RA. Archaea associated with human surfaces: not to be underestimated. FEMS Microbiol Rev. 2015;39(5):631–48.

Barr JJ, Auro R, Sam-Soon N, Kassegne S, Peters G, Bonilla N, Hatay M, Mourtada S, Bailey B, Youle M, et al. Subdiffusive motion of bacteriophage in mucosal surfaces increases the frequency of bacterial encounters. Proc Natl Acad Sci U S A. 2015;112(44):13675–80.

Barton ES, White DW, Cathelyn JS, Brett-McClellan KA, Engle M, Diamond MS, Miller VL, Virgin HW 4th. Herpesvirus latency confers symbiotic protection from bacterial infection. Nature. 2007;447(7142):326–9.

Basseri RJ, Basseri B, Pimentel M, Chong K, Youdim A, Low K, Hwang L, Soffer E, Chang C, Mathur R. Intestinal methane production in obese individuals is associated with a higher body mass index. Gastroenterol Hepatol (N Y). 2012;8(1):22–8.

Beller L, Matthijnssens J. What is (not) known about the dynamics of the human gut virome in health and disease. Curr Opin Virol. 2019;37:52–7.

Blais Lecours P, Marsolais D, Cormier Y, Berberi M, Hache C, Bourdages R, Duchaine C. Increased prevalence of Methanosphaera stadtmanae in inflammatory bowel diseases. PLoS One. 2014;9(2):e87734.

Bocian J, Januszkiewicz-Lewandowska D. [Epstein-Barr virus infection—life cycle, methods of diagnosis, associated diseases]. Postepy Hig Med Dosw (Online). 2011;65:286–98.

Boyd EF. Bacteriophage-encoded bacterial virulence factors and phage-pathogenicity island interactions. Adv Virus Res. 2012;82:91–118.

Brennan CA, Garrett WS. Gut microbiota, inflammation, and colorectal cancer. Annu Rev Microbiol. 2016;70:395–411.

Brugere JF, Borrel G, Gaci N, Tottey W, O'Toole PW, Malpuech-Brugere C. Archaebiotics: proposed therapeutic use of archaea to prevent trimethylaminuria and cardiovascular disease. Gut Microbes. 2014;5(1):5–10.

Cai M, Kandalai S, Tang X, Zheng Q. Contributions of human-associated archaeal metabolites to tumor microenvironment and carcinogenesis. Microbiol Spectr. 2022;10(2):e0236721.

Chen HP, Jiang JK, Chen CY, Chou TY, Chen YC, Chang YT, Lin SF, Chan CH, Yang CY, Lin CH, et al. Human cytomegalovirus preferentially infects the neoplastic epithelium of colorectal cancer: a quantitative and histological analysis. J Clin Virol. 2012;54(3):240–4.

Coker OO. Non-bacteria microbiome (virus, fungi, and archaea) in gastrointestinal cancer. J Gastroenterol Hepatol. 2022;37(2):256–62.

Coker OO, Dai Z, Nie Y, Zhao G, Cao L, Nakatsu G, Wu WK, Wong SH, Chen Z, Sung JJY, et al. Mucosal microbiome dysbiosis in gastric carcinogenesis. Gut. 2018;67(6):1024–32.

Coker OO, Nakatsu G, Dai RZ, Wu WKK, Wong SH, Ng SC, Chan FKL, Sung JJY, Yu J. Enteric fungal microbiota dysbiosis and ecological alterations in colorectal cancer. Gut. 2019;68(4):654–62.

Coker OO, Wu WKK, Wong SH, Sung JJY, Yu J. Altered gut archaea composition and interaction with bacteria are associated with colorectal cancer. Gastroenterology. 2020;159(4):1459–1470.e1455.

Deshpande NP, Riordan SM, Castano-Rodriguez N, Wilkins MR, Kaakoush NO. Signatures within the esophageal microbiome are associated with host genetics, age, and disease. Microbiome. 2018;6(1):227.

Domingues-Ferreira M, Grumach AS, Duarte AJD, De Moraes-Vasconcelos D. Esophageal cancer associated with chronic mucocutaneous candidiasis. Could chronic candidiasis lead to esophageal cancer? Med Mycol. 2009;47(2):201–5.

Elaskandrany M, Patel R, Patel M, Miller G, Saxena D, Saxena A. Fungi, host immune response, and tumorigenesis. Am J Physiol Gastrointest Liver Physiol. 2021;321(2):G213–22.

Febvre HP, Rao S, Gindin M, Goodwin NDM, Finer E, Vivanco JS, Lu S, Manter DK, Wallace TC, Weir TL, PHAGE Study. Effects of supplemental bacteriophage intake on inflammation and gut microbiota in healthy adults. Nutrients. 2019;11(3):666.

Fiers WD, Gao IH, Iliev ID. Gut mycobiota under scrutiny: fungal symbionts or environmental transients? Curr Opin Microbiol. 2019;50:79–86.

Gaitanis G, Magiatis P, Stathopoulou K, Bassukas ID, Alexopoulos EC, Velegraki A, Skaltsounis AL. AhR ligands, malassezin, and indolo[3,2-b]carbazole are selectively produced by Malassezia furfur strains isolated from seborrheic dermatitis. J Invest Dermatol. 2008;128(7):1620–5.

Gao R, Kong C, Li H, Huang L, Qu X, Qin N, Qin H. Dysbiosis signature of mycobiota in colon polyp and colorectal cancer. Eur J Clin Microbiol. 2017;36(12):2457–68.

Gribaldo S, Brochier-Armanet C. The origin and evolution of Archaea: a state of the art. Philos Trans R Soc Lond Ser B Biol Sci. 2006;361(1470):1007–22.

Hallen-Adams HE, Suhr MJ. Fungi in the healthy human gastrointestinal tract. Virulence. 2017;8(3):352–8.

Hibi M, Murakami M, Saito M, Hirano T, Taga T, Kishimoto T. Molecular cloning and expression of an IL-6 signal transducer, gp130. Cell. 1990;63(6):1149–57.

Hopcraft SE, Damania B. Tumour viruses and innate immunity. Philos Trans R Soc Lond Ser B Biol Sci. 2017;372(1732):20160267.

Huang J, Magnusson M, Torner A, Ye W, Duberg AS. Risk of pancreatic cancer among individuals with hepatitis C or hepatitis B virus infection: a nationwide study in Sweden. Br J Cancer. 2013;109(11):2917–23.

Iloeje UH, Yang HI, Jen CL, Su J, Wang LY, You SL, Lu SN, Chen CJ. Risk of pancreatic cancer in chronic hepatitis B virus infection: data from the REVEAL-HBV cohort study. Liver Int. 2010;30(3):423–9.

Jiang TT, Shao TY, Ang WXG, Kinder JM, Turner LH, Pham G, Whitt J, Alenghat T, Way SS. Commensal fungi recapitulate the protective benefits of intestinal bacteria. Cell Host Microbe. 2017;22(6):809–816.e804.

Kandler O, Konig H. Cell wall polymers in Archaea (Archaebacteria). Cell Mol Life Sci. 1998;54(4):305–8.

Kang HJ, Oh JH, Chun SM, Kim D, Ryu YM, Hwang HS, Kim SY, An J, Cho EJ, Lee H, et al. Immunogenomic landscape of hepatocellular carcinoma with immune cell stroma and EBV-positive tumor-infiltrating lymphocytes. J Hepatol. 2019;71(1):91–103.

Kernbauer E, Ding Y, Cadwell K. An enteric virus can replace the beneficial function of commensal bacteria. Nature. 2014;516(7529):94–8.

Kim JY, Whon TW, Lim MY, Kim YB, Kim N, Kwon MS, Kim J, Lee SH, Choi HJ, Nam IH, et al. The human gut archaeome: identification of diverse haloarchaea in Korean subjects. Microbiome. 2020;8(1):114.

Kirgan D, Manalo P, Hall M, McGregor B. Association of human papillomavirus and colon neoplasms. Arch Surg. 1990;125(7):862–5.

La Vecchia C, D'Avanzo B, Airoldi L, Braga C, Decarli A. Nitrosamine intake and gastric cancer risk. Eur J Cancer Prev. 1995;4(6):469–74.

Laghi L, Randolph AE, Chauhan DP, Marra G, Major EO, Neel JV, Boland CR. JC virus DNA is present in the mucosa of the human colon and in colorectal cancers. Proc Natl Acad Sci U S A. 1999;96(13):7484–9.

Lepp PW, Brinig MM, Ouverney CC, Palm K, Armitage GC, Relman DA. Methanogenic archaea and human periodontal disease. Proc Natl Acad Sci U S A. 2004;101(16):6176–81.

Li W, Wu BA, Zeng YM, Chen GC, Li XX, Chen JT, Guo YW, Li MH, Zeng Y. Epstein-Barr virus in hepatocellular carcinogenesis. World J Gastroenterol. 2004;10(23):3409–13.

Li YX, Zhang L, Simayi D, Zhang N, Tao L, Yang L, Zhao J, Chen YZ, Li F, Zhang WJ. Human papillomavirus infection correlates with inflammatory Stat3 signaling activity and IL-17 level in patients with colorectal cancer. PLoS One. 2015;10(2):e0118391.

Liu Q, Li F, Zhuang Y, Xu J, Wang J, Mao X, Zhang Y, Liu X. Alteration in gut microbiota associated with hepatitis B and non-hepatitis virus related hepatocellular carcinoma. Gut Pathog. 2019;11:1.

Lurie-Weinberger MN, Gophna U. Archaea in and on the human body: health implications and future directions. PLoS Pathog. 2015;11(6):e1004833.

Mahmoudvand S, Safaei A, Erfani N, Sarvari J. Presence of human papillomavirus DNA in colorectal cancer tissues in Shiraz, Southwest Iran. Asian Pac J Cancer Prev. 2015;16(17):7883–7.

Malik A, Sharma D, Malireddi RKS, Guy CS, Chang TC, Olsen SR, Neale G, Vogel P, Kanneganti TD. SYK-CARD9 signaling axis promotes gut fungi-mediated inflammasome activation to restrict colitis and colon cancer. Immunity. 2018;49(3):515–530.e515.

Malki MI, Gupta I, Fernandes Q, Aboulkassim T, Yasmeen A, Vranic S, Al Moustafa AE, Al-Thawadi HA. Co-presence of Epstein-Barr virus and high-risk human papillomaviruses in Syrian colorectal cancer samples. Hum Vaccin Immunother. 2020;16(10):2403–7.

Manzo-Avalos S, Saavedra-Molina A. Cellular and mitochondrial effects of alcohol consumption. Int J Environ Res Public Health. 2010;7(12):4281–304.

Maronek M, Link R, Monteleone G, Gardlik R, Stolfi C. Viruses in cancers of the digestive system: active contributors or idle bystanders? Int J Mol Sci. 2020;21(21):8133.

Massimino L, Lovisa S, Antonio Lamparelli L, Danese S, Ungaro F. Gut eukaryotic virome in colorectal carcinogenesis: is that a trigger? Comput Struct Biotechnol J. 2021;19:16–28.

Maucort-Boulch D, de Martel C, Franceschi S, Plummer M. Fraction and incidence of liver cancer attributable to hepatitis B and C viruses worldwide. Int J Cancer. 2018;142(12):2471–7.

McLaughlin-Drubin ME, Munger K. Viruses associated with human cancer. Biochim Biophys Acta. 2008;1782(3):127–50.

Meng C, Bai C, Brown TD, Hood LE, Tian Q. Human gut microbiota and gastrointestinal cancer. Genomics Proteomics Bioinformatics. 2018;16(1):33–49.

Mexia N, Gaitanis G, Velegraki A, Soshilov A, Denison MS, Magiatis P. Pityriazepin and other potent AhR ligands isolated from Malassezia furfur yeast. Arch Biochem Biophys. 2015;571:16–20.

Nakamura N, Lin HC, McSweeney CS, Mackie RI, Gaskins HR. Mechanisms of microbial hydrogen disposal in the human colon and implications for health and disease. Annu Rev Food Sci Technol. 2010;1:363–95.

Nakatsu G, Zhou H, Wu WKK, Wong SH, Coker OO, Dai Z, Li X, Szeto CH, Sugimura N, Lam TY, et al. Alterations in enteric virome are associated with colorectal cancer and survival outcomes. Gastroenterology. 2018;155(2):529–541.e525.

Patel DD, Kuchroo VK. Th17 cell pathway in human immunity: lessons from genetics and therapeutic interventions. Immunity. 2015;43(6):1040–51.

Perez JC. Fungi of the human gut microbiota: roles and significance. Int J Med Microbiol. 2021;311(3):151490.

Qiu Q, Li Y, Fan Z, Yao F, Shen W, Sun J, Yuan Y, Chen J, Cai L, Xie Y, et al. Gene expression analysis of human papillomavirus-associated colorectal carcinoma. Biomed Res Int. 2020;2020:5201587.

Ramezani A, Nolin TD, Barrows IR, Serrano MG, Buck GA, Regunathan-Shenk R, West RE 3rd, Latham PS, Amdur R, Raj DS. Gut colonization with methanogenic archaea lowers plasma trimethylamine N-oxide concentrations in apolipoprotein e−/− mice. Sci Rep. 2018;8(1):14752.

Ramirez-Garcia A, Rementeria A, Aguirre-Urizar JM, Moragues MD, Antoran A, Pellon A, Abad-Diaz-de-Cerio A, Hernando FL. Candida albicans and cancer: can this yeast induce cancer development or progression? Crit Rev Microbiol. 2016;42(2):181–93.

Rautemaa R, Hietanen J, Niissalo S, Pirinen S, Perheentupa J. Oral and oesophageal squamous cell carcinoma—a complication or component of autoimmune polyendocrinopathy-candidiasis-ectodermal dystrophy (APECED, APS-I). Oral Oncol. 2007;43(6):607–13.

Ringelhan M, O'Connor T, Protzer U, Heikenwalder M. The direct and indirect roles of HBV in liver cancer: prospective markers for HCC screening and potential therapeutic targets. J Pathol. 2015;235(2):355–67.

Roccarina D, Lauritano EC, Gabrielli M, Franceschi F, Ojetti V, Gasbarrini A. The role of methane in intestinal diseases. Am J Gastroenterol. 2010;105(6):1250–6.

Samonis G, Gikas A, Anaissie EJ, Vrenzos G, Maraki S, Tselentis Y, Bodey GP. Prospective evaluation of effects of broad-spectrum antibiotics on gastrointestinal yeast colonization of humans. Antimicrob Agents Chemother. 1993;37(1):51–3.

Santiago-Rodriguez TM, Hollister EB. Human virome and disease: high-throughput sequencing for virus discovery, identification of phage-bacteria dysbiosis and development of therapeutic approaches with emphasis on the human gut. Viruses. 2019;11(7):656.

Scholle F, Bendt KM, Raab-Traub N. Epstein-Barr virus LMP2A transforms epithelial cells, inhibits cell differentiation, and activates Akt. J Virol. 2000;74(22):10681–9.

Scinicariello F, Sato T, Lee CS, Hsu HC, Chan TS, Tyring SK. Detection of human papillomavirus in primary hepatocellular-carcinoma. Anticancer Res. 1992;12(3):763–6.

Seitz HK, Stickel F. Molecular mechanisms of alcohol-mediated carcinogenesis. Nat Rev Cancer. 2007;7(8):599–612.

Sherr CJ, McCormick F. The RB and p53 pathways in cancer. Cancer Cell. 2002;2(2):103–12.

Shkoporov AN, Clooney AG, Sutton TDS, Ryan FJ, Daly KM, Nolan JA, McDonnell SA, Khokhlova EV, Draper LA, Forde A, et al. The human gut virome is highly diverse, stable, and individual specific. Cell Host Microbe. 2019;26(4):527–541.e525.

Song QJ, Chen X, Hu WD, Mei GL, Yang XB, Wu H. Downregulation of Epstein-Barr virus-induced gene 3 is associated with poor prognosis of hepatocellular carcinoma after curative resection. Oncol Lett. 2018;15(5):7751–9.

Stoner GD, Gupta A. Etiology and chemoprevention of esophageal squamous cell carcinoma. Carcinogenesis. 2001;22(11):1737–46.

Su FH, Le TN, Muo CH, Te SA, Sung FC, Yeh CC. Chronic hepatitis B virus infection associated with increased colorectal cancer risk in Taiwanese population. Viruses. 2020;12(1):97.

Sun K, Jia K, Lv H, Wang SQ, Wu Y, Lei H, Chen X. EBV-positive gastric cancer: current knowledge and future perspectives. Front Oncol. 2020;10:583463.

Sung H, Ferlay J, Siegel RL, Laversanne M, Soerjomataram I, Jemal A, Bray F. Global cancer statistics 2020: GLOBOCAN estimates of incidence and mortality worldwide for 36 cancers in 185 countries. CA Cancer J Clin. 2021;71(3):209–49.

Syrjanen K, Pyrhonen S, Aukee S, Koskela E. Squamous cell papilloma of the esophagus: a tumour probably caused by human papilloma virus (HPV). Diagn Histopathol. 1982;5(4):291–6.

Wang LW, Jiang S, Gewurz BE. Epstein-Barr virus LMP1-mediated oncogenicity. J Virol. 2017;91(21):e01718–6.

Wang H, Chen XL, Liu K, Bai D, Zhang WH, Chen XZ, Hu JK, SIGES Research Group. Associations between gastric cancer risk and virus infection other than Epstein-Barr virus: a systematic review and meta-analysis based on epidemiological studies. Clin Transl Gastroenterol. 2020;11(7):e00201.

Weng MT, Chiu YT, Wei PY, Chiang CW, Fang HL, Wei SC. Microbiota and gastrointestinal cancer. J Formos Med Assoc. 2019;118(Suppl 1):S32–41.

Wong SH, Yu J. Gut microbiota in colorectal cancer: mechanisms of action and clinical applications. Nat Rev Gastroenterol Hepatol. 2019;16(11):690–704.

Wong SH, Zhao L, Zhang X, Nakatsu G, Han J, Xu W, Xiao X, Kwong TNY, Tsoi H, Wu WKK, et al. Gavage of fecal samples from patients with colorectal cancer promotes intestinal carcinogenesis in germ-free and conventional mice. Gastroenterology. 2017;153(6):1621–1633.e1626.

Xavier JB, Young VB, Skufca J, Ginty F, Testerman T, Pearson AT, Macklin P, Mitchell A, Shmulevich I, Xie L, et al. The cancer microbiome: distinguishing direct and indirect effects requires a systemic view. Trends Cancer. 2020;6(3):192–204.

Xi Y, Xu P. Global colorectal cancer burden in 2020 and projections to 2040. Transl Oncol. 2021;14(10):101174.

Xia L, Tan S, Zhou Y, Lin J, Wang H, Oyang L, Tian Y, Liu L, Su M, Wang H, et al. Role of the NFkappaB-signaling pathway in cancer. Onco Targets Ther. 2018;11:2063–73.

Xu W, Liu Z, Bao Q, Qian Z. Viruses, other pathogenic microorganisms and esophageal cancer. Gastrointest Tumors. 2015;2(1):2–13.

Yang J, Wu H, Wei S, Xiong H, Fu X, Qi Z, Jiang Q, Li W, Hu G, Yuan X, et al. HPV seropositivity joints with susceptibility loci identified in GWASs at apoptosis associated genes to increase the risk of Esophageal Squamous Cell Carcinoma (ESCC). BMC Cancer. 2014;14:501.

Yang JY, Kim MS, Kim E, Cheon JH, Lee YS, Kim Y, Lee SH, Seo SU, Shin SH, Choi SS, et al. Enteric viruses ameliorate gut inflammation via Toll-like receptor 3 and Toll-like receptor 7-mediated interferon-beta production. Immunity. 2016;44(4):889–900.

Yang Y, Jiang Z, Wu W, Ruan L, Yu C, Xi Y, Wang L, Wang K, Mo J, Zhao S. Chronic hepatitis virus infection are associated with high risk of gastric cancer: a systematic review and cumulative analysis. Front Oncol. 2021;11:703558.

Yang P, Zhang X, Xu R, Adeel K, Lu X, Chen M, Shen H, Li Z, Xu Z. Fungal microbiota dysbiosis and ecological alterations in gastric cancer. Front Microbiol. 2022;13:889694.

Zhang L, Wu J, Ling MT, Zhao L, Zhao KN. The role of the PI3K/Akt/mTOR signalling pathway in human cancers induced by infection with human papillomaviruses. Mol Cancer. 2015;14:87.

Zhang Z, Li J, Zheng W, Zhao G, Zhang H, Wang X, Guo Y, Qin C, Shi Y. Peripheral lymphoid volume expansion and maintenance are controlled by gut microbiota via RALDH+ dendritic cells. Immunity. 2016;44(2):330–42.

Zhang L, Guo G, Xu J, Sun X, Chen W, Jin J, Hu C, Zhang P, Shen X, Xue X. Human cytomegalovirus detection in gastric cancer and its possible association with lymphatic metastasis. Diagn Microbiol Infect Dis. 2017a;88(1):62–8.

Zhang D, Zhang W, Liu W, Mao Y, Fu Z, Liu J, Huang W, Zhang Z, An D, Li B. Human papillomavirus infection increases the chemoradiation response of esophageal squamous cell carcinoma based on P53 mutation. Radiother Oncol. 2017b;124(1):155–60.

Zhang YJ, Han Y, Sun YZ, Jiang HH, Liu M, Qi RQ, Gao XH. Extracellular vesicles derived from Malassezia furfur stimulate IL-6 production in keratinocytes as demonstrated in in vitro and in vivo models. J Dermatol Sci. 2019;93(3):168–75.

Zhong M, Xiong Y, Zhao J, Gao Z, Ma J, Wu Z, Song Y, Hong X. Candida albicans disorder is associated with gastric carcinogenesis. Theranostics. 2021;11(10):4945–56.

Zhu F, Willette-Brown J, Song NY, Lomada D, Song Y, Xue L, Gray Z, Zhao Z, Davis SR, Sun Z, et al. Autoreactive T cells and chronic fungal infection drive esophageal carcinogenesis. Cell Host Microbe. 2017;21(4):478–493.e477.

Chapter 7
The Role of Microbiome in Nonalcoholic Fatty Liver Disease

Hye Won Lee

Abstract Nonalcoholic fatty liver disease (NAFLD) includes simple steatosis, steatohepatitis, fibrosis, and cirrhosis. NAFLD can progress to more severe forms, including nonalcoholic steatohepatitis, liver fibrosis, and hepatocellular carcinoma. The gut–liver axis refers to the bidirectional relationship between the gut and liver. The gut microbiota is essential for host immunological, hormonal, and metabolic homeostasis. Dysbiosis increases intestinal permeability and delivers endotoxins to the portal vein to activate a wide range of inflammatory signaling pathways. This process results in the development of NAFLD. Various animal and human studies have provided evidence of a close relationship between NAFLD and the gut microbiota. In this chapter, we will look into the role of microbiome in NAFLD. It is expected that the use of intestinal antibiotics, adsorbents, and fecal transplantation will become possible therapeutics in the near future.

Keywords Gut microbiota · Liver · Nonalcoholic fatty liver disease

7.1 Introduction

Nonalcoholic fatty liver disease (NAFLD), including simple steatosis, steatohepatitis, fibrosis, and cirrhosis, is known to occur in association with metabolic risk factors. The human gut microbiota weighs approximately 1–2 kg and is an ecological community of microorganisms. About two-thirds of the blood supply to the liver comes from the intestine. This anatomical structure forms a connection axis between the intestine and the liver (gut–liver axis); thus, theoretically, the intestinal microbiome is closely related to the development of liver diseases. As for the mechanism of development, substances related to the occurrence of liver disease such as peptidoglycan and

H. W. Lee (✉)
Department of Internal Medicine, Insitute of Gastroenterology, Yonsei University College of Medicine, Seoul, South Korea
e-mail: lorry-lee@yuhs.ac

J. Yu (ed.), *Microbiome in Gastrointestinal Cancer*,
https://doi.org/10.1007/978-981-19-4492-5_7

endotoxin, are produced by intestinal bacteria and absorbed into the liver, causing damage to Kupffer cells or hepatocytes in the development of liver diseases.

The gut microbiota is essential for host immunological, hormonal, and metabolic homeostasis, however, the full understanding of the gut microbiota, including geographic, gender, and age-dependent changes, has yet to be established. Intestinal microbes play a key role in the pathogenesis of liver disease; thus, the close relationship between the gut and the intestines is an important factor in liver damage, as the liver receives most of the blood and nutrients from the intestine through the portal vein, as well as bacteria, damage-related metabolites and bacterial-derived substances. In addition, some gut microbes produce ammonia, ethanol and acetaldehyde, which are mainly metabolized in the liver and are associated with Kupffer cell and inflammatory cytokine activation. Inflammation and proliferation of intestinal bacteria, are defined as changes in the intestinal microflora (dysbiosis) whichincreases intestinal permeability and delivers endotoxins to the portal vein to activate a wide range of inflammatory signaling pathways, this, in turn, leads to the development of various liver problems, including NAFLD (Fig. 7.1).

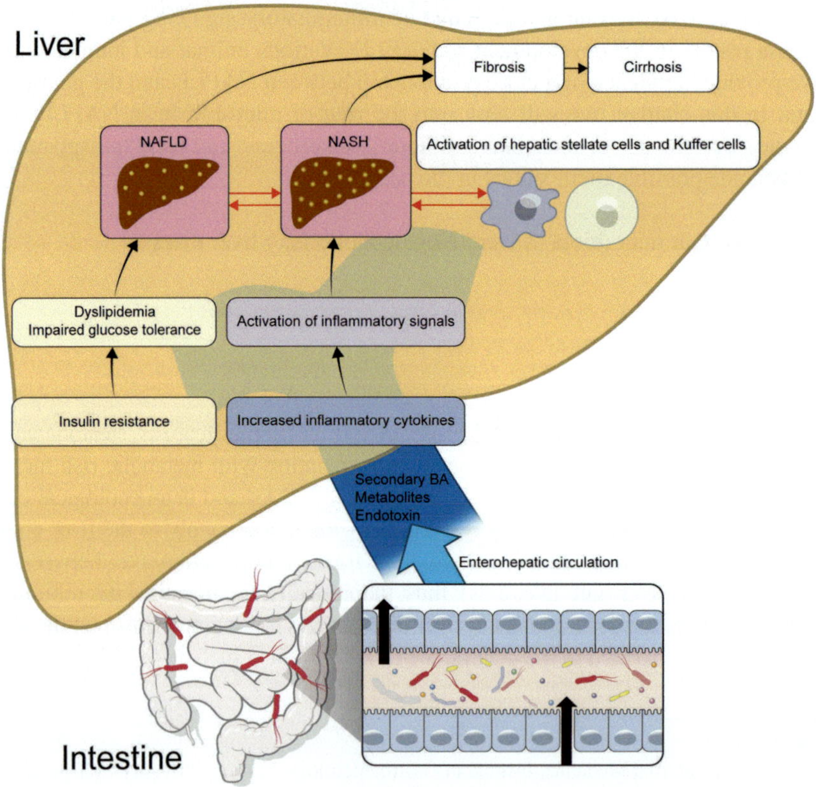

Fig. 7.1 Correlation between nonalcoholic fatty liver disease and the gut microbiome. This figure was modified based on the book titled "Digestive Diseases and Gut Microbiome" (Korean Society of Gastrointestinal Endoscopy, 2003). Abbreviations: *NAFLD,* nonalcoholic fatty liver disease; *NASH,* nonalcoholic steatohepatitis

7.2 Natural Course of NAFLD

NAFLD has been reported an increasing prevalence worldwide with an approximation of 25% globally to date, together with an increase incedence of obesity and type 2 diabetes (T2DM) (Henry et al. 2022), with the highest occurrence of 31.8% reported from the Middle East and South America and the lowest of 13.5% from Africa (Younossi et al. 2016). NAFLD can progress to more severe forms, including nonalcoholic steatohepatitis (NASH), liver fibrosis, and hepatocellular carcinoma (HCC). NAFLD is histologically defined when hepatic steatosis occurs in ≥5% of hepatocytes in the absence of other causes of liver disease and excess alcohol consumption. NASH consists of hepatic steatosis with inflammation and ballooning of hepatocytes. The incidence of NASH varies from 8.5 to 64.0% over a 3.0–6.6 year-follow-up period (Wong et al. 2010; Pais et al. 2013; McPherson et al. 2015). Liver fibrosis can progress faster in NASH than NAFLD. Specifically, the NAFLD progression is approximately 14.3 years to the next stage, whereas 7.1 years has been observed for NASH (Singh et al. 2015). Although the factors leading to the progression are not entirely clear, the presence of insulin resistance, T2DM, and visceral obesity are known risks for NASH progression. In addition, the incidence of liver cirrhosis and HCC associated with NAFLD is increasing. NAFLD can develop into HCC and is the third most common cause of HCC development in the United States (Mohamad et al. 2016; Younossi et al. 2015). NAFLD is related to a higher incidence of HCC compared to other etiologies, in the absence of advanced fibrosis or cirrhosis (Paradis et al. 2009; Yasui et al. 2011). The Veterans Administration cohort showed that ~13% of patients with HCC do not have cirrhosis; notably, NAFLD and its associated metabolic syndromes are risk factors for HCC in the absence of cirrhosis (Mittal et al. 2016).

7.3 Gut–Liver Axis

The gut–liver axis refers to the bidirectional relationship between the gut and the liver (Albillos et al. 2020; Safari and Gérard 2019), in which the reciprocal interaction is established by the portal vein that enables the transport of gut-derived products directly to the liver, leading to the liver feedback route of bile and antibody secretion to the intestine. The blood supply to the liver from the intestine includes metabolic products produced by the gut microbiome such as phenols, acetaldehyde, ammonia, peptidoglycan, and lipopolysaccharides (LPS) (Compare et al. 2012). The control of microbial communities is important for maintaining homeostasis of the gut–liver axis. High-fat diet changes the microbiome and impairs the intestinal barrier and the gut vascular barrier (Mouries et al. 2019). Consequently, it facilitates the portal influx of bacterial products, worsening non-hepatic inflammation and metabolic abnormalities. The liver has various kinds of immune cells. The liver, as a "first pass" organ, is exposed to the highest concentration of portal systemic products such as pathogen-associated molecular patterns (PAMPs), and is thus especially vulnerable to their effects. The innate immune system responds to the cell damage and pathogens via pattern recognition receptors (PRRs) that are expressed intracellularly or on the surface of hepatocytes (Bieghs and Trautwein 2014). The damage-associated molecular patterns (DAMPs) released by damaged cells or PAMPs are also recognized by the PRRs (Pedra et al. 2009). The function of toll-like receptors (TLRs) is to induce gene transcription that streamlines the response of the innate immune system.

7.4 Associations Between the Microbiome and NAFLD

7.4.1 Animal Studies

Animal studies and fecal transplantation experiments have provided evidence of a causal role between the gut microbiota and NAFLD development. Germ-free animal models have been used to investigate the consequences of the absence of gut microbiota (Safari and Gérard 2019). For example, in one study, the microbiome set up by mice that developed fasting hyperglycemia and insulinemia NAFLD development in recipient mice (Le Roy et al. 2013). In this model, *Lachnospiraceae bacterium 609* and *Barnesiella intestinihominis* were abundant, with a potency to induce NAFLD. Another study showed that germ-free animals are resistant to the obesity caused by different diets (Bäckhed et al. 2007); this finding was correlated with increased ANGPTL4 gene expression as well as the activity of AMP-activated protein kinase and its downstream target proteins, such as acetyl-CoA carboxylase. AMP-activated protein kinase plays a substantial role in the switch between the metabolism of glucose and lipids in various organs. However, the obesity resistance phenotype in germ-free mice was found to be associated with the sugar composition of the diet. Notably, germfree mice have an immature immune system and immunity compared to other animals (Le Roy et al. 2018). However, germ-free and conventional mice showed no difference in body weight gain with a low-fat diet (Fleissner et al. 2010); on the high-fat diet, the germ-free mice gained more body weight and body fat than conventional mice, with a lower energy expenditure. Finally, germ-free mice fed a Western diet showed significantly less body fat than germ-free mice on a high-fat diet, suggesting that the absence of gut microbiota does not generally protect the mice against diet-induced obesity (Fleissner et al. 2010).

Gut microbiota transplantation in germ-free mice has been used to assess the causality between microbiota composition and susceptibility to NAFLD. By transplanting gut microbiota from mice with or without NAFLD to germ-free mice, the tendency to develop NAFLD is transmissible by the gut microbiota. Additionally, the gut microbiota affects the lipid metabolism in the liver, regardless of obesity (Le Roy et al. 2013). Inflammasome-deficient mouse models have been used to investigate the possible role of the microbiome in NAFLD (Henao-Mejia et al. 2012). Gut microbiota changes due to NLRP6 and NLRP3 inflammasome deficiency have been related to aggravated hepatic steatosis and elevated tumor necrosis factor alpha (TNF-α) expression. Additionally, this phenotype is transferable, as evidenced by the results obtained by co-housing wild-type mice with inflammasome-deficient mice; this suggests that inflammasome-mediated dysbiosis is involved in NASH progression. Thus, these findings provide insight into the role of the gut microbiome in the development and progression of NAFLD.

7.4.2 Clinical Evidence

Clinical studies have revealed a direct association between NAFLD and the gut microbiome. When NAFLD patients were compared with healthy subjects, an altered signature was observed at the level of phylum (increased Proteobacteria), family (increased Enterobacteriaceae and decreased Rikenellaceae and Ruminococcaceae), and genera (increased *Escherichia, Dorea, Peptoniphilus*, and decreased *Anaeromyxobacter, Coprococcus, Eubacterium, Faecalibacterium,* and *Prevotella*) (Aron-Wisnewsky et al. 2020). NASH patients have a distinct gut microbiome compared to those with simple steatosis. Patients with NASH also showed altered microbial signatures at the level of phylum (increased Proteobacteria), family (increased Enterobacteriaceae and decreased Ruminococcaceae and Rikenellaceae), and general (increased *Dorea* and decreased *Faecalibacterium, Coprococcus,* and *Anaerosporobacter*) (Aron-Wisnewsky et al. 2020). A cross-sectional study demonstrated that NASH patients had a higher abundance of fecal Clostridium coccoides and a lower percentage of Bacteroidetes compared to those with steatosis (Mouzaki et al. 2013).

Recently, gut microbiome compositions were characterized via whole-genome shotgun sequencing of DNA extracted from stool samples to differentiate between NAFLD and advanced fibrosis (Loomba et al. 2017). Firmicutes was more prevalent in mild and moderate NAFLD, whereas Proteobacteria were more highly represented in patients with advanced fibrosis. At the species level, Bacteroides vulgatus was highly represented in both groups. Eubacterium rectale was frequently observed in NAFLD, whereas Escherichia coli was more abundant in advanced fibrosis. Ruminococcus obeum and E. rectale were significantly less abundant in advanced fibrosis than in NAFLD.

However, evaluation of the gut microbiota contribution in liver disease progression is limited and bacterial markers are frequently identified in a given study, yet not confirmed in independent cohorts. As the origin of liver disease is heterogeneous by nature, most studies in cirrhosis have included patients with different etiologies. An increased level of Bacteroides and a decreased level of Prevotella was observed in NASH patients with significant fibrosis (Boursier et al. 2016). However, some studies have shown controversial gut microbiome conditions. The role of gut microbiome dysbiosis on NASH progression is partially attributed to an increased susceptibility to intestinal permeability. As a result, some pro-inflammatory substances derived from gut microbiota can translocate to the portal vein and liver.

7.5 Gut Microbial Metabolites in NAFLD

The metabolites of the gut microbiome can modulate the pathogenesis of NAFLD. Most microbial metabolites are mainly derived from carbohydrate and protein fermentation (Song and Zhang 2022). Short-chain fatty acids (SCFAs) are one of the most common microbial metabolites derived from indigestible carbohydrates. SCFAs are beneficial to liver metabolism and are involved in NAFLD progression. A recent study showed that a kind of acetate from a commensal microbe suppresses NAFLD development by modulating hepatic FFAR2 signaling in the liver of high-fat-fed mice (Aoki et al. 2021). SCFA butyrate was able to attenuate NAFLD by regulating gut microbiota, intestinal tight junctions, hepatic glucagon-like peptide-1 receptor expression, and toll-like receptor 4 pathways (Baumann et al. 2020; Yang et al. 2020; Zhou et al. 2018). Decreased levels of butyrate production in NAFLD result in increased gut permeability, with an increased risk for bacterial and LPS translocation into the systemic circulation. Other SCFA members such as propionate can ameliorate the progression of NASH (Deng et al. 2020).

Also, there is an increased level of blood ethanol in patients with NAFLD (Engstler et al. 2016). The overproduction of ethanol produced by bacteria is responsible for hepatic inflammation in patients with NAFLD (Chen and Vitetta 2020). The level of alcohol-producing bacteria in the intestine and the concentration of blood ethanol is elevated in patients with NASH compared to those with NAFL (Zhu et al. 2013). This indicates that microbiome-derived ethanol is a contributing factor inducing the transition from simple steatosis into NASH. The gut microbiota has the capacity to convert primary bile acids into secondary bile acids. This ability is compromised due to the decreased abundance of related bacteria in patients with NAFLD (Chen et al. 2019). A decreased level of deconjugated bile acid can further decrease taurine production. Sequentially, it leads to hepatic steatosis and inflammation by targeting oxidative stress-related genes and fatty acid synthesis-associated genes (Miyata et al. 2020). In NAFLD, the abundance of bacteria that convert primary bile acids into secondary bile acids is reduced. The composition of the bile acid pool is important to maintain commensal bacterial community diversity. Farnesoid X receptor (FXR), the receptor of bile acids, is found to be downregulated in NAFLD (Chen et al. 2019). The decreased level of intestinal FXR reduces the secretion of fibroblast growth factor 15/19, both of which can reduce liver steatosis (Alvarez-Sola et al. 2017). Other gut microbial metabolites including amino acids and choline also reportedly modulate NAFLD (Chen and Vitetta 2020). The dysregulation of amino acids and choline contributes to lipid accumulation and chronic inflammation.

7.6 Gut Microbiome and NAFLD-Associated HCC

The etiologies of HCC in Asia are changing from viral to non-viral causes including NAFLD (Yip et al. 2022). The change in the gut microbiome can cause NAFLD-associated HCC. In a mouse experiment, high dietary cholesterol led to progression of steatosis, steatohepatitis, fibrosis, and HCC (Zhang et al. 2021). The microbiota composition clustered distinctly along stages of NAFLD (increased *Mucispirillum, Desulfovibrio, Anaerotruncus,* and *Desulfovibrionaceae* and decreased *Bifidobacterium* and *Bacteroides*). Dietary cholesterol induced gut bacterial metabolites were also altered as increased taurocholic acid and decreased 3-indolepropionic acid. In a metagenomic sequencing analysis, the results showed that the gut of NAFLD-HCC patients is enriched with five bacterial species (*Bacteroides caecimuris*, *Ruminococcus gnavus*, *Veillonella parvula*, *Bacteroides xylanisolvens*, and *Clostridium bolteae*) (Behary et al. 2021). All five bacterial species are SCFAs that produce bacteria with immunomodulatory activities.

7.7 Therapeutic Implications of the Gut Microbiota

7.7.1 Diet

Diet is an important factor for affecting change in gut microbiota (Pan and Zhang 2022). Lactobacillus species due to the high-fat diet can induce lipid metabolism by modulating that of bile acid. This means that diet can be used to re-establish healthy microbiota conditions to improve the pathological environment induced by unhealthy eating habits. A Western diet with high contents of red meat, fat, and fructose favors NAFLD development; whereas a Mediterranean diet, characterized by a low consumption of red meat, dairy products, and saturated fats and high intake of vegetables, fruits, nuts, and fish, is the most recommended dietary pattern for NAFLD prevention (Pan and Zhang 2022; Abenavoli et al. 2018).

7.7.2 Prebiotics

Prebiotics are defined as nondigestible food ingredients in the diet but that are subject to fermentation by gut microbiota (Chen and Vitetta 2020). Most prebiotics belong to carbohydrates, especially oligosaccharides, but they also include non-carbohydrate substances such as fatty acids, polyphenols, and phytochemicals. Oligosaccharides are composed of less than 10 sugar units, and may be contained in food or produced from ingested polysaccharides or low molecular weight sugars. Many studies have shown that various prebiotics can reduce NAFLD pathogenesis. Fructooligosaccharides (FOS) and inulin have been shown to improve NAFLD in various animal models. However, the mechanisms are not well understood relative to the changes that have been described for altered bacterial metabolites. FOS ameliorates parameters of NAFLD such as steatosis and inflammation (Takai et al. 2020). This improvement by FOS administration is associated with increased fecal SCFAs, including butyrate, propionate, and acetate; serum propionate is also increased more than twofold. These data suggest that FOS improves NAFLD through the restoration of the gut microbiota. The mechanisms could be associated with increased butyrate production, decreased endotoxemia, and decreased lipogenesis.

7.7.3 Probiotics

Probiotics, as defined by the World Health Organization, are live microorganisms that when administered in adequate amounts confer a health benefit on the host. The most used probiotics are from genera Lactobacillus, Bifidobacteria, and others (e.g., Streptococcus thermophilus and Saccharomyces yeast). Recently, butyrate-producing bacteria such as Lactobacillus rhamnosus GG (LGG) have been highly regarded. In a mouse model, LGG reduced gut inflammation by inhibiting the nuclear factor kappa B (NF-kB) signaling pathway (Ritze et al. 2014). The blood LPS levels were reduced due to increased gut barrier function by LGG. LGG decreased hepatic inflammation, as reflected by a reduction in TNF-α, interleukin (IL) 8 receptor, IL-1β mRNAs, and hepatic fat accumulation. A recent meta-analysis confirmed that probiotic administration has beneficial effects on improving body mass index, alanine aminotransferase, aspartate transaminase, gamma-glutamyl transpeptidase, insulin, homeostasis model assessment-insulin resistance, and total cholesterol levels, but not on fasting blood sugar, lipid profiles, or TNF-α (Xiao et al. 2019). In addition, VSL#3 supplementation, which is composed of eight bacterial strains that include Bifidobacteria (B. breve, B. longum, and B. infantis), Streptococcus thermophilus, L. plantarum, L. acidophilus, L. paracasei, and L. delbrueckii subsp. bulgaricus) has been investigated in patients with NAFLD (Alisi et al. 2014). VSL#3 has shown protective effects on NAFLD by inhibiting NF-kB signaling, reducing hepatic inflammation, and hepatic fat accumulation and by increasing insulin sensitivity (Alisi et al. 2014; Jena et al. 2020).

7.7.4 Synbiotics

A synbiotic is defined as the combination of probiotic bacteria with a prebiotic in the formulation. A synbiotic has the advantage of producing increased levels of butyrate through the action of the probiotic bacteria that provide materials for commensal bacteria to metabolize the prebiotic (Chen and Vitetta 2020). In a meta-analysis, probiotics and synbiotics were effective in the treatment of 782 patients with NAFLD (Hadi et al. 2019). In a mouse model of NAFLD using high-fat diet, treatments with Lactobacillus paracasei N1115, FOS, and their combination reduced hepatic steatosis (Yao et al. 2019). In patients with NASH, a synbiotic composed of Bifidobacterium longum and FOS improved aspartate aminotransferase, cholesterol, C-reactive protein,α, homeostasis model assessment of insulin resistance, serum endotoxin, steatosis, and NASH activity index levels (Malaguarnera et al. 2012). Based on these data, further clinical trials with probiotics and/or synbiotics are needed in patients with NAFLD.

7.8 Other Interventions

Other interventions targeting the microbiome include bacteriophages, synthetic live bacterial therapeutics, non-absorbable antibiotics, and fecal microbiota transplantation (FMT) (Albillos et al. 2020). Bacteriophages, viruses that specifically infect and kill bacteria, have been continually evolving to overcome the defense mechanisms developed by bacteria. Engineered probiotics may be uniquely designed to consume toxic metabolites in the intestine and convert them into non-toxic forms. Rifaximin, as the non-absorbable antibiotic with the most favorable safety profile, is currently being tested to target the microbiome in different clinical trials in chronic liver disease.

FMT was first introduced for the treatment of pseudomembranous colitis (Eiseman et al. 1958). Currently, it is being studied as a potential NAFLD treatment. Compared to probiotics and synbiotics, FMT can provide a wide range of commensal bacteria as well as other microbials that facilitate the maintenance of gut microbial ecology. Both animal studies and clinical trials have shown promising outcomes for FMT application in NAFLD. In an animal model of NAFLD, three groups of mice including a control, a high-fat diet group and a high-fat diet plus FMT group, were used to demonstrate the beneficial effects of FMT (Zhou et al. 2017). FMT from control mice reduced high-fat diet-induced steatohepatitis with decreased hepatic lipid accumulation, decreased pro-inflammatory cytokines, and increased anti-inflammatory cytokines as well as increased intestinal beneficial bacteria Christensenellaceae and Lactobacillus. Additionally, increased levels of intestinal butyrate, tight junction protein ZO-1, and decreased blood endotoxemia were reported.

7.9 Future Perspectives

NAFLD shows a close relationship with a wide range of diseases of gut microbiota. Currently, depending on the distribution of the intestinal microflora, it shows a unique pattern for each disease. Mechanism research using intestinal microbes in the developmental mechanism is in progress using omics, and diagnostic research using artificial intelligence related to big data is actively underway in the diagnosis process. In addition, treatments that address the imbalance of intestinal microflora or change it to a normal state are currently being studied, including the use of intestinal antibiotics, adsorbents, and fecal transplantation. It is expected that an effective NAFLD treatment is close at hand through this comprehensive effort.

The heterogeneous clinical features of NAFLD can be explained by the incorporation of various risk factors. Among them, a diverse spectrum of fatty liver disease is associated with an imbalance of the gut microbiota and other associated microbiota. Several animal and human studies have provided evidence of a close relationship between NAFLD and gut microbiota, and it is thought that more therapies targeting the gut microbiota will be explored. Additionally, precision medicine that targets individual gut microbiome environments is expected in the near future.

References

Abenavoli L, et al. Health benefits of Mediterranean diet in nonalcoholic fatty liver disease. Expert Rev Gastroenterol Hepatol. 2018;12(9):873–81.

Albillos A, de Gottardi A, Rescigno M. The gut-liver axis in liver disease: pathophysiological basis for therapy. J Hepatol. 2020;72(3):558–77.

Alisi A, et al. Randomised clinical trial: the beneficial effects of VSL#3 in obese children with non-alcoholic steatohepatitis. Aliment Pharmacol Ther. 2014;39(11):1276–85.

Alvarez-Sola G, et al. Fibroblast growth factor 15/19 (FGF15/19) protects from diet-induced hepatic steatosis: development of an FGF19-based chimeric molecule to promote fatty liver regeneration. Gut. 2017;66(10):1818–28.

Aoki R, et al. Commensal microbe-derived acetate suppresses NAFLD/NASH development via hepatic FFAR2 signalling in mice. Microbiome. 2021;9(1):188.

Aron-Wisnewsky J, et al. Gut microbiota and human NAFLD: disentangling microbial signatures from metabolic disorders. Nat Rev Gastroenterol Hepatol. 2020;17(5):279–97.

Bäckhed F, et al. Mechanisms underlying the resistance to diet-induced obesity in germ-free mice. Proc Natl Acad Sci U S A. 2007;104(3):979–84.

Baumann A, et al. Oral supplementation of sodium butyrate attenuates the progression of non-alcoholic steatohepatitis. Nutrients. 2020;12(4):951.

Behary J, et al. Gut microbiota impact on the peripheral immune response in non-alcoholic fatty liver disease related hepatocellular carcinoma. Nat Commun. 2021;12(1):187.

Bieghs V, Trautwein C. Innate immune signaling and gut-liver interactions in non-alcoholic fatty liver disease. Hepatobiliary Surg Nutr. 2014;3(6):377–85.

Boursier J, et al. The severity of nonalcoholic fatty liver disease is associated with gut dysbiosis and shift in the metabolic function of the gut microbiota. Hepatology. 2016;63(3):764–75.

Chen J, Vitetta L. Gut microbiota metabolites in NAFLD pathogenesis and therapeutic implications. Int J Mol Sci. 2020;21(15):5214.

Chen J, Thomsen M, Vitetta L. Interaction of gut microbiota with dysregulation of bile acids in the pathogenesis of nonalcoholic fatty liver disease and potential therapeutic implications of probiotics. J Cell Biochem. 2019;120(3):2713–20.

Compare D, et al. Gut-liver axis: the impact of gut microbiota on non alcoholic fatty liver disease. Nutr Metab Cardiovasc Dis. 2012;22(6):471–6.

Deng M, et al. SCFAs alleviated steatosis and inflammation in mice with NASH induced by MCD. J Endocrinol. 2020;245(3):425–37.

Eiseman B, et al. Fecal enema as an adjunct in the treatment of pseudomembranous enterocolitis. Surgery. 1958;44(5):854–9.
Engstler AJ, et al. Insulin resistance alters hepatic ethanol metabolism: studies in mice and children with non-alcoholic fatty liver disease. Gut. 2016;65(9):1564–71.
Fleissner CK, et al. Absence of intestinal microbiota does not protect mice from diet-induced obesity. Br J Nutr. 2010;104(6):919–29.
Hadi A, et al. Efficacy of synbiotic supplementation in patients with nonalcoholic fatty liver disease: a systematic review and meta-analysis of clinical trials: Synbiotic supplementation and NAFLD. Crit Rev Food Sci Nutr. 2019;59(15):2494–505.
Henao-Mejia J, et al. Inflammasome-mediated dysbiosis regulates progression of NAFLD and obesity. Nature. 2012;482(7384):179–85.
Henry L, Paik J, Younossi ZM. Review article: the epidemiologic burden of non-alcoholic fatty liver disease across the world. Aliment Pharmacol Ther. 2022;56(6):942–56.
Jena PK, et al. Probiotics VSL#3 are effective in reversing non-alcoholic steatohepatitis in a mouse model. Hepatobiliary Surg Nutr. 2020;9(2):170–82.
Le Roy T, et al. Intestinal microbiota determines development of non-alcoholic fatty liver disease in mice. Gut. 2013;62(12):1787–94.
Le Roy T, et al. Comparative evaluation of microbiota engraftment following fecal microbiota transfer in mice models: age, kinetic and microbial status matter. Front Microbiol. 2018;9:3289.
Loomba R, et al. Gut microbiome-based metagenomic signature for non-invasive detection of advanced fibrosis in human nonalcoholic fatty liver disease. Cell Metab. 2017;25(5):1054–1062.e5.
Malaguarnera M, et al. Bifidobacterium longum with fructo-oligosaccharides in patients with non alcoholic steatohepatitis. Dig Dis Sci. 2012;57(2):545–53.
McPherson S, et al. Evidence of NAFLD progression from steatosis to fibrosing-steatohepatitis using paired biopsies: implications for prognosis and clinical management. J Hepatol. 2015;62(5):1148–55.
Mittal S, et al. Hepatocellular carcinoma in the absence of cirrhosis in United States veterans is associated with nonalcoholic fatty liver disease. Clin Gastroenterol Hepatol. 2016;14(1):124–31.e1.
Miyata M, et al. Taurine attenuates hepatic steatosis in a genetic model of fatty liver disease. J Toxicol Sci. 2020;45(2):87–94.
Mohamad B, et al. Characterization of hepatocellular carcinoma (HCC) in non-alcoholic fatty liver disease (NAFLD) patients without cirrhosis. Hepatol Int. 2016;10(4):632–9.
Mouries J, et al. Microbiota-driven gut vascular barrier disruption is a prerequisite for non-alcoholic steatohepatitis development. J Hepatol. 2019;71(6):1216–28.
Mouzaki M, et al. Intestinal microbiota in patients with nonalcoholic fatty liver disease. Hepatology. 2013;58(1):120–7.
Pais R, et al. A systematic review of follow-up biopsies reveals disease progression in patients with non-alcoholic fatty liver. J Hepatol. 2013;59(3):550–6.
Pan Y, Zhang X. Diet and gut microbiome in fatty liver and its associated liver cancer. J Gastroenterol Hepatol. 2022;37(1):7–14.
Paradis V, et al. Hepatocellular carcinomas in patients with metabolic syndrome often develop without significant liver fibrosis: a pathological analysis. Hepatology. 2009;49(3):851–9.
Pedra JH, Cassel SL, Sutterwala FS. Sensing pathogens and danger signals by the inflammasome. Curr Opin Immunol. 2009;21(1):10–6.
Ritze Y, et al. Lactobacillus rhamnosus GG protects against non-alcoholic fatty liver disease in mice. PLoS One. 2014;9(1):e80169.
Safari Z, Gérard P. The links between the gut microbiome and non-alcoholic fatty liver disease (NAFLD). Cell Mol Life Sci. 2019;76(8):1541–58.
Singh S, et al. Fibrosis progression in nonalcoholic fatty liver vs nonalcoholic steatohepatitis: a systematic review and meta-analysis of paired-biopsy studies. Clin Gastroenterol Hepatol. 2015;13(4):643–54.e1–9; quiz e39–40.

Song Q, Zhang X. The role of gut-liver axis in gut microbiome dysbiosis associated NAFLD and NAFLD-HCC. Biomedicine. 2022;10(3):524.

Takai A, et al. Fructo-oligosaccharides ameliorate steatohepatitis, visceral adiposity, and associated chronic inflammation via increased production of short-chain fatty acids in a mouse model of non-alcoholic steatohepatitis. BMC Gastroenterol. 2020;20(1):46.

Wong VW, et al. Disease progression of non-alcoholic fatty liver disease: a prospective study with paired liver biopsies at 3 years. Gut. 2010;59(7):969–74.

Xiao MW, et al. Systematic review with meta-analysis: the effects of probiotics in nonalcoholic fatty liver disease. Gastroenterol Res Pract. 2019;2019:1484598.

Yang T, et al. Amelioration of non-alcoholic fatty liver disease by sodium butyrate is linked to the modulation of intestinal tight junctions in db/db mice. Food Funct. 2020;11(12):10675–89.

Yao F, et al. Effect of Lactobacillus paracasei N1115 and fructooligosaccharides in nonalcoholic fatty liver disease. Arch Med Sci. 2019;15(5):1336–44.

Yasui K, et al. Characteristics of patients with nonalcoholic steatohepatitis who develop hepatocellular carcinoma. Clin Gastroenterol Hepatol. 2011;9(5):428–33; quiz e50.

Yip TC, et al. Asian perspective on NAFLD-associated HCC. J Hepatol. 2022;76(3):726–34.

Younossi ZM, et al. Association of nonalcoholic fatty liver disease (NAFLD) with hepatocellular carcinoma (HCC) in the United States from 2004 to 2009. Hepatology. 2015;62(6):1723–30.

Younossi ZM, et al. Global epidemiology of nonalcoholic fatty liver disease-meta-analytic assessment of prevalence, incidence, and outcomes. Hepatology. 2016;64(1):73–84.

Zhang X, et al. Dietary cholesterol drives fatty liver-associated liver cancer by modulating gut microbiota and metabolites. Gut. 2021;70(4):761–74.

Zhou D, et al. Total fecal microbiota transplantation alleviates high-fat diet-induced steatohepatitis in mice via beneficial regulation of gut microbiota. Sci Rep. 2017;7(1):1529.

Zhou D, et al. Sodium butyrate reduces high-fat diet-induced non-alcoholic steatohepatitis through upregulation of hepatic GLP-1R expression. Exp Mol Med. 2018;50(12):1–12.

Zhu L, et al. Characterization of gut microbiomes in nonalcoholic steatohepatitis (NASH) patients: a connection between endogenous alcohol and NASH. Hepatology. 2013;57(2):601–9.

Chapter 8
Diet and Gut Microbiome in Gastrointestinal Cancer

Jia Yang and Jun Yu

Abstract Gastrointestinal (GI) cancer is one of the most prevalent and deadly cancer in the world. Recent studies have shown that gut microbiome is intensively involved in GI cancer especially in CRC development. Diet, as one of the key modulators of gut microbiome, could alter human gut microbiome and its associated metabolites rapidly and reproducibly. Dietary fat, fiber, and protein could induce microbial alteration to contribute to or protect against colorectal tumorigenesis. Hence, identification of gut microbiome alteration in CRC offers new possibility for treatment and prevention. In this chapter, we will take CRC as an example, demonstrate the influence of diets on gut microbiome that leads to predisposition to CRC, and will also discuss the mechanisms behind these microbial effects in contributing to CRC.

Keywords Diet · Gut microbiome · Metabolites · Gastrointestinal cancer

J. Yang
Department of Radiation Oncology, The Second Affiliated Hospital of Zhejiang University School of Medicine, Hangzhou, Zhejiang Province, China

J. Yu (✉)
Institute of Digestive Disease, Department of Medicine and Therapeutics, State Key Laboratory of Digestive Disease, Li Ka Shing Institute of Health Sciences, CUHK Shenzhen Research Institute, The Chinese University of Hong Kong, Hong Kong, China
e-mail: junyu@cuhk.edu.hk

J. Yu (ed.), *Microbiome in Gastrointestinal Cancer*,
https://doi.org/10.1007/978-981-19-4492-5_8

8.1 Introduction

Gastrointestinal (GI) cancer is one of the leading causes of death worldwide, with more than five million new cases and three million deaths are projected to occur in 2020 (Sung et al. 2021). Among all the GI cancers, colorectal cancer (CRC) is the most diagnosed and deadly cancer. CRC ranks third in terms of incidence, but second in terms of mortality. 1,880,725 new CRC cases are estimated to be diagnosed along with 915,880 associated deaths worldwide in 2020 (Sung et al. 2021). Notably, there is an approximately nine-fold variation in CRC incidence rates by world regions, with the highest rates in most developed regions including Europe, North America, and Australia/New Zealand and with the lowest rates in developing regions of Africa and South-Central Asia. Considering that nearly 90% of CRC cases are found to be sporadic (Doll and Peto 1981), geographic variation in CRC incidence is most likely attributed to diet and lifestyle factors, i.e., preferring an intake of animal-source foods rather than plant-based diet, sedentary lifestyle with decreased physical activity, heavy alcohol and cigarette consumption, and the consumption of red or processed meat (Siegel et al. 2020; World Cancer Research Fund, American Institute for Cancer Research 2018). This is further supported by a steadily rising trend in CRC incidence rates in transitioning countries which are under socioeconomic development and also dietary habits shift toward westernization (Arnold et al. 2017, 2020).

In recent decades, gut microbiome has been heavily investigated in various diseases including GI cancers. It is reported that gut microbial community is perturbed in patients with CRC or adenoma compared with healthy controls (Liang et al. 2017). Moreover, colonic mucosal microbiome has been also shifted continuously during tumorigenesis from normal mucosa to adenoma and adenocarcinoma (Nakatsu et al. 2015). Evidence showed that dysbiosis occurs when adenoma is developed, which is at very early stage of tumorigenesis, and deteriorates in adenocarcinoma stage (Nakatsu et al. 2015). Diet, as one of the most important factors, plays a crucial role in modulating gut microbial composition and function, and thus influences disease progression including GI cancers (Rothschild et al. 2018; Xu and Knight 2015). We previously reported that gut dysbiosis and gut metabolites dysregulation play an important role in CRC development induced by high fat diet (Yang et al. 2022). Dietary fat intake led to enrichments of pathogenic bacteria *Alistipes sp. Marseille-P5997* and *Alistipes sp. 5CPEGH6*, and depletion of probiotic *Parabacteroides distasonis*, during the development of CRC (Yang et al. 2022). Apart from fat, dietary fiber, cholesterol and protein could also induce gut microbial and metabolic alteration and eventually contribute to the pathogenesis of GI cancers including CRC (Wang et al. 2018) and liver cancer (Zhang et al. 2021; Singh et al. 2018). In contrast, other studies showed that intake of vegetables and fruits could effectively reduce the risk of CRC and liver cancer. These findings suggest that the important role of a balanced diet in preventing GI cancers. In this chapter, taking CRC as an example, we will discuss how diet composition impacts gut microbial ecology and leads to predisposition to GI cancers especially CRC.

8.2 Microbiome in Gastrointestinal Cancer

In the recent decade, gut microbiome has been intensively investigated and considered as a key role in mediating GI tumorigenesis especially CRC (Zhang et al. 2021; Yu et al. 2017). Colorectal tumorigenesis usually takes years even over a decade from normal mucosa to the formation of polyps and eventually adenocarcinoma (Clay et al. 2022). Studies have shown that gut dysbiosis has been involved in the early stage of colorectal tumorigenesis. Patients with benign polyps or adenoma have already shown features of gut dysbiosis with enrichments of *Eubacterium coprostanoligenes*, *Methanobrevibacter millerae*, *Christensenellaceae R-7 group sp.* and depletions of *Bifidobacterium longum*, *Anaerostipes hadrus*, *Lactococcus taiwanensis*, *Aminipila butyrica*, etc. (Wu et al. 2021) Moreover, gut dysbiosis deteriorates at CRC stage. Yu et al. performed metagenomic sequencing on stool samples from 128 individuals (74 patients with CRC and 54 control subjects) from China and found that CRC patient microbiomes exhibited reduced gene richness and gene alpha diversity (Yu et al. 2017).The principal component analysis (PCA) showed that the first and fifth principal components, which explained 6.6% and 3.2% of total variance, respectively, were significantly associated with CRC status (Yu et al. 2017). In another study on the combined analysis of 526 metagenomic samples from Hong Kong Chinese, Austrian, American, and German and French cohorts, although no significant difference in Shannon diversity index was observed between CRC patients and healthy controls, the diversity index decreased significantly in CRC cases compared to controls in the HK cohort. PCA identified significant differences in overall bacterial composition between cases and controls (Dai et al. 2018). Nakatsu et al. catalogued the mucosal microbial communities at different stages of colorectal tumorigenesis and discovered that a metacommunity predominated by oral microbial pathogens is associated with CRC. Furthermore, correlations of bacterial taxa indicated early signs of dysbiosis in adenoma, and co-exclusive relationships are subsequently more common in cancer, suggesting that a taxonomically defined microbial consortium is implicated in the development of CRC (Nakatsu et al. 2015). Altogether, this evidence suggested a sign of dysbiosis of the gut microbiome in colorectal tumorigenesis.

Based on the discovery of involvement of gut dysbiosis in colorectal tumorigenesis, gut microbiome has been used as a tool for the diagnosis of adenoma and CRC. In 2012, Kostic et al. found that *Fusobacterium (Fn)* was enriched in CRC tissues compared with normal tissues. Consistently, this finding was verified by the other study, which showed that overabundance of *Fn* in tumors tissues compared with matched normal samples and it is also positively associated with lymph node metastasis (Castellarin et al. 2012), indicating that Fn could be a potential diagnostic marker for CRC. Wong et al. discovered that the combination of Fn and fecal immunochemical test (FIT) showed superior sensitivity (92.3% vs 73.1%, $p < 0.001$) and area under the receiver-operating characteristic curve (AUC) (0.95 vs 0.86, $p < 0.001$) than stand-alone FIT in detecting CRC. This combined test also increased the sensitivity (38.6% vs 15.5%, $p < 0.001$) and AUC (0.65 vs 0.57, $p = 0.007$) for detecting advanced adenoma (Wong et al. 2017). Moreover, "M3," a combination of *Lachnoclostridium sp., Fusobacterium nucleatum (Fn),* and *Clostridium hathewayi (Ch),* was identified to be significantly increased from normal to adenoma to CRC. Fecal "m3" performed better than *Fn* in perspective of distinguishing adenoma from healthy controls, while *Fn* achieved better in the diagnosis of CRC (Liang et al. 2020). Therefore, these findings suggested that gut microbiome could be developed as a non-invasive and well-validated approach for detecting adenoma and CRC, and could be applied as a diagnostic and screening test for cancer detection and screening.

8.3 Diet Modulating Gut Microbiome to Influence Gastrointestinal Cancer

Accumulating evidence has demonstrated that western diet could contribute to colorectal tumorigenesis. Indeed, western-style diet, a combination of high levels of fat, sugar and low levels of dietary fiber, could alter gut microbial structure, induce gut metabolites dysregulation, impair gut barrier function, and eventually contribute to CRC formation (Yang et al. 2022). Given the intensive interaction between dietary components and gut microbiome, they both play crucial roles in the development of CRC.

8.4 Fat and Gut Microbiome in Gastrointestinal Cancer

As early as in 1973, Drasar and Irving discovered that colon cancer was highly associated with the intake of fat (Drasar and Irving 1973). This was the first time that the association between fat and CRC was established. Similarly, in 1990, the Nurses' Health Study revealed that a high intake of fat especially animal saturated and monounsaturated fat rather than vegetable fat, linoleic acid, or cholesterol, increased the risk of developing colon cancer (Willett et al. 1990). Although other human prospective cohort studies (Stemmermann et al. 1984; Giovannucci et al. 1994; Bostick et al. 1994; Goldbohm et al. 1994; Gaard et al. 1996; Chyou et al. 1996; Kato et al. 1997; Pietinen et al. 1999; Terry et al. 2001; Jarvinen et al. 2001; Flood et al. 2003; Brink et al. 2004; Lin et al. 2004; Oba et al. 2006; Weijenberg et al. 2007; Butler et al. 2009) did not reveal the equivalent findings, numerous animal studies have demonstrated that dietary fat could increase CRC risk through stimulating bile acids secretion, causing the regression of epithelium, damaging colonic mucosa, and impairing gut barrier function (Chomchai et al. 1974; Narisawa et al. 1974; Rijnkels et al. 1997).

Fat, as one of the most important components of our daily diets, could induce the secretion of bile acids from liver to the small intestine. With the fermentation of the gut microbiome, primary bile acids are deconjugated into secondary bile acids. Animal studies have already shown the relationship between fat and changes in gut microbiome and metabolites. Taira et al. reported that switching from a low-fat diet to a high fat diet in rats altered the microbiota composition with an increase in *Firmicutes* and a decrease in *Bacteroidetes* (Taira et al. 2015). Similarly, Guo et al. found that mice fed with a high fat diet had higher abundance of genus *Lactobacillus* and reduced abundances of genera *Turicibacter*, *Prevotella*, *Bacteroides*, and *Bifidobacteria* (Guo et al. 2017). High fat diet can also slightly increase total bile acids, particularly deoxycholic acid (DCA) and taurodeoxycholic acid (TDCA), which are both secondary bile acids which depend on the gut microbiome, in plasma and liver tissue (Lin et al. 2019). Mechanical studies have shown that the elevated bile acids could induce DNA damage, inflammation, and proliferation to the colonic epithelial cells. Farnesoid X receptor (FXR) is a nuclear receptor responsible for bile acids signaling. It is a master regulator of bile acid homeostasis, which mainly maintains bile acid concentrations in a normal range to prevent bile acid-associated cytotoxicity (Makishima et al. 1999; Parks et al. 1999; Wang et al. 1999). Furthermore, study has demonstrated that excess bile acid secretion induced by high fat diet, especially DCA and tauro-β-muricholic acid (T-βMCA), could antagonize intestinal FXR function, resulting in proliferation and DNA damage in Lgr5+ cells (Fu et al. 2019). Moreover, activation of intestinal FXR could restrict Lgr5+ cell growth and attenuate CRC development (Fu et al. 2019). This makes FXR a potential target to treat high fat diet or bile acid-associated CRC.

8.5 Fiber and Gut Microbiome in Gastrointestinal Cancer

Dietary fiber is usually derived from fruit, vegetables, and grains. In 1970s, Burkitt suggested that plant-based diet may protect against CRC based on his observation of the low incidence of CRC in Africa (Burkitt 1971). Similarly, Heilbrun et al. also discovered a significant negative association of dietary fiber and colon cancer risk among low fat intake men (Heilbrun et al. 1989). After that, numerous evidence has shown the same perspectives (Nomura et al. 2007; McCullough et al. 2003).

Dietary fiber, as a key modulator of gut microbiome, is one of the determinants of microbial species diversity. A study investigated the microbial profiling of vegetarians, vegans and controls consuming an omnivorous diet, and revealed a significant reduction in *Enterobacteriaceae* in vegans compared with omnivorous controls while vegetarians placed between vegans and controls (Zimmer et al. 2012). De Filippo et al. discovered that children from rural Africa were exclusively colonized by *Treponema species, Butyrivibrio, Prevotella,* and *Xylanibacter* with increased utilization of cellulose and xylose, and increased synthesis of short chain fatty acids (SCFAs) (De Filippo et al. 2010). Similarly, Ou et al. measured differences in gut microbiome and their metabolites in African Americans who were in high risk of developing CRC and in rural native Africans who were of lower risk, and reported that the microbiome composition showed significant difference with a dominance of *Bacteroides* in African Americans and *Prevotella* in native Africans (Ou et al. 2013). Native Africans had a more abundant butyrate producing bacteria population with higher expression levels of microbial genes encoding for methanogenesis and hydrogen sulfide production than African Americans, who had higher levels of expression of microbial genes encoding for secondary bile acid production. Higher abundance of SCFAs were found in native African subjects, which was consistent with their lower risk of developing CRC (Ou et al. 2013). Moreover, a follow-up dietary intervention study of 2-week food exchanges in African Americans and rural Africans showed increased butyrogenesis and saccharolytic fermentation, suppressed secondary bile acid synthesis and colonocytes proliferation in the African Americans while increased secondary bile acid production and colonocytes proliferation in the native Africans (O'Keefe et al. 2015). In mechanism, study has shown that fiber derived metabolites SCFAs especially butyrate could promote the apoptosis of colonocytes, suppress oncogene expression through blocking histone deacetylases (Steliou et al. 2012), and activate gluconeogenesis through a cAMP-dependent manner (De Vadder et al. 2014).

Although accumulating evidence supports that fiber and butyrate protect against CRC, there are other voices against it. Several human cohort studies did not reveal the benefit of fiber in reducing CRC risk (Butler et al. 2008; Mai et al. 2003; Sanjoaquin et al. 2004; Michels et al. 2005; Otani et al. 2006; Kabat et al. 2008). In a population-based prospective cohort study conducted among Chinese women in urban Shanghai, no obvious association between fiber intake and CRC risk was observed (Shin et al. 2006). Similarly, two cohort studies conducted in Northern European population discovered that intake of dietary fiber was not associated with decreased risk of CRC (Gaard et al. 1996; Pietinen et al. 1999). Furthermore, our unpublished data showed that extreme high level of soluble fiber such as inulin and guar gum could promote colorectal tumorigenesis in both *Apc* min mice and AOM-induced CRC mice. Similarly, Singh et al. reported that soluble fibers including inulin, pectin, and fructooligosaccharide were found to induce hepatic carcinoma via dysregulated gut microbiota in mice (Singh et al. 2018). In this study, it is found that prolonged exposure to butyrate could promote hepatocyte proliferation and lead to liver fibrosis (Singh et al. 2018). Gut fermentation inhibition and soluble fiber exclusion could attenuate and prevent HCC development (Singh et al. 2018). Furthermore, butyrate was also shown to promote colorectal tumorigenesis in a mouse model with *Apc* gene and mismatch repair gene Msh2 mutations (Belcheva et al. 2014). Hence, more cohort studies with high level of different sources of fiber intervention are warranted in the near future.

8.6 Protein and Gut Microbiome in Gastrointestinal Cancer

In contrast to fermentation of complex carbohydrates and bile acid metabolism, proteolytic fermentation is quantitatively smaller, which attributes to the high efficiency of protein digestion and absorption in the small intestine, resulting in a much smaller amount of protein entering the colon for fermentation (Silvester and Cummings 1995). However, there are some exceptional cases particularly when large amounts of protein are adopted. Beaumont et al. reported that large amounts of protein intake induced no alteration to gut microbiome, but induced a change in bacterial metabolism with increased amino acid degradation, which was positively promoted by phylum *Firmicutes* (*Clostridiales, Christensenellaceae, Ruminococcaceae,* and *Oscillospira*) and *Bacteroidetes* phylum (*Odoribacter* and *Butyricimonas*) (Beaumont et al. 2017). The major products of protein fermentation are nitrogenous and sulfur metabolites, for instance, ammonia, nitrites, amines, hydrogen sulfide (Windey et al. 2012). Evidence has shown that excess nitrogenous and sulfur metabolites could cause damage to the epithelial cells in the gut, including inflammation and even tumorigenesis (Sodring et al. 2015). Moreover, recent study has shown that higher sulfur microbial diet scores were associated with increased risk for early-onset adenomas, suggesting a role for dietary interactions with gut sulfur-metabolizing bacteria in early-onset colorectal carcinogenesis, possibly beginning in adolescence (Nguyen et al. 2021).

Besides fiber, fat, and protein, there are various other kinds of compositions existing in diet that may contribute to gut microbial metabolism, but currently, evidence is much limited. More studies are warranted to investigate the relation between diet and microbial metabolism.

8.7 Diet and Microbiome Regulation to Prevent Gastrointestinal Cancer

Accumulating evidence has supported the view that diet and its associated gut microbiome play an important role in initiation and development of CRC. For instance, western-style diet with high fat is associated with increased CRC risk while grains and vegetables may help reduce CRC risk. Meanwhile, dietary intervention could reshape gut microbiota and alter the diet residues entering the colon. Thus, it makes diet and microbiome regulation a promising strategy in CRC prevention. With the evidence available now, a balanced diet is strongly suggested. Meanwhile, it is not encouraged to take too much animal fat frequently, especially through excessive cooking methods like grilling and barbecuing. Instead, fish, poultry, and milk consumption are encouraged.

Beneficial bacteria could also confer health benefit to the gut. Growing evidence has suggested that probiotics and their metabolites could inhibit CRC development. For example, *Streptococcus thermophilus*, which is identified to be depleted in patients with colorectal cancer (CRC) by shotgun metagenomic sequencing, inhibits colorectal tumorigenesis through secreting β-Galactosidase (Li et al. 2021). Furthermore, *Lactobacillus gallinarum*, another depleted bacterium in CRC patients, could protect against CRC through producing indole-3-lactic acid (ILA) which displayed anti-CRC growth in vitro and inhibited intestinal tumorigenesis in vivo (Sugimura et al. 2021).

Apart of dietary prevention and probiotics, antibiotic therapy may act as a way to prevent from colorectal tumorigenesis. Study has shown that antibiotics could alleviate high fat diet-associated CRC development (Yang et al. 2022). However, antibiotics also led to the depletion of most microbial species, thus may bring other health concerns. Yet, it is still not recommended for CRC prevention.

8.8 Conclusion

In this book chapter, the impacts of different diets on the gut microbiome in colorectal tumorigenesis are explored. Both cohort studies and animal experiments have shown different diet-associated signatures of gut microbiome alterations in colorectal tumorigenesis, and these signatures are of high potential to serve as non-invasive diagnostic biomarkers. However, more large-scale studies are warranted to ensure their accuracy. In conclusion, the gut microbiome plays a key role in the development of colorectal tumorigenesis; hence, direct modulation of gut microbiome by dietary intervention could be an ideal and feasible way for CRC treatment and prevention.

References

Arnold M, Sierra MS, Laversanne M, et al. Global patterns and trends in colorectal cancer incidence and mortality. Gut. 2017;66:683–91.

Arnold M, Abnet CC, Neale RE, et al. Global burden of 5 major types of gastrointestinal cancer. Gastroenterology. 2020;159:335–349.e15.

Beaumont M, Portune KJ, Steuer N, et al. Quantity and source of dietary protein influence metabolite production by gut microbiota and rectal mucosa gene expression: a randomized, parallel, double-blind trial in overweight humans. Am J Clin Nutr. 2017;106:1005–19.

Belcheva A, Irrazabal T, Robertson SJ, et al. Gut microbial metabolism drives transformation of MSH2-deficient colon epithelial cells. Cell. 2014;158:288–99.

Bostick RM, Potter JD, Kushi LH, et al. Sugar, meat, and fat intake, and non-dietary risk factors for colon cancer incidence in Iowa women (United States). Cancer Causes Control. 1994;5:38–52.

Brink M, Weijenberg MP, de Goeij AFPM, et al. Fat and K-ras mutations in sporadic colorectal cancer in the Netherlands cohort study. Carcinogenesis. 2004;25:1619–28.

Burkitt DP. Epidemiology of cancer of the colon and rectum. Cancer. 1971;28:3–13.

Butler LM, Wang R, Koh WP, et al. Prospective study of dietary patterns and colorectal cancer among Singapore Chinese. Br J Cancer. 2008;99:1511–6.

Butler LM, Wang R, Koh WP, et al. Marine n-3 and saturated fatty acids in relation to risk of colorectal cancer in Singapore Chinese: a prospective study. Int J Cancer. 2009;124:678–86.

Castellarin M, Warren RL, Freeman JD, et al. Fusobacterium nucleatum infection is prevalent in human colorectal carcinoma. Genome Res. 2012;22:299–306.

Chomchai C, Bhadrachari N, Nigro ND. The effect of bile on the induction of experimental intestinal tumors in rats. Dis Colon Rectum. 1974;17:310–2.

Chyou PH, Nomura AMY, Stemmermann GN. A prospective study of colon and rectal cancer among Hawaii Japanese men. Ann Epidemiol. 1996;6:276–82.

Clay SL, Fonseca-Pereira D, Garrett WS. Colorectal cancer: the facts in the case of the microbiota. J Clin Invest. 2022;132:e155101.
Dai Z, Coker OO, Nakatsu G, et al. Multi-cohort analysis of colorectal cancer metagenome identified altered bacteria across populations and universal bacterial markers. Microbiome. 2018;6:70.
De Filippo C, Cavalieri D, Di Paola M, et al. Impact of diet in shaping gut microbiota revealed by a comparative study in children from Europe and rural Africa. Proc Natl Acad Sci U S A. 2010;107:14691–6.
De Vadder F, Kovatcheva-Datchary P, Goncalves D, et al. Microbiota-generated metabolites promote metabolic benefits via gut-brain neural circuits. Cell. 2014;156:84–96.
Doll R, Peto R. The causes of cancer: quantitative estimates of avoidable risks of cancer in the United States today. J Natl Cancer Inst. 1981;66:1191–308.
Drasar BS, Irving D. Environmental factors and cancer of the colon and breast. Br J Cancer. 1973;27:167–72.
Flood A, Velie EM, Sinha R, et al. Meat, fat, and their subtypes as risk factors for colorectal cancer in a prospective cohort of women. Am J Epidemiol. 2003;158:59–68.
Fu T, Coulter S, Yoshihara E, et al. FXR regulates intestinal cancer stem cell proliferation. Cell. 2019;176:1098–1112.e18.
Gaard M, Tretli S, Loken EB. Dietary factors and risk of colon cancer: a prospective study of 50,535 young Norwegian men and women. Eur J Cancer Prev. 1996;5:445–54.
Giovannucci E, Rimm EB, Stampfer MJ, et al. Intake of fat, meat, and fiber in relation to risk of colon-cancer in men. Cancer Res. 1994;54:2390–7.
Goldbohm RA, Vandenbrandt PA, Vantveer P, et al. A prospective cohort study on the relation between meat consumption and the risk of colon-cancer. Cancer Res. 1994;54:718–23.
Guo XL, Li JC, Tang RY, et al. High fat diet alters gut microbiota and the expression of Paneth cell-antimicrobial peptides preceding changes of circulating inflammatory cytokines. Mediat Inflamm. 2017;2017:9474896.
Heilbrun LK, Nomura A, Hankin JH, et al. Diet and colorectal cancer with special reference to fiber intake. Int J Cancer. 1989;44:1–6.
Jarvinen R, Knekt P, Hakulinen T, et al. Dietary fat, cholesterol and colorectal cancer in a prospective study. Br J Cancer. 2001;85:357–61.
Kabat GC, Shikany JM, Beresford SA, et al. Dietary carbohydrate, glycemic index, and glycemic load in relation to colorectal cancer risk in the Women's Health Initiative. Cancer Causes Control. 2008;19:1291–8.
Kato I, Akhmedkhanov A, Koenig K, et al. Prospective study of diet and female colorectal cancer: the New York University Women's Health Study. Nutr Cancer. 1997;28:276–81.
Li Q, Hu W, Liu WX, et al. Streptococcus thermophilus inhibits colorectal tumorigenesis through secreting beta-galactosidase. Gastroenterology. 2021;160:1179–1193.e14.
Liang Q, Chiu J, Chen Y, et al. Fecal bacteria act as novel biomarkers for noninvasive diagnosis of colorectal cancer. Clin Cancer Res. 2017;23:2061–70.
Liang JQ, Li T, Nakatsu G, et al. A novel faecal Lachnoclostridium marker for the non-invasive diagnosis of colorectal adenoma and cancer. Gut. 2020;69:1248–57.
Lin J, Zhang SM, Cook NR, et al. Dietary fat and fatty acids and risk of colorectal cancer in women. Am J Epidemiol. 2004;160:1011–22.
Lin H, An YP, Tang HR, et al. Alterations of bile acids and gut microbiota in obesity induced by high fat diet in rat model. J Agric Food Chem. 2019;67:3624–32.
Mai V, Flood A, Peters U, et al. Dietary fibre and risk of colorectal cancer in the breast cancer detection demonstration project (BCDDP) follow-up cohort. Int J Epidemiol. 2003;32:234–9.
Makishima M, Okamoto AY, Repa JJ, et al. Identification of a nuclear receptor for bile acids. Science. 1999;284:1362–5.
McCullough ML, Robertson AS, Chao A, et al. A prospective study of whole grains, fruits, vegetables and colon cancer risk. Cancer Causes Control. 2003;14:959–70.

Michels KB, Fuchs CS, Giovannucci E, et al. Fiber intake and incidence of colorectal cancer among 76,947 women and 47,279 men. Cancer Epidemiol Biomark Prev. 2005;14:842–9.
Nakatsu G, Li XC, Zhou HK, et al. Gut mucosal microbiome across stages of colorectal carcinogenesis. Nat Commun. 2015;6:8727.
Narisawa T, Magadia NE, Weisburger JH, et al. Promoting effect of bile-acids on colon carcinogenesis after intrarectal instillation of N-methyl-N'-nitro-N-nitrosoguanidine in rats. J Natl Cancer Inst. 1974;53:1093–7.
Nguyen LH, Cao Y, Hur J, et al. The sulfur microbial diet is associated with increased risk of early-onset colorectal cancer precursors. Gastroenterology. 2021;161:1423–1432.e4.
Nomura AM, Hankin JH, Henderson BE, et al. Dietary fiber and colorectal cancer risk: the multiethnic cohort study. Cancer Causes Control. 2007;18:753–64.
O'Keefe SJ, Li JV, Lahti L, et al. Fat, fibre and cancer risk in African Americans and rural Africans. Nat Commun. 2015;6:6342.
Oba S, Shimizu N, Nagata C, et al. The relationship between the consumption of meat, fat, and coffee and the risk of colon cancer: a prospective study in Japan. Cancer Lett. 2006;244:260–7.
Otani T, Iwasaki M, Ishihara J, et al. Dietary fiber intake and subsequent risk of colorectal cancer: the Japan Public Health Center-based prospective study. Int J Cancer. 2006;119:1475–80.
Ou J, Carbonero F, Zoetendal EG, et al. Diet, microbiota, and microbial metabolites in colon cancer risk in rural Africans and African Americans. Am J Clin Nutr. 2013;98:111–20.
Parks DJ, Blanchard SG, Bledsoe RK, et al. Bile acids: natural ligands for an orphan nuclear receptor. Science. 1999;284:1365–8.
Pietinen P, Malila N, Virtanen M, et al. Diet and risk of colorectal cancer in a cohort of Finnish men. Cancer Causes Control. 1999;10:387–96.
Rijnkels JM, Hollanders VM, Woutersen RA, et al. Interaction of dietary fat and of a vegetables/fruit mixture on 1,2-dimethylhydrazine- or N-methyl-N'-nitro-N-nitrosoguanidine-induced colorectal cancer in rats. Cancer Lett. 1997;114:297–8.
Rothschild D, Weissbrod O, Barkan E, et al. Environment dominates over host genetics in shaping human gut microbiota. Nature. 2018;555:210–5.
Sanjoaquin MA, Appleby PN, Thorogood M, et al. Nutrition, lifestyle and colorectal cancer incidence: a prospective investigation of 10 998 vegetarians and non-vegetarians in the United Kingdom. Br J Cancer. 2004;90:118–21.
Shin A, Li H, Shu XO, et al. Dietary intake of calcium, fiber and other micronutrients in relation to colorectal cancer risk: results from the Shanghai Women's Health Study. Int J Cancer. 2006;119:2938–42.
Siegel RL, Miller KD, Goding Sauer A, et al. Colorectal cancer statistics, 2020. CA Cancer J Clin. 2020;70:145–64.
Silvester KR, Cummings JH. Does digestibility of meat protein help explain large-bowel cancer risk. Nutr Cancer. 1995;24:279–88.
Singh V, Yeoh BS, Chassaing B, et al. Dysregulated microbial fermentation of soluble fiber induces cholestatic liver cancer. Cell. 2018;175:679–694.e22.
Sodring M, Oostindjer M, Egelandsdal B, et al. Effects of hemin and nitrite on intestinal tumorigenesis in the A/J Min/plus mouse model. PLoS One. 2015;10:e0122880.
Steliou K, Boosalis MS, Perrine SP, et al. Butyrate histone deacetylase inhibitors. Biores Open Access. 2012;1:192–8.
Stemmermann GN, Nomura AM, Heilbrun LK. Dietary fat and the risk of colorectal cancer. Cancer Res. 1984;44:4633–7.
Sugimura N, Li Q, Chu ESH, et al. Lactobacillus gallinarum modulates the gut microbiota and produces anti-cancer metabolites to protect against colorectal tumourigenesis. Gut. 2021;71(10):2011–21.
Sung H, Ferlay J, Siegel RL, et al. Global cancer statistics 2020: GLOBOCAN estimates of incidence and mortality worldwide for 36 cancers in 185 countries. CA Cancer J Clin. 2021;71:209–49.

Taira T, Yamaguchi S, Takahashi A, et al. Dietary polyphenols increase fecal mucin and immunoglobulin A and ameliorate the disturbance in gut microbiota caused by a high fat diet. J Clin Biochem Nutr. 2015;57:212–6.

Terry P, Bergkvist L, Holmberg L, et al. No association between fat and fatty acids intake and risk of colorectal cancer. Cancer Epidemiol Biomark Prev. 2001;10:913–4.

Wang HB, Chen J, Hollister K, et al. Endogenous bile acids are ligands for the nuclear receptor FXR BAR. Mol Cell. 1999;3:543–53.

Wang B, Rong X, Palladino END, et al. Phospholipid remodeling and cholesterol availability regulate intestinal stemness and tumorigenesis. Cell Stem Cell. 2018;22:206–220.e4.

Weijenberg MP, Luchtenborg M, de Goeij AF, et al. Dietary fat and risk of colon and rectal cancer with aberrant MLH1 expression, APC or KRAS genes. Cancer Causes Control. 2007;18:865–79.

Willett WC, Stampfer MJ, Colditz GA, et al. Relation of meat, fat, and Fiber intake to the risk of colon cancer in a prospective-study among women. N Engl J Med. 1990;323:1664–72.

Windey K, De Preter V, Verbeke K. Relevance of protein fermentation to gut health. Mol Nutr Food Res. 2012;56:184–96.

Wong SH, Kwong TNY, Chow TC, et al. Quantitation of faecal fusobacterium improves faecal immunochemical test in detecting advanced colorectal neoplasia. Gut. 2017;66:1441–8.

World Cancer Research Fund, American Institute for Cancer Research. The Continuous Update Project Expert Report. Diet, nutrition, physical activity and cancer: colorectal cancer. 2018.

Wu Y, Jiao N, Zhu R, et al. Identification of microbial markers across populations in early detection of colorectal cancer. Nat Commun. 2021;12:3063.

Xu Z, Knight R. Dietary effects on human gut microbiome diversity. Br J Nutr. 2015;113 Suppl:S1–5.

Yang J, Wei H, Zhou Y, et al. High-fat diet promotes colorectal tumorigenesis through modulating gut microbiota and metabolites. Gastroenterology. 2022;162:135–149.e2.

Yu J, Feng Q, Wong SH, et al. Metagenomic analysis of faecal microbiome as a tool towards targeted non-invasive biomarkers for colorectal cancer. Gut. 2017;66:70–8.

Zhang X, Coker OO, Chu ES, et al. Dietary cholesterol drives fatty liver-associated liver cancer by modulating gut microbiota and metabolites. Gut. 2021;70:761–74.

Zimmer J, Lange B, Frick JS, et al. A vegan or vegetarian diet substantially alters the human colonic faecal microbiota. Eur J Clin Nutr. 2012;66:53–60.

Chapter 9
Diet Modulates Gut Microbiome and Metabolites in Non-alcoholic Fatty Liver Diseases

Yasi Pan and Xiang Zhang

Abstract Non-alcoholic fatty liver disease (NAFLD) is the most prevalent chronic liver disease globally. NAFLD is a spectrum disease ranging from simple steatosis, non-alcoholic steatohepatitis (NASH), fibrosis/cirrhosis to hepatocellular carcinoma (HCC). Although the mechanism of NAFLD progression to HCC is obscure, increasing evidence suggested that gut microbiome and its metabolites play an important role. Diet is one of the strongest factors that could change gut microbiota composition. Diet could rapidly and reproducibly change the human gut microbiome and modulate multiple metabolic pathways. Dietary cholesterol, fiber, fat, or carbohydrate could reshape the microbiome composition to contribute to the progression of NASH and NAFLD-HCC. Hence, the identification of gut–liver axis elements that are primarily impaired in NASH and NAFLD-HCC opens up new avenues for therapeutic intervention. In this book chapter, we first covered the role of the gut microbiome and microbial metabolites in the pathogenesis and progression of NAFLD and NAFLD-HCC. The impacts of various dietary components, such as cholesterol, fat, sugar, protein, and fiber on the gut microbiome which contribute to susceptibility to NASH and NAFLD-HCC are also explored. We finally summarized the article by discussing potential therapeutic implication of diet and microbiome modulation in fatty liver and liver cancer.

Keywords Diet · Gut microbiome · Non-alcoholic steatohepatitis · Hepatocellular carcinoma

Y. Pan · X. Zhang (✉)
Institute of Digestive Disease and the Department of Medicine and Therapeutics, State Key Laboratory of Digestive Disease, Li Ka Shing Institute of Health Sciences, The Chinese University of Hong Kong, Hong Kong, China
e-mail: jenniferzhang@link.cuhk.edu.hk; yasipan@link.cuhk.edu.hk

J. Yu (ed.), *Microbiome in Gastrointestinal Cancer*,
https://doi.org/10.1007/978-981-19-4492-5_9

Abbreviations

DCA	Deoxycholic acid
FMT	Fecal microbiota transplantation
FXR	Farnesoid X receptor
HCC	Hepatocellular carcinoma
LPS	Lipopolysaccharide
NAFLD	Non-alcoholic fatty liver disease
NASH	Non-alcoholic steatohepatitis
PAMPs	Pathogen-associated molecular patterns
PUFA	Polyunsaturated fatty acids
SCFAs	Short chain fatty acids
TMAVA	N,N,N-trimethyl-5-aminovaleric acid
VLDL	Very low-density lipoprotein

9.1 Introduction

Non-alcoholic fatty liver disease (NAFLD) is an increasingly important disease worldwide due to the sedentary lifestyle and overnutrition (Younossi et al. 2016). The prevalence of NAFLD in the Middle East was reported to be the highest (32%), followed by South America (31%), Asia (27%), and Europe (23%), whereas Africa has the lowest prevalence (13%) (Lonardo et al. 2016). In general, the number of NAFLD cases has been rapidly increasing in developed regions or countries where people are more likely to have unhealthy lifestyles and suffer from metabolic disorders including obesity, diabetes, and hypertriglyceridemia which are well-acknowledged risk factors of NAFLD. The prevalence of NAFLD in patients with type 2 diabetes was 47.3–63.7%, while 80% of obese people suffer from NAFLD (Polyzos et al. 2019; Younossi et al. 2019a). Notably, some people with a healthy body mass index can still develop NAFLD which is often described as non-obese or lean NAFLD, suggesting that other factors such as overall caloric intake, body fat distribution, physical activity, and genetic composition may also contribute to the onset NAFLD (Ye et al. 2020). In 2020, International experts have proposed a new definition—metabolic dysfunction-associated fatty liver disease (MAFLD), which is defined as the evidence of hepatic steatosis and one of the following criteria, obesity, type 2 diabetes, or other evidence of metabolic dysregulation (Eslam et al. 2020a, b). However, a debate raised considering that changing nomenclature may affect the drug development in pharmaceutical industry and provide limited clinical benefit. Therefore, we keep using the term NAFLD in the current chapter.

NAFLD comprised of a spectrum of diseases from simple steatosis, steatohepatitis (NASH), fibrosis/cirrhosis, which may further develop to hepatocellular carcinoma (HCC) (Chalasani et al. 2018). About 10% of patients with NAFLD gradually develop cirrhotic complications and the end-stage HCC in 10–20 years after diagnosis, one of the most common cancer malignancies worldwide (Ekstedt et al. 2015). Although the incidence of HCC is relatively low, it is expected to increase sharply in the near future due to the substantial number of NAFLD cases. NASH-associated liver mortality is expected to increase more than double in the next decade due to epidemics of obesity and diabetes (Estes et al. 2018; Zhang 2018).

Gut microbiome has been considered one of the driving roles in host digestion and metabolic processes (Ho et al. 2015). Recently, accumulated evidence has demonstrated the crucial influence of gut microbiome in organs beyond the intestine (Ezzaidi et al. 2019). Liver is the primary recipient of gut microbes-derived products via portal vein, taking up 70% of the blood supply of liver, thus showing the crucial and extensive communication between intestine and liver (Saeedi et al. 2020). Evidence supported that gut microbiome contributes to several liver diseases, such as oxidative liver injury (Saeedi et al. 2020), steatosis (Hoyles et al. 2018), NASH (Wong et al. 2013a; Naudin et al. 2020), cirrhosis (Qin et al. 2014), and HCC (Ma et al. 2018; Ponziani et al. 2019). And diet could reshape our gut microbiome. We previously reported that high-cholesterol diet promotes NASH and NAFLD-related liver cancer (NAFLD-HCC) through microbiome dysbiosis and gut metabolite alteration (Zhang et al. 2021). In addition to cholesterol, dietary fiber, fat, protein, and sugar have important impacts on the microbial diversity and microbiome composition. These alterations might lead to the pathogenesis of inflammatory liver disease including NASH and NAFLD-HCC (Makki et al. 2018; Berna and Romero-Gomez 2020). Conversely, intake of vegetables, fruits, and vitamin K could effectively reduce the risk of NAFLD development (Chan et al. 2015; Han et al. 2014). These findings suggest the importance of a balanced diet for preventing the development of NAFLD. Here, we discuss how dietary composition affects gut microbial ecology and contributes to susceptibility to NASH and liver cancer.

9.2 Microbiome and Gut Barrier Dysfunction in NAFLD

Gut microbiota dysbiosis is one of the driving forces in the development of a variety of liver diseases, including simple steatosis, NASH, and NAFLD-HCC (Moschen et al. 2013). Indeed, steatosis patients already exhibit features of gut dysbiosis with reduced microbial diversity and enrichments in certain species related to insulin resistance, such as *Acidaminococcus*, *Escherichia spp.*, and *Bacteroides spp.* (Hoyles et al. 2018; Pedersen et al. 2016). Gut dysbiosis is also found in NASH, NASH-cirrhosis and NAFLD-HCC. NASH patients had increased abundance of *Parabacteroides,* while the abundance of *Faecalibacterium* and *Anaerosporobacter* were reduced (Wong et al. 2013a). NASH-cirrhosis patients displayed a higher abundance of *Enterobacteriaceae* and *Streptococcus* and reduced abundance of *Akkermansia*. NASH-HCC patients showed the enrichment of *Bacteroides* and *Ruminococcacea*e, while *Bifidobacterium* was depleted (Ponziani et al. 2019). Both *Akkermansia* and *Bifidobacterium* play protective roles in liver injury, and their depletions could enhance inflammation in intestine and liver to contribute to liver

(Wu et al. 2017; Fang et al. 2017). Metagenomic sequencing analysis showed that five bacterial species, *Bacteroides caecimuris, Ruminococcus gnavus*, *Veillonella parvula, Bacterodies xylanisolvens,* and *Clostridium bolteae,* were enriched in the gut of NAFLD-HCC patients, and all of them are correlated with immunomodulatory activities (Behary et al. 2021). Moreover, other studies demonstrated that *Bacteroides and Ruminococcus* are associated with inflammation and pro-inflammatory markers (Ponziani et al. 2019; Behary et al. 2021). Therefore, these findings clearly indicate that gut microbiome dysbiosis is involved in different stages of NAFLD progression. However, it should be noted that the gut microbiome is influenced by various environmental factors, thus results among microbial profiling studies can be greatly varied.

Gut barrier dysfunction is a key mechanistic factor in microbiome-driven NASH progression. Microbial commensals are components of gut barrier that prevent pathogenic microbes from entering the portal vein (Chopyk and Grakoui 2020). Toxic metabolites produced by gut microbes may impair gut barrier function. Once the gut barrier is disrupted, bacteria and pathogen-associated molecular patterns (PAMPs) including lipopolysaccharides (LPS) can translocate to liver through the leaky gut, thereby activating pathogen recognition receptors and inducing immune response to promote NASH and HCC progression (Chopyk and Grakoui 2020; Dapito et al. 2012). Indeed, mice with intestinal permeability defects develop more severe steatohepatitis with increased steatosis, lobular inflammation, hepatocellular ballooning, and fibrosis (Rahman et al. 2016). Recent study reported that impaired gut barrier function, which allows bacterial translocation to the liver, is an early event in the progression of NASH (Mouries et al. 2019).

Besides of gut microbes, bacterial DNA was also detected in liver tissues of NAFLD patients with direct correlation with disease severity (Sookoian et al. 2020). In particular, *Peptostreptococcaceae, Verrucomicrobia, Actinobacteria,* and *Gamma Proteobacteria* in liver tissue were closely associated with the severity of NAFLD. These results indicate that translocation of gut bacteria could be detrimental to liver as well as hepatopathogenesis. Nevertheless, investigation of microbes in liver tissues is currently at an early stage with inadequate evidence proving their contribution to the development of NAFLD, NASH, or other liver diseases. Further studies are therefore needed to clarify whether bacteria could be cultivated from a NASH liver and how intrahepatic bacterial components are involved in the pathophysiology of NASH and NAFLD-HCC.

9.3 Microbial Metabolites in NAFLD

Microbial metabolites, including amino acids, SCFAs, and bile acids, play an important role in the development of NAFLD and NAFLD-HCC (Zhao et al. 2020a). For instance, non-diabetic obese women with hepatic steatosis were found to have dysregulated aromatic and branched-chain amino acid metabolism (Hoyles et al. 2018). N,N,N-trimethyl-5-aminovaleric acid, a metabolite of intestinal microbes metabolized from trimethyllysine, could reduce carnitine synthesis and fatty acid oxidation, thereby exacerbating NAFLD development (Zhao et al. 2020a).

Bile acid is a key component in gut–liver axis. Bile acid receptor (farnesoid X receptor) activator obeticholic acid could significantly ameliorate fibrosis and disease severity of NASH patients in a phase 3 clinical trial (Younossi et al. 2019b). In general, primary bile acids secreted from liver are unconjugated by gut microbes, and these unconjugated bile acids are reabsorbed to form secondary bile acid and sent back to liver for detoxification (Jia et al. 2018). Gut dysbiosis especially enrichment of *Clostridium* in obesity and NASH could induce the secretion of deoxycholic acid (DCA), a secondary bile acid that is famous to cause DNA damage (Yoshimoto et al. 2013). Increased DCA in liver could also provoke senescence-associated secretory phenotype to promote the secretion of various inflammatory and tumor-promoting factors, thus further boosting HCC development (Yoshimoto et al. 2013).

SCFAs comprised of formate, acetate, propionate, and butyrate. Of note, reports on the abundance and function of SCFAs in NAFLD and its related diseases have been controversial. A study involving 72 biopsy-proven NAFLD and 14 NAFLD-fibrosis patients demonstrated that fecal abundances of SCFAs are significantly different in these two groups: enriched acetate and formate in NAFLD patients, whereas butyrate and propionate were increased in NAFLD-fibrosis group (Loomba et al. 2017). However, another study revealed that fecal formate, acetate, and butyrate were all significantly increased in NAFLD-HCC patients compared with NAFLD-cirrhosis patients and healthy controls (Behary et al. 2021). Butyrate has been reported to protect against diet-induced NASH development in mice (Jin et al. 2015), while acetate could induce de novo lipogenesis through activating lipogenic genes (Gao et al. 2016). Nevertheless, diet and other environmental factors may greatly contribute to the result inconsistency among different results. Further mechanistic studies need to be performed to clarify the role of SCFAs in NAFLD and its related liver disease.

9.4 Diet Modulates Gut Microbiome to Influence NAFLD

Accumulating evidence has shown that gut microbiome could promote western diet-induced systemic pathologies. In turn, western-style diet, a dietary combination with high contents of sugar, fat, protein, and cholesterol and low in fiber, could alter the gut microbiome (David et al. 2014). Given the interaction between diet and gut microbiome, they are both crucial factors for the development of NASH and NAFLD-HCC (Fig. 9.1).

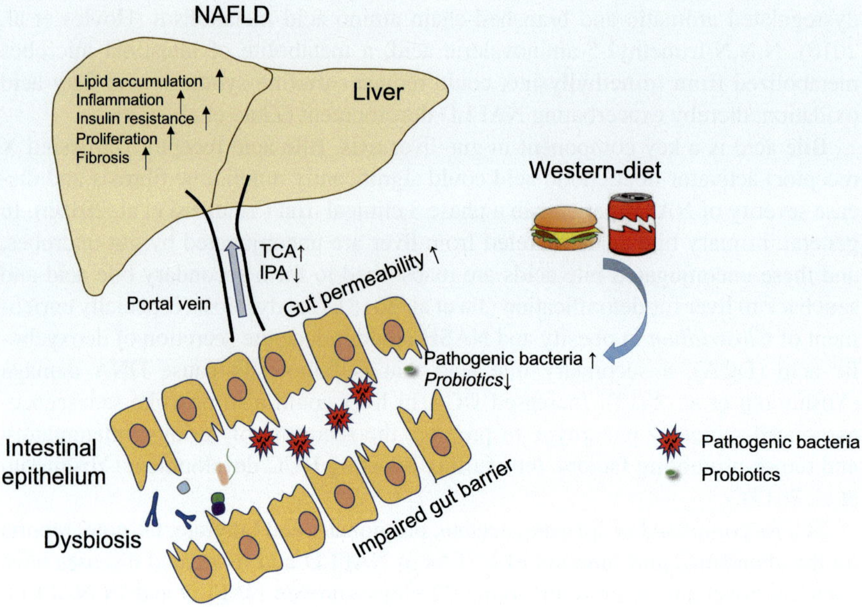

Fig. 9.1 The Western diet is characterized by increased intake of red meat, high-fat, and high-fructose diets. Western diets high in fat, cholesterol, protein, or sugar lead to gut microbiota dysbiosis, decreased probiotics, increased pathogenic bacteria, altered metabolites, and increased gut permeability, resulting in impaired gut barrier. Translocated bacteria and toxic metabolites induce lipid accumulation, inflammation, insulin resistance, and tumorigenesis, thereby promoting the development of NAFLD and its associated HCC. TCA, Taurocholic acid; IPA, 3-indolepropionic acid

9.4.1 Cholesterol and Gut Microbiome in NASH and NAFLD-HCC

Epidemiology statistics have reported the significant positive correlation between cholesterol intake and the risk of cirrhosis and liver cancer (Ioannou et al. 2009). Preclinical studies also showed that animals (including mice, rats, and rabbits) with consumption of high-cholesterol diet have increased incidence of fatty liver (Wouters et al. 2008; Lai et al. 2016; Liaw et al. 2014). Mechanically, excess cholesterol is usually stored in intracellular oil droplets in the form of cholesteryl esters. At the same time, the synthesis of triglycerides which is conducive to the formation of very low-density lipoprotein (VLDL) is also stimulated. However, if VLDL cannot be effectively composed, cholesterol and triglycerides are secreted into the circulation, causing lipids to accumulate in liver cells. Therefore, it is expected that excess intake of cholesterol could increase the chance of fatty liver development. As cholesterol intake is closely associated with elevated risk of NAFLD, reducing the content of cholesterol in diet is extremely important in NAFLD prevention.

In our previous study, for the first time we showed that dietary cholesterol plays a crucial role in NASH-HCC progression by modulating gut microbiome, of which cholesterol-modulated gut microbiome could induce steatohepatitis and liver cells proliferation in germ-free mice (Zhang et al. 2021). High-cholesterol diet increased abundances of *Mucispirillum, Desulfovibrio, Anaerotruncus,* and *Desulfovibrionaceae*; while probiotic *Bifidobacterium* and *Bacteroides* were depleted. Consistently, high-cholesterol diet increased serum level of taurocholic acid and decreased 3-indolepropionic acid which enter the liver through portal vein and regulate NAFLD-HCC. When transplanting feces from high-cholesterol fed mice into germ-free mice, hepatic inflammation, lipid accumulation, and hepatocyte proliferation were successfully triggered (Zhang et al. 2021). Hence, these results implicate that without an intact gut microbiome, the effect of cholesterol to induce metabolic disease could be different or even totally abolished. In another study by Kubeck et al., they found that germ-free mice receiving cholesterol-rich based high-fat diet could completely reverse diet-induced obesity, suggesting that dietary cholesterol protects germ-free mice from obesity through the absence of gut microbiome (Kubeck et al. 2016). When investigating the metabolic fate of dietary cholesterol, gut *Clostridium* was found to have a positive correlation with bile acid level (Kubeck et al. 2016). Collectively, dietary cholesterol plays a crucial role in NASH and NAFLD-HCC development through modulating gut microbiome.

On the other hand, gut microbiome could also regulate cholesterol homeostasis. Antibiotic treatment decreases the circulating and hepatic cholesterol levels, indicating the crucial role of gut microbiome in cholesterol metabolism (Le Roy et al. 2019). Moreover, research by Kenny and colleagues identified a group of coprostanol-forming microbes, which converse cholesterol to sterol coprostanol and reduce gut and serum cholesterol levels (Kenny et al. 2020). Therefore, cholesterol and gut microbiome interact with each other and contribute to NAFLD progression.

9.4.2 Fat and Gut Microbiome in NASH and NAFLD-HCC

Recent studies indicated that fat could have diverse effects on NAFLD and NASH. Most studies showed evidence that high-fat diet triggered NAFLD via various possible mechanisms, including mitochondrial dysfunction (Zhang et al. 2015), increasing inflammatory responses (Wang et al. 2015), endoplasmic reticulum stress (Lebeaupin et al. 2018), and gut microbiota dysbiosis (Le Roy et al. 2013; Kashtanova et al. 2018). However, research also provided evidence that diets enriched with omega-3 polyunsaturated fatty acids (PUFA) prevented the development of insulin resistance (Storlien et al. 1987), ameliorated hepatic steatosis (Sekiya et al. 2003), and decreased intrahepatic triglyceride storage (Levy et al. 2004) in obese rodents. But in human, overconsumption of PUFA and saturated fatty acids could significantly promote fat accumulation in liver (Zelber-Sagi et al. 2007; Rosqvist et al. 2014). While in contrast, another study involving 355 individuals showed that PUFA supplementation could in turn decrease liver fat accumulation (Parker et al. 2012). Hence, although preclinical studies have shown benefits of fat consumption in the prevention of fatty liver diseases, more in-depth investigation is necessary to confirm these effects in human.

The crosstalk between dietary fat and gut microbiome has long been of interest. A large-scale dietary intervention study involving 88 human subjects provided evidence that high-fat diet could reduce microbial diversity and richness (Fava et al. 2013). Mechanically, administration of high-fat diet significantly reduces abundances of dominant members of the gut microbiome in mice such as *Bacteroides spp.*, *Eu. rectale-Cl. coccoides* group and *Bifidobacterium*, and induces insulin resistance in bacterial lipopolysaccharide (LPS)-dependent manner (Cani et al. 2007). In another animal study, mice treated with high-fat diet showed enrichment of *Enterobacterales*, which was correlated with the obese phenotype (Mujico et al. 2013). However, supplementing oleic acid-derived compounds to these mice could restore bacterial diversity (increased *Enterobacterales* and decreased *Bifidobacterium spp.*) and counteract microbiome imbalance caused by high-fat diet (Mujico et al. 2013). Similar findings were also reported in other studies (Robertson et al. 2018; Lam et al. 2015), suggesting that certain fatty acids could have protective roles against obesity through altering the gut microbiome. Indeed, supplementation of different types of fats can lead to diverse changes in the gut microbiome. A clinical trial was conducted with supplementation of different types of high-fat diet to 25 subjects at risk of metabolic syndrome. Diets rich in monounsaturated fatty acids (e.g., conventional canola oil, oleic canola oil) showed significant enrichment of *Parabacteroides*, while PUFA-rich diets (a blend of corn/safflower oil or flax/safflower oil) favored high abundance of *Isobaculum* (Pu et al. 2016). Recent study from our group showed that high-fat diet increased *Alistipes sp. Marseille-P5997 and Alistipes sp. 5CPEGH6* accompanied with elevated metabolite lysophosphatidic acid, and depleted probiotic *Parabacteroides distasonis* (Yang et al. 2022). Of note, there is not much known about the functional and mechanistic roles of these altered gut microbiome, thus further in-depth investigation of these microbes in the development of obesity and NAFLD is needed. In summary, extensive study is needed to identify specific types of fat as well as gut microbes that are associated with risk of NAFLD, and reduction in total fat intake is still too early to be the simple solution for NAFLD and NASH patients.

9.4.3 Sugar and Gut Microbiome in NASH and NAFLD-HCC

Dietary sugar is usually obtained from sucrose, high-fructose corn syrup and sugary beverages, which all have been shown to have particular tendency to induce NAFLD in epidemiological (Ouyang et al. 2008; Mosca et al. 2017; Hamza et al. 2016; O'Sullivan et al. 2014) and preclinical studies (Softic et al. 2017; Cho et al. 2021; Roncal-Jimenez et al. 2011; Sanchez-Lozada et al. 2010). While fructose metabolism that takes place in mouse gut could disrupt intestinal barrier to increase permeability (Cho et al. 2021; Johnson et al. 2013), thereby contributing to the development of NAFLD. Indeed, when treated mice with antibiotics, fatty liver could be improved by reducing endotoxemia (Bergheim et al. 2008). Dietary fructose could also reshape the gut microbial community to favor NAFLD development. Bouriser et al. observed that the severity of human NAFLD is associated with the changes in metabolic functions of gut microbiome with increased abundance of *Bacteroides* in NASH (Boursier et al. 2016), of which *Bacteroides* was shown to have strong positive correlation with fecal content of raffinose and stachyose (containing glucose and fructose) (Boursier et al. 2016; Jensen et al. 2018). In another study, Kathryn and colleagues found that fructose consumption triggers hepatic de novo lipogenesis depending on the microbes-mediated metabolism of fructose to produce acetate, which is then consumed in lipogenic pools of acetyl-CoA (Zhao et al. 2020b). Gut microbes also produce other SCFAs such as butyrate, which has been confirmed as a contributor to hepatic lipogenesis (den Besten et al. 2013). Taken together, the convincing evidence demonstrated that sugar especially fructose intake increases the risk of NAFLD development. Nevertheless, extensive clinical trials and mechanistic studies are urgently needed to confirm the direct interaction between dietary fructose and gut microbiome.

9.4.4 Protein and Gut Microbiome in NAFLD and NAFLD-HCC

Dietary protein is essential nutrient for human. It could ferment bacterial metabolites in the colon (Geypens et al. 1997) and modify colon luminal content and epithelial cell morphology in rat (Andriamihaja et al. 2010). Recently, Tan et al. identified increased abundance of *Actinobacteria* and *Bifidobacterium* in the small intestine of high protein-fed mice. The gut microbiota-derived extracellular vesicles by dietary protein promote host sIgA production, inducing host-microbiota mutualism. Lang et al. confirmed the association of high protein intake and gut microbiota alteration. They found low abundance of *Bacteroides* in subjects with high-fat diet intake, which is correlated with more activate and severe NAFLD (Lang et al. 2020). However, the in-depth mechanism of how high protein and amino acid play a detrimental role to NAFLD through gut microbiome dysbiosis need further investigation.

9.4.5 Fiber and Gut Microbiome in NASH and NAFLD-HCC

Based on its solubility in water, fiber can be divided into soluble fibers (e.g., pectin, inulin) and insoluble cellulose (e.g., cellulose). Dietary fiber could induce the production of SCFA-producing bacteria which may suppress metabolic syndrome (Zhao et al. 2018). Recent evidence revealed that fiber consumption could play a crucial role in NAFLD—not only as a part of balanced diet, but also involved in the modulation of gut microbiome. Gut microbes ferment dietary soluble fibers into SCFAs (Canfora et al. 2019), playing an important role in metabolic function. In particular, inulin-type fructans prebiotics could increase abundances of probiotic *Bifidobacterium* and *Faecalibacterium* in obese women to improve host metabolism (Dewulf et al. 2013). In a randomized clinical trial, dietary fiber intake significantly improved hepatic steatosis and liver function by ameliorating intestinal permeability of 32 NAFLD patients (Krawczyk et al. 2018). A high-fiber diet also enriched beneficial microbes (e.g., *Bifidobacteria*), depleted potential detrimental microbes, and reduced the ratio of *Firmicutes/Bacteroides* in both humans and mice (Yang et al. 2020). Another cross-sectional study showed that daily ingestion of 16 g of oligofructose, one of soluble prebiotic dietary fiber, improved hepatic enzymes and insulin levels in NASH patients (Daubioul et al. 2005; Parnell et al. 2012). Whereas Cantero et al. (2017) reported that consumption of insoluble fibers (≥7.5 g/day), rather than soluble fibers could also ameliorate hepatic steatosis and NAFLD.

However, the effects of fiber consumption on host metabolism could be varied among individuals (Healey et al. 2017). To address this issue, a preclinical study colonized mice with feces collected from different human subjects with supplementation of any one type of fiber (cellulose, inulin, pectin, or assorted fiber). As expected, mice harboring diverse human-derived microbiomes resulted in different metabolic outcomes even though they were fed with the same dietary fiber. Hence, dietary fiber could benefit certain microbiome but not all microbiome composition (Healey et al. 2017). Dietary fiber was also found to have disturbing effects. *Singh* et al. reported that soluble fiber inulin could induce HCC in a microbiome-dependent manner (Singh et al. 2018), of which high-fat high-inulin diet led to gut dysbiosis with enrichments of fiber-fermenting bacteria and *Proteobacteria.* Thus, supplementation of foods with high content of fermentable fibers should be approached with great caution as it may in turn increase the risk of HCC. In general, one-fits-all fiber supplementation is unlikely to have consistent effect among individuals, therefore indicating that clinicians need to consider whether fiber supplementation could optimize treatment outcomes. Another critical issue is that, to date, no studies have shown solid evidence to confirm whether patients with advanced NAFLD could be benefited from high-fiber intake.

9.5 Modulation of Diet and Microbiome in Preventing NAFLD and NAFLD-HCC

Although being prevalent, western diet with high contents of red meat, fat, and fructose favors the development of NAFLD. While the Mediterranean diet, characterized by low consumption of red meat, dairy products and saturated fats and high intakes of vegetables, fruits, nuts, and fish, is the most recommended dietary pattern for NAFLD prevention. Beneficial bacteria could also directly confer health benefits to host, thus approaches that aim to change the indigenous gut microbiome or their derived metabolites have been constantly studied (Suez et al. 2019). Growing evidence suggested that probiotics especially *Lactobacillus* could inhibit the development of chronic liver diseases. For example, gut-resident *Lactobacillus* could activate the transcription factor Nrf2 in liver to protect against oxidative injury (Saeedi et al. 2020). Lactococcus lactis subspecies cremoris protected mice from NASH by reducing serum cholesterol level and increasing glucose tolerance (Naudin et al. 2020). While in human, treatment of probiotics formula containing *Lactobacillus acidophilus* could reduce liver fat accumulation and liver injury in NASH patients (Wong et al. 2013b). Prebiotics is another approach for gut microbiome modification which has shown its therapeutic potential in NAFLD patients by reducing body mass index, hepatic enzymes, and serum cholesterol level (Loman et al. 2018). Preclinical mechanistic studies suggested that dietary supplementation of prebiotics could improve NAFLD by modulating gut microbiome and attenuating insulin resistance and liver fat accumulation (Parnell et al. 2012).

Both NAFLD and NAFLD-HCC patients display signatures of gut dysbiosis signature with enrichments of opportunistic pathobionts. To deplete these detrimental microbes, FMT has been recently emerged as an alternative therapeutic option which includes transplantation of feces from a healthy donor to the recipient patient. FMT has achieved a big success against inflammatory bowel disease with receiving FDA approval for treatment of recurrent *Clostridium difficile* infection. In comparison, much less FMT studies were carried on NAFLD patients. A few pieces of evidence showed that FMT could improve the gut microenvironment, reduce intestinal permeability and liver lipid accumulation, and improve insulin resistance (Nicolas et al. 2017). In another animal study, transplanting feces obtained from patients with steatosis (grade 3, >66%) into recipient mice resulted in initiation of hepatic lipid accumulation (Hoyles et al. 2018), indicating the importance of a pathological microbiota for NAFLD development and progression. By contrast, transplanting feces of lean human donors increase insulin sensitivity in mice with metabolic syndrome, suggesting the feasibility and potential of FMT against NAFLD (Vrieze et al. 2012). Apart of probiotics and FMT, antibiotic therapy may act as a way. But employing antibiotics may lead to altering ranges of microbial species. Yet, whether NAFLD patients could benefit from it needs further evaluation.

9.6 Conclusion

In this chapter, the impacts of different diets on the gut microbiome in NASH and its associated disease progression are explored. Both animal experiments and clinical data have shown different diet-associated signatures of gut microbiome signatures in NASH and NAFLD-HCC, and these signatures could potentially serve as non-invasive diagnostic biomarkers for diagnosis. However, the identified signatures need to be extensively evaluated in large-scale randomized clinical trials to ensure their accuracy. Meanwhile, although accumulated clinical evidence confirmed the association of gut dysbiosis with NAFLD, NASH, and NAFLD-HCC, the actual mechanistic links are far from well-established. In summary, the gut microbiome is an essential element involved in NAFLD pathogenesis or disease prevention, hence direct modulation of gut microbiome by dietary intervention could be an ideal and feasible option for NASH patients for disease management.

Acknowledgement National Natural Science Foundation of China (No. 82103355; 82272619; 82222901), RGC-General Research Fund (14117422), Health and Medical Research Fund, Hong Kong (No. 08191336).

Conflict of Interest None.

References

Andriamihaja M, et al. Colon luminal content and epithelial cell morphology are markedly modified in rats fed with a high-protein diet. Am J Physiol Gastrointest Liver Physiol. 2010;299(5):G1030–7.

Behary J, et al. Gut microbiota impact on the peripheral immune response in non-alcoholic fatty liver disease related hepatocellular carcinoma. Nat Commun. 2021;12(1):187.

Bergheim I, et al. Antibiotics protect against fructose-induced hepatic lipid accumulation in mice: role of endotoxin. J Hepatol. 2008;48(6):983–92.

Berna G, Romero-Gomez M. The role of nutrition in non-alcoholic fatty liver disease: Pathophysiology and management. Liver Int. 2020;40(Suppl 1):102–8.

Boursier J, et al. The severity of nonalcoholic fatty liver disease is associated with gut dysbiosis and shift in the metabolic function of the gut microbiota. Hepatology. 2016;63(3):764–75.

Canfora EE, et al. Gut microbial metabolites in obesity, NAFLD and T2DM. Nat Rev Endocrinol. 2019;15(5):261–73.

Cani PD, et al. Metabolic endotoxemia initiates obesity and insulin resistance. Diabetes. 2007;56(7):1761–72.

Cantero I, et al. Fruit fiber consumption specifically improves liver health status in obese subjects under energy restriction. Nutrients. 2017;9(7):667.

Chalasani N, et al. The diagnosis and management of nonalcoholic fatty liver disease: practice guidance from the American Association for the Study of Liver Diseases. Hepatology. 2018;67(1):328–57.

Chan R, et al. Diet-quality scores and prevalence of nonalcoholic fatty liver disease: a population study using proton-magnetic resonance spectroscopy. PLoS One. 2015;10(9):e0139310.

Cho YE, et al. Fructose promotes leaky gut, endotoxemia, and liver fibrosis through ethanol-inducible cytochrome P450-2E1-mediated oxidative and nitrative stress. Hepatology. 2021;73(6):2180–95.

Chopyk DM, Grakoui A. Contribution of the intestinal microbiome and gut barrier to hepatic disorders. Gastroenterology. 2020;159(3):849–63.

Dapito DH, et al. Promotion of hepatocellular carcinoma by the intestinal microbiota and TLR4. Cancer Cell. 2012;21(4):504–16.

Daubioul CA, et al. Effects of oligofructose on glucose and lipid metabolism in patients with nonalcoholic steatohepatitis: results of a pilot study. Eur J Clin Nutr. 2005;59(5):723–6.

David LA, et al. Diet rapidly and reproducibly alters the human gut microbiome. Nature. 2014;505(7484):559–63.

den Besten G, et al. Gut-derived short-chain fatty acids are vividly assimilated into host carbohydrates and lipids. Am J Physiol Gastrointest Liver Physiol. 2013;305(12):G900–10.

Dewulf EM, et al. Insight into the prebiotic concept: lessons from an exploratory, double blind intervention study with inulin-type fructans in obese women. Gut. 2013;62(8):1112–21.
Ekstedt M, et al. Fibrosis stage is the strongest predictor for disease-specific mortality in NAFLD after up to 33 years of follow-up. Hepatology. 2015;61(5):1547–54.
Eslam M, et al. A new definition for metabolic dysfunction-associated fatty liver disease: an international expert consensus statement. J Hepatol. 2020a;73(1):202–9.
Eslam M, et al. MAFLD: a consensus-driven proposed nomenclature for metabolic associated fatty liver disease. Gastroenterology. 2020b;158(7):1999–2014.e1.
Estes C, et al. Modeling NAFLD disease burden in China, France, Germany, Italy, Japan, Spain, United Kingdom, and United States for the period 2016-2030. J Hepatol. 2018;69(4):896–904.
Ezzaidi N, et al. New insights and therapeutic implication of gut microbiota in non-alcoholic fatty liver disease and its associated liver cancer. Cancer Lett. 2019;459:186–91.
Fang D, et al. Bifidobacterium pseudocatenulatum LI09 and Bifidobacterium catenulatum LI10 attenuate D-galactosamine-induced liver injury by modifying the gut microbiota. Sci Rep. 2017;7(1):8770.
Fava F, et al. The type and quantity of dietary fat and carbohydrate alter faecal microbiome and short-chain fatty acid excretion in a metabolic syndrome 'at-risk' population. Int J Obes. 2013;37(2):216–23.
Gao X, et al. Acetate functions as an epigenetic metabolite to promote lipid synthesis under hypoxia. Nat Commun. 2016;7:11960.
Geypens B, et al. Influence of dietary protein supplements on the formation of bacterial metabolites in the colon. Gut. 1997;41(1):70–6.
Hamza RT, et al. Dietary fructose intake in obese children and adolescents: relation to procollagen type III N-terminal peptide (P3NP) and non-alcoholic fatty liver disease. J Pediatr Endocrinol Metab. 2016;29(12):1345–52.
Han JM, et al. Associations between intakes of individual nutrients or whole food groups and non-alcoholic fatty liver disease among Korean adults. J Gastroenterol Hepatol. 2014;29(6):1265–72.
Healey GR, et al. Interindividual variability in gut microbiota and host response to dietary interventions. Nutr Rev. 2017;75(12):1059–80.
Ho JT, Chan GC, Li JC. Systemic effects of gut microbiota and its relationship with disease and modulation. BMC Immunol. 2015;16:21.
Hoyles L, et al. Molecular phenomics and metagenomics of hepatic steatosis in non-diabetic obese women. Nat Med. 2018;24(7):1070–80.
Ioannou GN, et al. Association between dietary nutrient composition and the incidence of cirrhosis or liver cancer in the United States population. Hepatology. 2009;50(1):175–84.
Jensen T, et al. Fructose and sugar: a major mediator of non-alcoholic fatty liver disease. J Hepatol. 2018;68(5):1063–75.
Jia W, Xie G, Jia W. Bile acid-microbiota crosstalk in gastrointestinal inflammation and carcinogenesis. Nat Rev Gastroenterol Hepatol. 2018;15(2):111–28.
Jin CJ, et al. Supplementation of sodium butyrate protects mice from the development of non-alcoholic steatohepatitis (NASH). Br J Nutr. 2015;114(11):1745–55.
Johnson RJ, et al. Fructokinase, fructans, intestinal permeability, and metabolic syndrome: an equine connection? J Equine Vet Sci. 2013;33(2):120–6.
Kashtanova DA, et al. Gut microbiota in patients with different metabolic statuses: Moscow study. Microorganisms. 2018;6(4):98.
Kenny DJ, et al. Cholesterol metabolism by uncultured human gut bacteria influences host cholesterol level. Cell Host Microbe. 2020;28(2):245–257.e6.
Krawczyk M, et al. Gut permeability might be improved by dietary fiber in individuals with nonalcoholic fatty liver disease (NAFLD) undergoing weight reduction. Nutrients. 2018;10(11):1793.
Kubeck R, et al. Dietary fat and gut microbiota interactions determine diet-induced obesity in mice. Mol Metab. 2016;5(12):1162–74.
Lai YS, et al. Electronegative LDL is linked to high-fat, high-cholesterol diet-induced nonalcoholic steatohepatitis in hamsters. J Nutr Biochem. 2016;30:44–52.

Lam YY, et al. Effects of dietary fat profile on gut permeability and microbiota and their relationships with metabolic changes in mice. Obesity (Silver Spring). 2015;23(7):1429–39.

Lang S, et al. High protein intake is associated with histological disease activity in patients with NAFLD. Hepatol Commun. 2020;4(5):681–95.

Le Roy T, et al. Intestinal microbiota determines development of non-alcoholic fatty liver disease in mice. Gut. 2013;62(12):1787–94.

Le Roy T, et al. The intestinal microbiota regulates host cholesterol homeostasis. BMC Biol. 2019;17(1):94.

Lebeaupin C, et al. Endoplasmic reticulum stress signalling and the pathogenesis of non-alcoholic fatty liver disease. J Hepatol. 2018;69(4):927–47.

Levy JR, Clore JN, Stevens W. Dietary n-3 polyunsaturated fatty acids decrease hepatic triglycerides in Fischer 344 rats. Hepatology. 2004;39(3):608–16.

Liaw YW, et al. A vaccine targeted at CETP alleviates high fat and high cholesterol diet-induced atherosclerosis and non-alcoholic steatohepatitis in rabbit. PLoS One. 2014;9(12):e111529.

Loman BR, et al. Prebiotic and probiotic treatment of nonalcoholic fatty liver disease: a systematic review and meta-analysis. Nutr Rev. 2018;76(11):822–39.

Lonardo A, et al. Global epidemiology of nonalcoholic fatty liver disease: meta-analytic assessment of prevalence, incidence, and outcomes. Hepatology. 2016;64(4):1388–9.

Loomba R, et al. Gut microbiome-based metagenomic signature for non-invasive detection of advanced fibrosis in human nonalcoholic fatty liver disease. Cell Metab. 2017;25(5):1054–1062.e5.

Ma C, et al. Gut microbiome-mediated bile acid metabolism regulates liver cancer via NKT cells. Science. 2018;360(6391):eaan5931.

Makki K, et al. The impact of dietary fiber on gut microbiota in host health and disease. Cell Host Microbe. 2018;23(6):705–15.

Mosca A, et al. Serum uric acid concentrations and fructose consumption are independently associated with NASH in children and adolescents. J Hepatol. 2017;66(5):1031–6.

Moschen AR, Kaser S, Tilg H. Non-alcoholic steatohepatitis: a microbiota-driven disease. Trends Endocrinol Metab. 2013;24(11):537–45.

Mouries J, et al. Microbiota-driven gut vascular barrier disruption is a prerequisite for non-alcoholic steatohepatitis development. J Hepatol. 2019;71(6):1216–28.

Mujico JR, et al. Changes in gut microbiota due to supplemented fatty acids in diet-induced obese mice. Br J Nutr. 2013;110(4):711–20.

Naudin CR, et al. Lactococcus lactis subspecies cremoris elicits protection against metabolic changes induced by a western-style diet. Gastroenterology. 2020;159(2):639–651.e5.

Nicolas S, et al. Transfer of dysbiotic gut microbiota has beneficial effects on host liver metabolism. Mol Syst Biol. 2017;13(3):921.

O'Sullivan TA, et al. Lower fructose intake may help protect against development of nonalcoholic fatty liver in adolescents with obesity. J Pediatr Gastroenterol Nutr. 2014;58(5):624–31.

Ouyang X, et al. Fructose consumption as a risk factor for non-alcoholic fatty liver disease. J Hepatol. 2008;48(6):993–9.

Parker HM, et al. Omega-3 supplementation and non-alcoholic fatty liver disease: a systematic review and meta-analysis. J Hepatol. 2012;56(4):944–51.

Parnell JA, et al. The potential role of prebiotic fibre for treatment and management of non-alcoholic fatty liver disease and associated obesity and insulin resistance. Liver Int. 2012;32(5):701–11.

Pedersen HK, et al. Human gut microbes impact host serum metabolome and insulin sensitivity. Nature. 2016;535(7612):376–81.

Polyzos SA, Kountouras J, Mantzoros CS. Obesity and nonalcoholic fatty liver disease: from pathophysiology to therapeutics. Metabolism. 2019;92:82–97.

Ponziani FR, et al. Hepatocellular carcinoma is associated with gut microbiota profile and inflammation in nonalcoholic fatty liver disease. Hepatology. 2019;69(1):107–20.

Pu S, et al. Interactions between obesity status and dietary intake of monounsaturated and polyunsaturated oils on human gut microbiome profiles in the Canola Oil Multicenter Intervention Trial (COMIT). Front Microbiol. 2016;7:1612.

Qin N, et al. Alterations of the human gut microbiome in liver cirrhosis. Nature. 2014;513(7516):59–64.

Rahman K, et al. Loss of junctional adhesion molecule A promotes severe steatohepatitis in mice on a diet high in saturated fat, fructose, and cholesterol. Gastroenterology. 2016;151(4):733–746.e12.

Robertson RC, et al. Maternal omega-3 fatty acids regulate offspring obesity through persistent modulation of gut microbiota. Microbiome. 2018;6(1):95.

Roncal-Jimenez CA, et al. Sucrose induces fatty liver and pancreatic inflammation in male breeder rats independent of excess energy intake. Metabolism. 2011;60(9):1259–70.

Rosqvist F, et al. Overfeeding polyunsaturated and saturated fat causes distinct effects on liver and visceral fat accumulation in humans. Diabetes. 2014;63(7):2356–68.

Saeedi BJ, et al. Gut-resident lactobacilli activate hepatic Nrf2 and protect against oxidative liver injury. Cell Metab. 2020;31(5):956–968.e5.

Sanchez-Lozada LG, et al. Comparison of free fructose and glucose to sucrose in the ability to cause fatty liver. Eur J Nutr. 2010;49(1):1–9.

Sekiya M, et al. Polyunsaturated fatty acids ameliorate hepatic steatosis in obese mice by SREBP-1 suppression. Hepatology. 2003;38(6):1529–39.

Singh V, et al. Dysregulated microbial fermentation of soluble fiber induces cholestatic liver cancer. Cell. 2018;175(3):679–694.e22.

Softic S, et al. Divergent effects of glucose and fructose on hepatic lipogenesis and insulin signaling. J Clin Invest. 2017;127(11):4059–74.

Sookoian S, et al. Intrahepatic bacterial metataxonomic signature in non-alcoholic fatty liver disease. Gut. 2020;69(8):1483–91.

Storlien LH, et al. Fish oil prevents insulin resistance induced by high-fat feeding in rats. Science. 1987;237(4817):885–8.

Suez J, et al. The pros, cons, and many unknowns of probiotics. Nat Med. 2019;25(5):716–29.

Vrieze A, et al. Transfer of intestinal microbiota from lean donors increases insulin sensitivity in individuals with metabolic syndrome. Gastroenterology. 2012;143(4):913–916.e7.

Wang J, et al. Modulation of gut microbiota during probiotic-mediated attenuation of metabolic syndrome in high fat diet-fed mice. ISME J. 2015;9(1):1–15.

Wong VW, et al. Molecular characterization of the fecal microbiota in patients with nonalcoholic steatohepatitis—a longitudinal study. PLoS One. 2013a;8(4):e62885.

Wong VW, et al. Treatment of nonalcoholic steatohepatitis with probiotics. A proof-of-concept study. Ann Hepatol. 2013b;12(2):256–62.

Wouters K, et al. Dietary cholesterol, rather than liver steatosis, leads to hepatic inflammation in hyperlipidemic mouse models of nonalcoholic steatohepatitis. Hepatology. 2008;48(2):474–86.

Wu W, et al. Protective effect of Akkermansia muciniphila against immune-mediated liver injury in a mouse model. Front Microbiol. 2017;8:1804.

Yang Q, et al. Role of dietary nutrients in the modulation of gut microbiota: a narrative review. Nutrients. 2020;12(2):381.

Yang J, et al. High-fat diet promotes colorectal tumorigenesis through modulating gut microbiota and metabolites. Gastroenterology. 2022;162:135–149.e2.

Ye Q, et al. Global prevalence, incidence, and outcomes of non-obese or lean non-alcoholic fatty liver disease: a systematic review and meta-analysis. Lancet Gastroenterol Hepatol. 2020;5(8):739–52.

Yoshimoto S, et al. Obesity-induced gut microbial metabolite promotes liver cancer through senescence secretome. Nature. 2013;499(7456):97–101.

Younossi ZM, et al. Global epidemiology of nonalcoholic fatty liver disease-Meta-analytic assessment of prevalence, incidence, and outcomes. Hepatology. 2016;64(1):73–84.

Younossi ZM, et al. The global epidemiology of NAFLD and NASH in patients with type 2 diabetes: a systematic review and meta-analysis. J Hepatol. 2019a;71(4):793–801.

Younossi ZM, et al. Obeticholic acid for the treatment of non-alcoholic steatohepatitis: interim analysis from a multicentre, randomised, placebo-controlled phase 3 trial. Lancet. 2019b;394(10215):2184–96.

Zelber-Sagi S, et al. Long term nutritional intake and the risk for non-alcoholic fatty liver disease (NAFLD): a population based study. J Hepatol. 2007;47(5):711–7.
Zhang X. NAFLD related-HCC: the relationship with metabolic disorders. Adv Exp Med Biol. 2018;1061:55–62.
Zhang H, et al. Effects of dietary energy level on lipid metabolism-related gene expression in subcutaneous adipose tissue of Yellow breed x Simmental cattle. Anim Sci J. 2015;86(4):392–400.
Zhang X, et al. Dietary cholesterol drives fatty liver-associated liver cancer by modulating gut microbiota and metabolites. Gut. 2021;70(4):761–74.
Zhao L, et al. Gut bacteria selectively promoted by dietary fibers alleviate type 2 diabetes. Science. 2018;359(6380):1151–6.
Zhao M, et al. TMAVA, a metabolite of intestinal microbes, is increased in plasma from patients with liver steatosis, inhibits gamma-butyrobetaine hydroxylase, and exacerbates fatty liver in mice. Gastroenterology. 2020a;158(8):2266–2281.e27.
Zhao S, et al. Dietary fructose feeds hepatic lipogenesis via microbiota-derived acetate. Nature. 2020b;579(7800):586–91.

Chapter 10
Host–Microbiome Interactions in Gastrointestinal Cancers

Jun Sun

Abstract A dynamic and highly competitive microbial community inhabits in the gastrointestinal (GI) tract. These microbes include bacteria, viruses, fungi, and archaea. The host–microbial interactions play critical roles in health and disease. From the host side, the innate and adaptive immunities are the keys for maintaining the hemostasis. From the microbial side, the strategies to overcome the host defenses include secreting effectors and manipulating metabolites. GI cancers are modulated by the host factors (e.g., gene polymorphisms in regulating the inflammatory response), microbial factors (e.g., bacterial effectors), and environmental factors (e.g., lifestyle and food). However, there are some common pathophysiological mechanisms that involve in the development of cancer. In the current chapter, we will focus on the host–microbial interactions by discussing key signaling pathways and bacterial factors in the development of gastrointestinal cancers. We will discuss a single pathogen and the microbiome as a community. Better understanding the dynamic interactions between host and microbe will provide novel insights into the GI cancer prevention, diagnosis, and treatment.

Keywords Bacteria · Bacterial effector · Beta-catenin · Colon cancer · Esophageal cancer · Fungi · Fecal microbiota transplant · Inflammation · Microbiome · Gastric cancer · Gallbladder cancer · Liver cancer · Pancreatic cancer · P53 · Virus

J. Sun (✉)
Division of Gastroenterology and Hepatology, Department of Medicine, University of Illinois at Chicago, Chicago, IL, USA

Department of Microbiology/Immunology, University of Illinois at Chicago, Chicago, IL, USA

University of Illinois Cancer Center, Chicago, IL, USA

Jesse Brown VA Medical Center, Chicago, IL, USA
e-mail: junsun7@uic.edu

J. Yu (ed.), *Microbiome in Gastrointestinal Cancer*,
https://doi.org/10.1007/978-981-19-4492-5_10

10.1 Introduction

The gastrointestinal tract is associated with a dynamic microbial community. The normal gut microbiota contribute to host nutrient metabolism, xenobiotic and drug metabolism, barrier function, immunomodulation, and protection against pathogens. The microbial distribution from the esophagus to the rectum varies spatially and temporally throughout the individual's lifespan. Emerging evidence suggests that imbalanced gut microbiome or pathogens induces changes in the GI environment that lead to tumorigenesis. GI cancers include esophageal cancer, stomach cancer (gastric cancer), small intestine cancer, colorectal cancer (CRC), anal cancer, liver cancer, gallbladder cancer, and pancreatic cancer. The roles of microbes in tumorigenesis also vary spatially depending on the location and function of microbiomes. The microbe-related damage in GI cancers is modulated by the host factors (e.g., gene variation), microbial factors (e.g., bacterial effectors), and environmental factors (e.g., lifestyle and food). However, there are some common pathophysiological mechanisms that involve host–microbial interactions.

Here, we will discuss the roles of host–microbial interactions in GI cancers. From the host side, the innate and adaptive immunities are the keys for maintaining the hemostasis. From the microbial side, the strategies to overcome the host defenses include secreting effectors and manipulating metabolites. There are also microbe–microbe interactions that influence host physiology and microbial community. The complex interactions among bacteria, immune response, and environmental factors have been investigated in gastric cancer, but more and more research suggest that bacteria play a critical role in other GI cancers. We will focus on the key signaling pathways in the host and bacterial factors in the development of various GI cancers. We not only discussed single pathogens but also microbiome as a community in the development of cancer. By better understanding the mechanisms and microbial contributions to GI cancers, we can develop accurate diagnosis and new strategies that treat or prevent GI cancers.

10.2 The Microbes and the Hallmarks of GI Cancers

The hallmarks constitute an organizing principle for rationalizing the complexities of cancer, based on Hanahan's and Weinberg's review in 2000 (Hanahan and Weinberg 2000) and the updated version in 2011 (Hanahan and Weinberg 2011). During the multistep development of tumors, these are six biological capabilities acquired: sustaining proliferative signaling, evading growth suppressors, resisting cell death, enabling replicative immortality, inducing angiogenesis, and activating invasion and metastasis (Hanahan and Weinberg 2000). Two emerging hallmarks are reprogramming of energy metabolism and evading immune destruction (Hanahan and Weinberg 2011). Underlying these hallmarks are genome instability, which generates the genetic diversity that expedites their acquisition, and inflammation, which fosters multiple hallmark functions. Tumors contain a repertoire of recruited, ostensibly normal cells that contribute to the acquisition of hallmark traits by creating the "tumor microenvironment." (Hanahan and Weinberg 2011). Enteric microbes contribute to the multistep development of tumors and make the microenvironment in favor of the tumor growth in the development of GI cancers.

We have presented the progress in the bacterial infection and microbiome in various cancers in a recent book "Inflammation, infection, and microbiome in cancers: evidence, mechanisms, and implications" (Sun 2021). Using the hallmarks of cancer as a framework, Bleich et al. discussed the microbiome and hallmarks of cancer, mainly for the CRC. Microbiota promote tumorigenesis in the intestine through crosstalk with the host, interactions between other microbes in relation to carcinogenesis (Bleich and Arthur 2021). In general, host–microbe interactions and the microbe–microbe interactions influence host physiology and microbial community dynamics in the gastrointestinal tract. Microbes influence host through physical and chemical interactions and signaling. There is constant communication and feedback between members of microbial community and the host (Bleich and Arthur 2021).

In the following sections, we will mainly discuss the DNA damage, inflammation, the host pathways manipulated by microbes, and the roles of microbial products and microbiome in the development of GI cancers. We focus on the bacteria and bacterial effectors, whereas summarizing the roles of viruses and fungi in GI cancers. Finally, we will discuss the diagnosis and therapeutic targets based on the microbes and cancer hall markers.

10.3 DNA Damage

About 20% of human cancers are linked to infection by virus, bacteria, or parasites (Parkin 2006). Early precancerous lesions in patient samples, as well as specific oncogene activation in experimental tumor models, have shown the formation of DNA double-strand breaks (DSBs) and the activation of DNA-damage checkpoints (Discussed in a recent review Sun, 2021 #149). Virus is known to integrate itself into the human genome. For example, Hepatitis B virus (HBV) is an enveloped DNA virus that can cause hepatocellular carcinoma (HCC). HBV integrates itself into the human genome and replicates within liver cells. The malignant transformation of liver cells caused mutations of genes (e.g., p53 and beta-catenin) (Tornesello et al. 2013). The X gene of HBV (HBx) is the most common open reading frame integrated into the host genome in HCC and the integrated HBx is frequently mutated. Mutant HBx proteins still retain their ability to bind to p53, and attenuate DNA repair, and *p53*-mediated apoptosis (Hussain et al. 2007). However, majority of the research focused on viral infection and cancer; limited topics of bacterial infection in cancer are mainly about *H. pylori*.

In vitro, *H. pylori* has shown the ability to induce host cellular DNA damage directly. Efficient repair of *H. pylori*-induced DSBs was apparent after antibiotic treatment to kill the bacteria, but prolonged infection led to residual unrepaired breaks and negatively affected cell viability (Toller et al. 2011). *H. pylori* also induces mitochondrial DNA (mtDNA) mutagenesis which seems to enhance oxidative stress and contribute to gastric cancer development (Machado et al. 2009).

Nougayrede et al. reported that *Escherichia* coli induces DNA double-strand breaks (Nougayrede et al. 2006). A recent study provides etiological evidence for *E. coli.* colibactin in human cancer. The genomic contexts of colibactin-induced DSBs were enriched for an AT-rich hexameric sequence motif, associated with distinct DNA-shape characteristics (Dziubanska-Kusibab et al. 2020). The exact double-strand break loci corresponded with mutational hot spots in cancer genomes, reminiscent of a trinucleotide signature previously identified in healthy colorectal epithelial cells (Dziubanska-Kusibab et al. 2020).

Salmonella enterica is a Gram-negative intracellular pathogen to humans and animals. *Salmonella* ser. Typhi carriers had increased risk of gallbladder cancer. A meta-analysis of 22 studies by Koshiol et al demonstrated the summary odds ratios (OR) of 4.6 and 5 for gallbladder cancer (Koshiol et al. 2016). The level of anti-*Salmonella* flagellin antibody was higher in CRC and pre-cancer cases than controls in the US and the Netherlands (Kato et al. 2013). Based on the study in the Netherlands analyzing cancer registry and public health surveillance data, there was an increased incidence of colorectal cancer (CRC), compared with the general population, among residents who were reported for enteric salmonellosis caused by *Salmonella Enteritidis (*Mughini-Gras et al. 2018*). Salmonella* Typhi induces systematic salmonellosis. The typhoid toxin activated the host DNA damage in vitro (Ibler et al. 2019). *Salmonella* Typhi typhoid toxin exhausted the RPA response to DNA replication stress, thus driving senescence *and Salmonella* infection. More studies are needed to study *Salmonella Enteritidis* and DNA damage and the *Salmonella* infection using experimental models or human organoids (Sun 2022).

A recent study reported CRC-promoting bacteria *H. hathewayi* with epigenetic regulation of TSGs in host cells (Xia et al. 2020). *H. hathewayi* and *Streptococcus spp.* significantly correlated with CDX2 and MLH1 promoter hypermethylation, respectively. Moreover, *F. nucleatum* and *H. hathewayi* upregulated DNA methyltransferase. In vivo, *H. hathewayi* inoculation promoted colonic epithelial cell proliferation in germ-free and conventional mice.

Gut microbiome stimulates reactive oxygen species (ROS) (Dziubanska-Kusibab et al. 2020) by immune cells (Iida et al. 2013). ROS is known to enhance the DNA damage caused by oxaliplatin, blocking DNA replication and transcription, and resulting in cell death. Disruption of the microbiota impairs the response of subcutaneous tumors to CpG-oligonucleotide immunotherapy and platinum chemotherapy (Iida et al. 2013).

10.4 Inflammation and Infection

Inflammation has been identified as a significant factor in the development of GI tumor malignancies. Inflammation is a double-edged sword. Host uses inflammation to get rid of pathogens during infection, whereas microbes adopt the chronic inflammatory environment for their benefits to invade and survive in the host cells.

There is no report on a single strain of pathogen that directly cause inflammation in the esophagus. Emerging evidence from microbiome studies showed that *Fusobacterium nucleatum* in esophageal cancer tissue is associated with prognosis (Yamamura et al. 2016). Yamamura et al. identified "cytokine-cytokine receptor interaction" and revealed the increased genes of specific chemokines (e.g., CCL20) in the esophageal cancer. The role of the oral and gut microbiome in esophageal cancer has been well discussed in several papers (Baba et al. 2017; Peters et al. 2017).

Gastric cancer is an inflammation- and infection-associated cancer in which persistent *Helicobacter pylori* (*H. pylori*)-related acute-on-chronic inflammation. *H. pylori* plays an essential role in the development of atrophic gastritis, which represents pathways in multistep intestinal-type gastric carcinogenesis. Not every individual with *H. pylori* developed gastric cancer. The severity of gastric damage and eventual clinical outcome of *H. pylori* infection are determined by a combination of host genetic and bacterial virulence factors (reviewed by Engstrand and Graham 2020; Ando et al. 2006). CagA is delivered into gastric epithelial cells by the bacterial type IV secretion system. CagA deregulates the SHP2 oncoprotein and is divided into the East Asian and Western types (Yamaoka et al. 1999). Patients with East Asian cagA-positive strains had higher risk of gastric cancer than those with cagA-negative or Western cagA -positive strains. Among host genetic factors contributing to the disease outcome, inflammatory cytokines IFN-G AA favors cagA-positive *H. pylori* infection, TNF-A TT for duodenal ulcer, whereas IL-10 TT is more common in intestinal metaplasia gastric cancer (Zambon et al. 2005).

CRC progression begins when healthy tissue develops into the precancerous polyps or adenoma in the colon (Hannigan et al. 2018). Colonic carcinogenesis involves a progressive accumulation of mutations in a genetically susceptible host leading to eventual cellular autonomy (Vogelstein and Kinzler 2004). Patients with chronic intestinal inflammation, such as inflammatory bowel disease (IBD), are at higher risk of CRC. Bacterial-induced tumorigenesis in CRC is exerted by induction of intestinal inflammation which characterized by infiltration of myeloid immune cells and the release of inflammatory cytokines, and by direct genotoxic activity (Sun 2022; Massimino et al. 2021). Intestinal inflammation targets CRC-inducing activity of the microbiota and the key player in the process is mucosa-associated polyketide synthase (pks) (+) *E. coli* (Arthur et al. 2012). Monocolonization with the commensal *E. coli* NC101 promoted invasive carcinoma in azoxymethane (AOM)-treated IL10(−/−) mice. IL-10 operates on innate and adaptive immune mechanisms to suppress the intestinal inflammation. IL-10−/− mice spontaneously develop colitis starting at 2–3 months of age. Deletion of the pks genotoxic island from *E. coli NC101* decreased tumor multiplicity and invasion in AOM/IL10(−/−) mice, without altering intestinal inflammation. Mucosa-associated pks(+) *E. coli* were found in a significantly high percentage of IBD and CRC patients. Intestinal inflammation could promote tumorigenesis by altering microbial composition and inducing the expansion of microbes with genotoxic capabilities.

The presence of bacteria in the gut appears to be of crucial importance in the pathogenesis of CRC. However, not all bacterial proteins will enhance inflammation in the host. *Salmonella* AvrA in an anti-inflammation protein secreted through the type three secretion system of *Salmonella* for its long-term survival and promoting tumorigenesis by activating the beta-catenin pathway (Lu et al. 2010, 2012, 2014, 2016). This activity is consistent with the natural history of *Salmonella* in hosts, where the bacteria elicit transient inflammation but do not destroy epithelial cells (Jones et al. 2008). *Salmonella* AvrA possesses acetyltransferase activity toward specific mitogen-activated protein kinase kinases (MAPKKs) and potently inhibits c-Jun N-terminal kinase (JNK) and NF-κB signaling pathways (Sun 2009, 2022; Jones et al. 2008).

Enterococcus faecalis is an intestinal pathobiont contributing to liver damage in alcoholic liver disease. Chronic liver disease enables *Enterococcus faecalis* colonization and internalization in hepatocytes to promote liver carcinogenesis (Iida et al. 2021). It also suggested the role of liver–gut–microbial axis in tumorigenesis of liver cancer. The development of liver cancer is vs. the inflammation–fibrosis–cirrhosis–cancer axis. Increased TNF by monocytes in mesenteric lymph nodes constitutes one of the main factors increasing gut permeability and bacterial translocation. It is supported by the evidence that anti-TNF-alpha antibody downregulated bacterial translocation in rats with cirrhosis and ascites (Frances et al. 2007).

Salmonella infection increases the risk of gallbladder cancer (GBC). The recurrent cycles of gallbladder epithelium damage and repair enable a chronic inflammatory environment that promotes progressive morphological impairment through a metaplasia–dysplasia–carcinoma with cumulative genome instability and inactivation of TP53 (Espinoza et al. 2016). TP53 is mutated in over 50% of gallbladder cancer cases and seems to be the earliest and one of the most important carcinogenic pathways. Increased cell turnover and oxidative stress promote early alteration of TP53, cell cycle deregulation, apoptosis, and replicative senescence (Espinoza et al. 2016). In India, gallbladder cancer correlated with higher prevalence of chronic S. Typhi carriers defined by antibodies against S. typhi (ViAb) in patient serum (Nath et al. 2008). GBC in India has unique mutations and is marked by S. typhi DNA (Scanu et al. 2015).

An increased risk of pancreatic cancer is associated with chronic pancreatitis. The combined increase in genomic damage and cellular proliferation strongly promotes malignant transformation of pancreatic cells (Farrow and Evers 2002). However, direct role of pathogen infection and cause of local inflammation other than pancreatitis are still unknown. Epidemiological data suggest that *H. pylori* may be a risk factor for pancreatic cancer, and more recently, data suggest that periodontal disease, and *Porphyromonas gingivalis*, a pathogen for periodontal disease, may play a role in pancreatic carcinogenesis (As reviewed by Michaud 2013).

Taken together, like many common cancers, GI cancer is developed as a consequence of chronic inflammation and/or infectious. Imbalanced gut microbiome or pathogens induces altered enteric environment, thus leading to local mucosal inflammation and tumorigenesis.

10.5 Microbial Manipulation of the Key Pathways in the Host

There are key pathways involved the initiation and early stage of GI cancers. For example, the sequential accumulation of mutations in specific genes, including APC, beta-catenin, and p53, drives the transition from healthy colonic epithelia through increasingly dysplastic adenoma to CRC (Smith et al. 2002). Host genetic factors should also play a critical role in microbe-induced outcomes of general GI cancers.

In fact, most *H. pylori*-infected people develop no significant disease, remaining asymptomatic throughout their lives. In gastric *H. pylori*-infected patients, atrophy grade varies even among patients with East Asian *cagA*-positive strains (Azuma et al. 2004). This outcome could not be explained by bacterial virulence factors alone; rather, host genetic factors and environmental factors should be considered.

A previous study has demonstrated that the difference of GBC samples collected in India and the Netherlands is associated with *Salmonella* infection (Scanu et al. 2015), Indian patients with benign gallbladder diseases (benign, 39.6%; $n = 187$), or GBC (carcinoma, 74.1%; $n = 54$). Carcinomas from both countries were positive for Cytokeratin-8 (a secretory epithelial differentiation marker) and TP53 (shown by a strong nuclear signal as mutated inactive TP53 aggregates). Interestingly, c-MYC presented strongly nuclear staining in 9/10 Indian samples, whereas only 1/6 patient samples from the Netherlands contained a small number of positive cells. The other five Dutch patients did not show c-MYC staining. It indicated that Indian GBC tumors associated with *Salmonella* are different from the Netherlands. The c-myc is a target gene of the beta-catenin pathway to control cell growth and proliferation. In colon cancer, mutations in the tumor suppressor APC usually occur first. A recent study has shown that the APC gene was frequently affected by *E. coli* colibactin (Dziubanska-Kusibab et al. 2020).

Acetylation of p53 has been shown to increase its stability and transcriptional activities (Reed and Quelle 2015). Bacterial regulation of p53 was first discovered in *Salmonella* infected cells and an animal model (Wu et al. 2010). We are the first to report that bacterial AvrA is able to target acetylation of p53 for the bacterial survival using the human intestinal epithelial cell lines and infected animal models (Wu et al. 2010). Bacterial degradation of p53 was later reported in the *Helicobacter pylori*-infected gastric epithelial cells (Wei et al. 2010) and CagA protein induces degradation of p53 protein in a p14ARF-dependent manner (Wei et al. 2015).

The innate immune response is known to be nonspecific as the first line of defense against infective agents and initiates antigen presentation. The intracellular innate pathogen recognition receptors (PRRs) are present in kinds of immune cells, such as macrophages, monocytes, and epithelial cells, and are crucial points for innate immune response (Metzger et al. 2018). It is tightly controlled to avoid detrimental immune responses against harmless commensals and allows the generation of effective immune responses against invasive pathogens, such as bacteria and virus, by sensing microbes by PRRs in the intestinal mucosa or other body surfaces. As a subgroup of PRRs, toll-like receptors (TLRs) recognize microbial molecules, like lipopolysaccharides (LPS), viral nucleoid, and proteins. In monocytes and epidermal keratinocytes, germ-free (GF) mice developed liver tumors less frequently than their specific-pathogen-free (SPF) counterparts, partially due to decreased TLR4 signaling by the intestinal microbiota (Dapito et al. 2012). Vitamin D receptor (VDR) regulates the TLRs through 1α,25(OH)2D (Gruber-Bzura 2018). Our recent findings indicate the significantly alteration of PRRs, including upregulated TLR3, TLR7, and NOD2 (NLRs) in mice lacking VDR in myeloid cells, compared with VDR^{LoxP} control mice (Zhang et al. 2021). Moreover, deficiency of host factor (e.g., vitamin/VDR deficiency), dysbiosis, and bacterial invasion impaired the innate immunity and anti-microbial function of Paneth cells in the intestine (Wu et al. 2015; Lu et al. 2021), thus increasing the risk of chronical intestinal inflammation and cancer (Zhang et al. 2020).

Cytokines, ROS, and mediators of the inflammatory pathway (e.g., NF-κB, STAT, and COX-2) have been shown to increase cell cycling, cause loss of tumor suppressor function, and stimulate oncogene expression. Sustained inflammation induced by microbes may contribute to the development of cancer by continuous activation of MYD88 (Elinav et al. 2013). *Salmonella* could translocate from the intestine to gallbladder for the long-term infection (Lu et al. 2010). *Salmonella* infection of gallbladder organoids induced cell transformation (Scanu et al. 2015). *Salmonella* manipulated the host signaling pathways (e.g., activation of MAPK and AKT pathways) to provoke cellular transformation in carcinoma (Scanu et al. 2015). The STAT-3 is involved in the bacterial inflammation and tumorigenesis, reviewed in a previous paper (Lu et al. 2017).

Bacteria target the cellular structure of host cells to invade and survive. *Salmonella Enteritidis* and *Salmonella* Typhimurium are reported to alter the intestinal permeability through tight junctions in the epithelial cells (Zhang et al. 2014, 2015). The mechanism of *Salmonella* AvrA to enhance the tight junctions and inhibit inflammation is through the JNK pathway (Lin et al. 2016). The roles of bacterial infection in cancer have been discussed in the recent reviews (Sun 2022; Zha et al. 2019), interested readers could have further read.

The direct infection-related damage is modulated by the host's response to the inflammatory stimuli, environment (e.g., vitamin D deficiency, sun exposure), and lifestyle, such as food balance between the intake of cancer promoting agents (e.g., red meat) and cancer preventing agents (e.g., phyto-nutrients) (Engstrand and Graham 2020; Ando et al. 2006; Sun and Kato 2016; Wirbel et al. 2019; Yang and Yu 2018; Song et al. 2020). Thus, to predict the GI cancer risk and to provide prevention and treatment, multiple factors should be considered (Fig. 10.1).

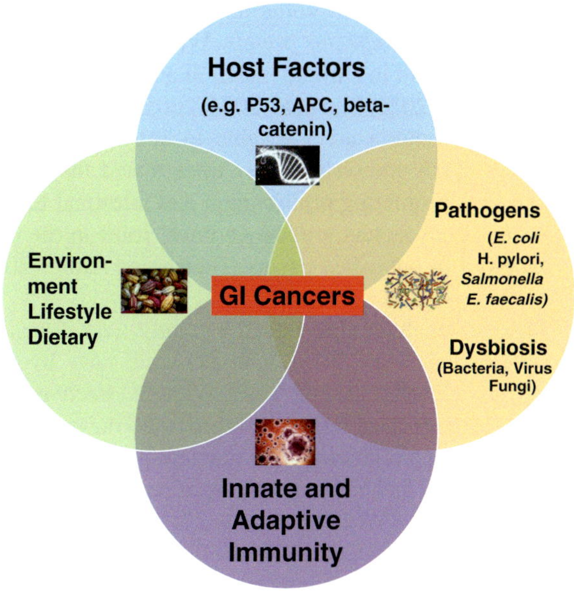

Fig. 10.1 The development of GI cancers. The development of GI cancers is a combination of host genetic factors, microbial virulence factors, immunity, and environmental and lifestyle factors that determine the severity of mucosal damage and the eventual clinical outcome of chronic inflammation and/or infection. Accumulating evidence suggests that imbalanced gut microbiome or pathogens induces altered enteric environment (e.g., inflammation, DNA damage, and hyperproliferation), thus increasing risks of tumorigenesis

10.6 Microbial Factors Contribute to GI Tumorigenesis

Effective *H. pylori* eradication along with a natural decrease in infection due to improved living conditions has resulted in declining gastric cancer rates in Western countries, although it remains a significant cause of morbidity and mortality in other parts of the world. While the genes in *cag* PAI are the most strongly virulence-related among those reported to date, other genes have also been reported as candidates that determine outcome in *H. pylori*-infected persons. Studies that identify further bacterial as well as host genetic factors that place the patient at greatest risk of disease progression will enhance better screening strategies, and improve the control of *H. pylori* infection in affected subjects (Engstrand and Graham 2020; Ando et al. 2006).

E. coli (Pkc+) carries the genomic island responsible for colibactin synthesis or produces other genotoxins to promote cancer (Dziubanska-Kusibab et al. 2020). *Salmonella* lacking type three secretion system (TTSS) (*ΔprgH*) failed to induce colon carcinomas in mice, suggesting that *Salmonella* manipulation of host cells is critical in the development of cancer (Scanu et al. 2015). *B. fragilis* toxin stimulated the translocation of ß-catenin to nuclei. Subsequently, induced c-myc transcription and translation for persistent cellular proliferation (Wu et al. 2003). We have demonstrated that *Salmonella TTSS effector protein* AvrA activates ß-catenin signaling and its upstream regulator Wnt in chronic infection and development of CRC (Zha et al. 2019; Silbergleit et al. 2020; Sun et al. 2004, 2005; Ye et al. 2007; Zhang et al. 2012). AvrA-expressing bacteria are also able to activate the STAT3 pathway. *Salmonella* expressing AvrA transcriptionally upregulated the activity of STAT3 and its target genes, thus promoting proliferation and intestinal tumorigenesis (Lu et al. 2016). Other bacterial factors are shown novel roles in the development of cancer as well, reviewed in published papers (Bleich and Arthur 2021; Silbergleit et al. 2020).

Chronic liver diseases include viral infections, fatty liver disease (FLD), alcoholic liver disease (Wirbel et al. 2019), non-alcoholic fatty liver disease, non-alcoholic steatohepatitis (NASH), and cirrhosis. Without effective treatments, these liver diseases can lead to liver cancer. Dysbiosis promotes the progression of inflammation and cancer by leakage of microbial products, e.g., deoxycholic acid (DCA), LPS, and unmethylated CpG DNA. These microbial products promote liver inflammation, fibrosis, and cirrhosis (Yu and Schwabe 2017). In CRC, there are reduced butyrate producing bacteria (Song et al. 2020) and enhanced production of secondary bile acids from metagenomes. It indicates a metabolic link between cancer-associated microbes and diet (Wirbel et al. 2019). Identifying new microbial products and understanding their functions will open new avenues studying interaction of the microbes and host cells and their novel roles in carcinogenesis.

10.7 Diagnosis and Therapeutic Targets Based on the Microbial Cancer Hall Markers

The microbiota is a potential biomarker of diagnosis or clinical outcome of GI cancers. By elucidating the mechanisms and microbial contributions to the development and progression of GI cancers, we will develop new diagnosis and therapeutics that treat or prevent GI cancers. Yu et al. have the first metagenomic profiling study of CRC fecal microbiomes and validate microbial biomarkers in ethnically different cohorts. Besides confirming known associations of *Fusobacterium nucleatum* and *Peptostreptococcus stomatis* with CRC, this study found significant associations with several species, including *Parvimonas micra* and *Solobacterium moorei*. They identified 20 microbial gene markers that differentiated CRC and control microbiomes and validated 4 markers in the Danish cohort. This study independently validated selected biomarkers, suggesting the affordable non-invasive early diagnostic biomarkers for CRC (Yu et al. 2017). Wirbel et al. (2019) did eight geographically and technically diverse fecal metagenomic studies of CRC, highlighting the globally generalizable potential for using fecal metagenomic biomarkers for early diagnosis of CRC (Wirbel et al. 2019).

Antibiotics, probiotics, prebiotics, and fecal microbiota transplant (FMT) can modify the microbiome. It is known that gut microbiota impacts the efficacy of chemotherapy and immunotherapy of cancers, given the intertwined nature of the microbiota and the immune system. A recent review of the up-to-date findings on the influence of gut microbiota on three common immunotherapies including adoptive cell transfer, immune checkpoint blockade, and CpG-oligodeoxynucleotide therapy (Lau et al. 2021).

10.8 Future Direction

Except bacteria, viruses, and fungi, subsets of microbiome are another important component of the microbial community. Their roles have been actively studied in the context of GI cancers (Engstrand and Graham 2020; Stern et al. 2019; Nakatsu et al. 2018). Fungal component of the pancreatic microbiome (known as the mycobiome) is also altered in CRC (Coker et al. 2019) and pancreatic ductal adenocarcinoma (Aykut et al. 2019). In fact, an abundance of a specific fungal genus actually promotes the disease. Studies on fungi in gastric microbiology were prominent in the nineteenth century, and their potential role in disease pathogenesis has yet to be addressed using modern techniques (Engstrand and Graham 2020).

Modulation of gut microbiota by probiotics, prebiotics, or using antagonists of microbial products can improve barrier function, inhibit chronic inflammation, and reduce the risk of carcinogenesis. The research progress also urges for a rethinking on the use of certain bacteria in patients: e.g., colibactin-producing *E. coli* as probiotics and *Salmonella* as a stimulator of immune responses in the cancer therapy. We must learn more about the physiological conditions, under which bacteria could cause mutations and whether only certain age groups or population are affected. FMT could turn cancer immunotherapy non-responders into responders, based on two recent studies in melanoma patients (Baruch et al. 2021; Davar et al. 2021). FMT promotes response in immunotherapy-refractory in melanoma patients. However, GI cancers have their unique microenvironment and immune responses. Better understanding the diverse ways that the microbiota contributes to carcinogenesis will open new possibilities for the diagnosis, prevention, and personalized treatment of GI cancers.

Funding Support This work was supported by the U.S. National Institutes of Health grant NIDDK R01 DK105118, R01DK114126, DOD BC160450P1/GRANT12929009, and the VA Merit Award 1 I01BX004824-01. The study sponsors play no role in the study design, data collection, analysis, and interpretation of data. The contents do not represent the views of the United States Department of Veterans Affairs or the United States Government.

References

Ando T, Goto Y, Maeda O, Watanabe O, Ishiguro K, Goto H. Causal role of Helicobacter pylori infection in gastric cancer. World J Gastroenterol. 2006;12(2):181–6.

Arthur JC, Perez-Chanona E, Muhlbauer M, Tomkovich S, Uronis JM, Fan TJ, et al. Intestinal inflammation targets cancer-inducing activity of the microbiota. Science. 2012;338(6103):120–3.

Aykut B, Pushalkar S, Chen R, Li Q, Abengozar R, Kim JI, et al. The fungal mycobiome promotes pancreatic oncogenesis via activation of MBL. Nature. 2019;574(7777):264–7.

Azuma T, Yamazaki S, Yamakawa A, Ohtani M, Muramatsu A, Suto H, et al. Association between diversity in the Src homology 2 domain--containing tyrosine phosphatase binding site of Helicobacter pylori CagA protein and gastric atrophy and cancer. J Infect Dis. 2004;189(5):820–7.

Baba Y, Iwatsuki M, Yoshida N, Watanabe M, Baba H. Review of the gut microbiome and esophageal cancer: pathogenesis and potential clinical implications. Ann Gastroenterol Surg. 2017;1(2):99–104.

Baruch EN, Youngster I, Ben-Betzalel G, Ortenberg R, Lahat A, Katz L, et al. Fecal microbiota transplant promotes response in immunotherapy-refractory melanoma patients. Science. 2021;371(6529):602–9.

Bleich RM, Arthur JC. Microbiome and the hallmarks of cancer. In: Sun J, editor. Inflammation, infection, and microbiome in cancers. Physiology in health and disease. Cham: Springer; 2021.

Coker OO, Nakatsu G, Dai RZ, Wu WKK, Wong SH, Ng SC, et al. Enteric fungal microbiota dysbiosis and ecological alterations in colorectal cancer. Gut. 2019;68(4):654–62.

Dapito DH, Mencin A, Gwak GY, Pradere JP, Jang MK, Mederacke I, et al. Promotion of hepatocellular carcinoma by the intestinal microbiota and TLR4. Cancer Cell. 2012;21(4):504–16.

Davar D, Dzutsev AK, McCulloch JA, Rodrigues RR, Chauvin JM, Morrison RM, et al. Fecal microbiota transplant overcomes resistance to anti-PD-1 therapy in melanoma patients. Science. 2021;371(6529):595–602.

Dziubanska-Kusibab PJ, Berger H, Battistini F, Bouwman BAM, Iftekhar A, Katainen R, et al. Colibactin DNA-damage signature indicates mutational impact in colorectal cancer. Nat Med. 2020;26(7):1063–9.

Elinav E, Nowarski R, Thaiss CA, Hu B, Jin C, Flavell RA. Inflammation-induced cancer: crosstalk between tumours, immune cells and microorganisms. Nat Rev Cancer. 2013;13(11):759–71.

Engstrand L, Graham DY. Microbiome and gastric cancer. Dig Dis Sci. 2020;65(3):865–73.

Espinoza JA, Bizama C, Garcia P, Ferreccio C, Javle M, Miquel JF, et al. The inflammatory inception of gallbladder cancer. Biochim Biophys Acta. 2016;1865(2):245–54.

Farrow B, Evers BM. Inflammation and the development of pancreatic cancer. Surg Oncol. 2002;10(4):153–69.

Frances R, Chiva M, Sanchez E, Gonzalez-Navajas JM, Llovet T, Zapater P, et al. Bacterial translocation is downregulated by anti-TNF-alpha monoclonal antibody administration in rats with cirrhosis and ascites. J Hepatol. 2007;46(5):797–803.

Gruber-Bzura B. Vitamin D and influenza—prevention or therapy? Int J Mol Sci. 2018;19(8):2419.

Hanahan D, Weinberg RA. The hallmarks of cancer. Cell. 2000;100(1):57–70.

Hanahan D, Weinberg RA. Hallmarks of cancer: the next generation. Cell. 2011;144(5):646–74.

Hannigan GD, Duhaime MB, Ruffin MT, Koumpouras CC, Schloss PD. Diagnostic potential and interactive dynamics of the colorectal cancer virome. mBio. 2018;9(6):e02248–18.

Hussain SP, Schwank J, Staib F, Wang XW, Harris CC. TP53 mutations and hepatocellular carcinoma: insights into the etiology and pathogenesis of liver cancer. Oncogene. 2007;26(15):2166–76.

Ibler AEM, ElGhazaly M, Naylor KL, Bulgakova NA, El-Khamisy SF, Humphreys D. Typhoid toxin exhausts the RPA response to DNA replication stress driving senescence and Salmonella infection. Nat Commun. 2019;10(1):4040.

Iida N, Dzutsev A, Stewart CA, Smith L, Bouladoux N, Weingarten RA, et al. Commensal bacteria control cancer response to therapy by modulating the tumor microenvironment. Science. 2013;342(6161):967–70.
Iida N, Mizukoshi E, Yamashita T, et al. Chronic liver disease enables gut Enterococcus faecalis colonization to promote liver carcinogenesis. Nat Cancer. 2021;2:1039–54.
Jones RM, Wu H, Wentworth C, Luo L, Collier-Hyams L, Neish AS. Salmonella AvrA coordinates suppression of host immune and apoptotic defenses via JNK pathway blockade. Cell Host Microbe. 2008;3(4):233–44.
Kato I, Boleij A, Kortman GA, Roelofs R, Djuric Z, Severson RK, et al. Partial associations of dietary iron, smoking and intestinal bacteria with colorectal cancer risk. Nutr Cancer. 2013;65(2):169–77.
Koshiol J, Wozniak A, Cook P, Adaniel C, Acevedo J, Azocar L, et al. Salmonella enterica serovar Typhi and gallbladder cancer: a case-control study and meta-analysis. Cancer Med. 2016;5(11):3310–235.
Lau HCH, Sung JJ, Yu J. Gut microbiota: impacts on gastrointestinal cancer immunotherapy. Gut Microbes. 2021;13(1):1–21.
Lin Z, Zhang YG, Xia Y, Xu X, Jiao X, Sun J. Salmonella enteritidis effector AvrA stabilizes intestinal tight junctions via the JNK pathway. J Biol Chem. 2016;291(52):26837–49.
Lu R, Wu S, Liu X, Xia Y, Zhang YG, Sun J. Chronic effects of a Salmonella type III secretion effector protein AvrA in vivo. PLoS One. 2010;5(5):e10505.
Lu R, Liu X, Wu S, Xia Y, Zhang YG, Petrof EO, et al. Consistent activation of the beta-catenin pathway by Salmonella type-three secretion effector protein AvrA in chronically infected intestine. Am J Physiol Gastrointest Liver Physiol. 2012;303(10):G1113–25.
Lu R, Wu S, Zhang YG, Xia Y, Liu X, Zheng Y, et al. Enteric bacterial protein AvrA promotes colonic tumorigenesis and activates colonic beta-catenin signaling pathway. Oncogenesis. 2014;3:e105.
Lu R, Wu S, Zhang Y-g, Xia Y, Zhou Z, Kato I, et al. Salmonella protein AvrA activates the STAT3 Signaling pathway in colon cancer. Neoplasia. 2016;18(5):307–16.
Lu R, Zhang YG, Sun J. STAT3 activation in infection and infection-associated cancer. Mol Cell Endocrinol. 2017;451:80–7.
Lu R, Zhang Y, Xia Y, Zhang J, Kaser A, Blumberg R, et al. Paneth cell alertness to pathogens maintained by vitamin D receptors. Gastroenterology. 2021;160(4):1269–83.
Machado AM, Figueiredo C, Touati E, Maximo V, Sousa S, Michel V, et al. Helicobacter pylori infection induces genetic instability of nuclear and mitochondrial DNA in gastric cells. Clin Cancer Res. 2009;15(9):2995–3002.
Massimino L, Lovisa S, Antonio Lamparelli L, Danese S, Ungaro F. Gut eukaryotic virome in colorectal carcinogenesis: is that a trigger? Comput Struct Biotechnol J. 2021;19:16–28.
Metzger RN, Krug AB, Eisenächer K. Enteric virome sensing—its role in intestinal homeostasis and immunity. Viruses. 2018;10(4):146.
Michaud DS. Role of bacterial infections in pancreatic cancer. Carcinogenesis. 2013;34(10):2193–7.
Mughini-Gras L, Schaapveld M, Kramers J, Mooij S, Neefjes-Borst EA, van Pelt W, et al. Increased colon cancer risk after severe Salmonella infection. PLoS One. 2018;13(1):e0189721.
Nakatsu G, Zhou H, Wu WKK, Wong SH, Coker OO, Dai Z, et al. Alterations in enteric virome are associated with colorectal cancer and survival outcomes. Gastroenterology. 2018;155(2):529–41.e5.
Nath G, Singh YK, Kumar K, Gulati AK, Shukla VK, Khanna AK, et al. Association of carcinoma of the gallbladder with typhoid carriage in a typhoid endemic area using nested PCR. J Infect Dev Ctries. 2008;2(4):302–7.
Nougayrede JP, Homburg S, Taieb F, Boury M, Brzuszkiewicz E, Gottschalk G, et al. Escherichia coli induces DNA double-strand breaks in eukaryotic cells. Science. 2006;313(5788):848–51.
Parkin DM. The global health burden of infection-associated cancers in the year 2002. Int J Cancer. 2006;118(12):3030–44.

Peters BA, Wu J, Pei Z, Yang L, Purdue MP, Freedman ND, et al. Oral microbiome composition reflects prospective risk for esophageal cancers. Cancer Res. 2017;77(23):6777–87.

Reed SM, Quelle DE. p53 acetylation: regulation and consequences. Cancers. 2015;7(1):30–69.

Scanu T, Spaapen RM, Bakker JM, Pratap CB, Wu LE, Hofland I, et al. Salmonella manipulation of host signaling pathways provokes cellular transformation associated with gallbladder carcinoma. Cell Host Microbe. 2015;17(6):763–74.

Silbergleit M, Vasquez AA, Miller CJ, Sun J, Kato I. Oral and intestinal bacterial exotoxins: potential linked to carcinogenesis. Prog Mol Biol Transl Sci. 2020;171:131–93.

Smith G, Carey FA, Beattie J, Wilkie MJ, Lightfoot TJ, Coxhead J, et al. Mutations in APC, Kirsten-ras, and p53--alternative genetic pathways to colorectal cancer. Proc Natl Acad Sci U S A. 2002;99(14):9433–8.

Song M, Chan AT, Sun J. Influence of the gut microbiome, diet, and environment on risk of colorectal cancer. Gastroenterology. 2020;158(2):322–40.

Stern J, Miller G, Li X, Saxena D. Virome and bacteriome: two sides of the same coin. Curr Opin Virol. 2019;37:37–43.

Sun J. Pathogenic bacterial proteins and their anti-inflammatory effects in the eukaryotic host. Antiinflamm Antiallergy Agents Med Chem. 2009;8(3):214–27.

Sun J. Inflammation, infection, and microbiome in cancers: evidence, mechanisms, and implications. 2021.

Sun J. Impact of bacterial infection and intestinal microbiome on colorectal cancer development. Chin Med J. 2022;135(4):400–8.

Sun J, Kato I. Gut microbiota, inflammation and colorectal cancer. Genes Dis. 2016;3(2):130–43.

Sun J, Hobert ME, Rao AS, Neish AS, Madara JL. Bacterial activation of beta-catenin signaling in human epithelia. Am J Physiol Gastrointest Liver Physiol. 2004;287(1):G220–7.

Sun J, Hobert ME, Duan Y, Rao AS, He TC, Chang EB, et al. Crosstalk between NF-kappaB and beta-catenin pathways in bacterial-colonized intestinal epithelial cells. Am J Physiol Gastrointest Liver Physiol. 2005;289(1):G129–37.

Toller IM, Neelsen KJ, Steger M, Hartung ML, Hottiger MO, Stucki M, et al. Carcinogenic bacterial pathogen Helicobacter pylori triggers DNA double-strand breaks and a DNA damage response in its host cells. Proc Natl Acad Sci U S A. 2011;108(36):14944–9.

Tornesello ML, Buonaguro L, Tatangelo F, Botti G, Izzo F, Buonaguro FM. Mutations in TP53, CTNNB1 and PIK3CA genes in hepatocellular carcinoma associated with hepatitis B and hepatitis C virus infections. Genomics. 2013;102(2):74–83.

Vogelstein B, Kinzler KW. Cancer genes and the pathways they control. Nat Med. 2004;10(8):789–99.

Wei J, Nagy TA, Vilgelm A, Zaika E, Ogden SR, Romero-Gallo J, et al. Regulation of p53 tumor suppressor by Helicobacter pylori in gastric epithelial cells. Gastroenterology. 2010;139(4):1333–43.

Wei J, Noto JM, Zaika E, Romero-Gallo J, Piazuelo MB, Schneider B, et al. Bacterial CagA protein induces degradation of p53 protein in a p14ARF-dependent manner. Gut. 2015;64(7):1040–8.

Wirbel J, Pyl PT, Kartal E, Zych K, Kashani A, Milanese A, et al. Meta-analysis of fecal metagenomes reveals global microbial signatures that are specific for colorectal cancer. Nat Med. 2019;25(4):679–89.

Wu S, Morin PJ, Maouyo D, Sears CL. Bacteroides fragilis enterotoxin induces c-Myc expression and cellular proliferation. Gastroenterology. 2003;124(2):392–400.

Wu S, Ye Z, Liu X, Zhao Y, Xia Y, Steiner A, et al. Salmonella typhimurium infection increases p53 acetylation in intestinal epithelial cells. Am J Physiol Gastrointest Liver Physiol. 2010;298(5):G784–94.

Wu S, Zhang Y-G, Lu R, Xia Y, Zhou D, Petrof EO, et al. Intestinal epithelial vitamin D receptor deletion leads to defective autophagy in colitis. Gut. 2015;64(7):1082–94.

Xia X, Wu WKK, Wong SH, Liu D, Kwong TNY, Nakatsu G, et al. Bacteria pathogens drive host colonic epithelial cell promoter hypermethylation of tumor suppressor genes in colorectal cancer. Microbiome. 2020;8(1):108.

Yamamura K, Baba Y, Nakagawa S, Mima K, Miyake K, Nakamura K, et al. Human microbiome Fusobacterium nucleatum in esophageal cancer tissue is associated with prognosis. Clin Cancer Res. 2016;22(22):5574–81.

Yamaoka Y, El-Zimaity HM, Gutierrez O, Figura N, Kim JG, Kodama T, et al. Relationship between the cagA 3′ repeat region of Helicobacter pylori, gastric histology, and susceptibility to low pH. Gastroenterology. 1999;117(2):342–9.

Yang J, Yu J. The association of diet, gut microbiota and colorectal cancer: what we eat may imply what we get. Protein Cell. 2018;9(5):474–87.

Ye Z, Petrof EO, Boone D, Claud EC, Sun J. Salmonella effector AvrA regulation of colonic epithelial cell inflammation by deubiquitination. Am J Pathol. 2007;171(3):882–92.

Yu LX, Schwabe RF. The gut microbiome and liver cancer: mechanisms and clinical translation. Nat Rev Gastroenterol Hepatol. 2017;14(9):527–39.

Yu J, Feng Q, Wong SH, Zhang D, Liang QY, Qin Y, et al. Metagenomic analysis of faecal microbiome as a tool towards targeted non-invasive biomarkers for colorectal cancer. Gut. 2017;66(1):70–8.

Zambon CF, Basso D, Navaglia F, Belluco C, Falda A, Fogar P, et al. Pro- and anti-inflammatory cytokines gene polymorphisms and Helicobacter pylori infection: interactions influence outcome. Cytokine. 2005;29(4):141–52.

Zha L, Garrett S, Sun J. Salmonella infection in chronic Inflammation and gastrointestinal cancer. Diseases. 2019;7(1):28.

Zhang YG, Wu S, Xia Y, Chen D, Petrof EO, Claud EC, et al. Axin1 prevents Salmonella invasiveness and inflammatory response in intestinal epithelial cells. PLoS One. 2012;7(4):e34942.

Zhang YG, Wu S, Xia Y, Sun J. Salmonella-infected crypt-derived intestinal organoid culture system for host-bacterial interactions. Physiol Rep. 2014;2(9):e12147.

Zhang Y, Wu S, Ma J, Xia Y, Ai X, Sun J. Bacterial protein AvrA stabilizes intestinal epithelial tight junctions via blockage of the C-Jun N-terminal kinase pathway. Tissue Barriers. 2015;3(1–2):e972849.

Zhang YG, Lu R, Wu S, Chatterjee I, Zhou D, Xia Y, et al. Vitamin D receptor protects against dysbiosis and tumorigenesis via the JAK/STAT pathway in intestine. Cell Mol Gastroenterol Hepatol. 2020;10(4):729–46.

Zhang J, Zhang Y, Xia Y, Sun J. Imbalance of the intestinal virome and altered viral-bacterial interactions caused by a conditional deletion of the vitamin D receptor. Gut Microbes. 2021;13(1):1957408.

Chapter 11
Gut Microbiome and Immune Responses in Gastrointestinal Cancer

Robyn Laube and Ken Liu

Abstract The immune system plays an integral role in both the prevention and development of gastrointestinal malignancies. This effect is partially mediated via the gut microbiome, which ordinarily maintains a bidirectional homeostatic balance with the immune system. In addition to influencing the development of inflammation and malignancy, the microbiome can also affect the response to anti-cancer therapies and development of immune-mediated toxicities. Modulation of the gut microbiome via diet, antibiotics, probiotics and faecal microbiota transplantation are therefore also able to influence the course of a malignancy. Continued research in this field will pave the way towards the development of personalised medicine utilising individual microbial analysis to inform treatment decisions and enhance patient prognoses.

Keywords Microbiome · Gastrointestinal malignancy, colorectal cancer Hepatocellular carcinoma · Immune system · Faecal microbiota transplantation Immunotherapy · Checkpoint inhibitor · Probiotics

R. Laube
Faculty of Medicine and Health Sciences, Macquarie University, Sydney, NSW, Australia

Department of Gastroenterology, Macquarie University Hospital, Sydney, NSW, Australia

K. Liu (✉)
AW Morrow Gastroenterology and Liver Centre, Royal Prince Alfred Hospital, Sydney, NSW, Australia

Faculty of Medicine, University of Sydney, Sydney, NSW, Australia

Centenary Institute, University of Sydney, Sydney, NSW, Australia
e-mail: ken.liu@health.nsw.gov.au

J. Yu (ed.), *Microbiome in Gastrointestinal Cancer*,
https://doi.org/10.1007/978-981-19-4492-5_11

11.1 Introduction

Over the past decade, the significance of the gut microbiome in many conditions has been increasingly recognised. The microbiome is most intimately related to gastrointestinal and liver pathologies, such as inflammatory bowel disease (IBD), primary sclerosing cholangitis, non-alcoholic fatty liver disease and gastrointestinal cancers. The microbiome and its manipulation influence many pathways in the body, including metabolic, oncogenic and immune systems. There is an intricate crosstalk between the host immune system and microbiome. This delicate relationship can easily be unbalanced, contributing to carcinogenesis. The immune system plays a crucial role in influencing the initiation and development of cancers, and hence is one of the primary targets of anti-cancer therapy. The initial success of immune checkpoint inhibitors in melanoma has triggered significant interest in harnessing and manipulating immune responses for the treatment of other advanced cancers, including gastrointestinal malignancies. This chapter reviews the role of the gut microbiome and host immune response in gastrointestinal malignancies, including therapeutic methods to modulate the natural history of these cancers.

11.2 Importance of Immune Responses in Gastrointestinal Cancers

11.2.1 Cancer Pathogenesis

The immune system can contribute to both the prevention and initiation of cancers. In a process named 'cancer immunoediting', cancer cells interact with immune cells in three phases: elimination, equilibrium and escape (O'Donnell et al. 2019). During elimination, immune surveillance by the innate and adaptive immune cells identifies tumour-specific antigens on cancer cells and then eliminates these cells. During equilibrium, any remaining cancer cells which were not eliminated undergo replication, producing new cells with potentially greater ability to resist immune defences. These cancer cells can then either revert to elimination or progress to the escape phase. The escape phase refers to cancer cells which have evaded immune control to replicate and form clinically detectable cancers. Multiple physiological processes can contribute to this phase, such as defects in the immune system in the tumour microenvironment (O'Donnell et al. 2019). Immunosuppressive states, either due to primary or secondary aetiologies, facilitate the development of cancers via impairing this immunosurveillance process.

The immune system can also influence cancer development through the pro-tumourigenic microenvironment, which is established to promote cancer development. This is characterised by the presence of inflammatory cells (particularly immature myeloid cells, macrophages and pro-inflammatory CD4+ T-lymphocytes) and mesenchymal tissue enmeshed with the proliferating tumour cells. Cancer cells drive the development of this immunosuppressive microenvironment through cytokines and growth factor signalling, enabling themselves to evade immune surveillance and proliferate (Francescone et al. 2014; Zhang et al. 2020). For example, in colorectal cancers (CRC), tumour-associated macrophages secrete CCL17, CCL18 and CCL21 to recruit both Th2 and naïve lymphocytes into the microenvironment, and CCL20 to recruit T-regulatory cells, creating a local immunosuppressive environment for the developing cancer (Erreni et al. 2011; Liu et al. 2011). Patients with hepatocellular carcinoma (HCC) have an immunosuppressive tumour microenvironment with structurally and functionally abnormal immune and vascular cells (Santhakumar et al. 2020). This includes an increased expression of T-regulatory lymphocytes in the microenvironment as well as in peripheral blood, and reduced CD8+ T-lymphocytes, all of which contribute to HCC development (Ormandy et al. 2005).

Cancer development can also be driven by chronic inflammation, which is thought to provoke the development of up to 20% of all tumours (Grivennikov 2012). This occurs via several mechanisms, including production of cytokines and growth factors which directly increase proliferation and growth of pre-malignant and malignant cells, or via modulating the tumour microenvironment to induce more immunosuppressive action (Greten and Grivennikov 2019). CRC is particularly susceptible, as local inflammation (for example active IBD) allows for increased gut permeability which induces production of pro-inflammatory and angiogenic cytokines, inflammation, and subsequent tumour progression (Francescone et al. 2014). Inflammation can also trigger turnover of non-malignant host cells to create space for proliferation of malignant cells, for example in HCC which almost universally occurs in the setting of underlying chronic inflammation (Greten and Grivennikov 2019).

11.2.2 Prognostication and Treatment of Cancer

As well as influencing the development of cancers, the immune system has prognostic utility and can guide therapeutic decisions in oncology (Dienstmann et al. 2017). In CRC, increased tumour inflammatory infiltrate signifies a better survival and greater response to chemotherapy (Wilkinson et al. 2021). For example, tumour infiltrating lymphocytes (TILs) are more prevalent in CRCs with wild-type KRAS or BRAF oncogenes and in CRCs with deficient DNA mismatch repair (MMR) status, and this portends a better survival (Sinicrope et al. 2016). Additionally, higher titres of M2 macrophages, natural killer cells and CD8+ T-lymphocytes within the tumour microenvironment are associated with a better CRC prognosis, as crosstalk between these latter two cell types intensifies the antigen-driven T cell responses (Coppola et al. 2015). The immunoscore uses the CD8+ T-lymphocyte and memory T-lymphocyte density to produce a score from 0 to 4, which has been validated for predicting survival in CRC (Wilkinson et al. 2021). Immunoscore has a greater prognostic ability than the traditional tumour/node/metastasis system, and

Table 11.1 Approaches to cancer immunotherapy (Zhang et al. 2020; Waldman et al. 2020)

Therapeutic approach	Example targets	Mechanism
Checkpoint inhibitors	– PD-1 (programmed cell death-1) – PD-ligand 1/2 (programmed cell death ligand 1/2) – CTLA-4 – BTLA (B and T cell lymphocyte attenuator)	Stimulate an inhibitory molecule or inhibit a stimulatory molecule which is expressed on the tumour and/or immune cells in the microenvironment, thereby promoting apoptosis of tumour cells and other anti-cancer effects
Cytokines	– IL-2 (interleukin 2) – Interferon alpha 2b	Introduce iatrogenic cytokines to stimulate inhibitory components of the immune response against the tumour
Costimulatory receptor agonists	– OX40 – 4-1BB – CD28	Activate surface receptors on immune cells to stimulate their anti-cancer activity
Adoptive immune cell therapy	– CAR-T (chimeric antigen receptor T cells) – CAR-NK (chimeric antigen receptor natural killer cells)	Individualised therapy; modifying patient immune cells ex-vivo to increase their reactivity against target antigens
Cancer vaccines	– BCG (Bacillus Calmette–Guerin)	Harness the immune system to eliminate malignant cells

can predict CRCs which will benefit from adjuvant chemotherapy (score 2–4) versus those that will not benefit (score 0–1) (Wilkinson et al. 2021).

Cancer immunotherapy provides a modality by which to harness this interaction between the immune system and cancer cells to achieve a therapeutic benefit. The various approaches of cancer immunotherapy are outlined in Table 11.1.

11.3 Immunity-Microbiota Crosstalk

11.3.1 Influence of the Microbiome on the Immune System

The relationship between the microbiota and immune system starts developing at the time of birth when the neonate is exposed to commensal organisms in the birth canal. Live microbes, immune cells and IgA in breastmilk and colostrum shape the development of the infant's gut microbiota and their immune response to these microbes. For example, maternal IgA binds to microbial and nutritional antigens in the infant's gut, subsequently preventing immune activation and sensitisation (Marcobal et al. 2010). Animal studies have demonstrated that mice raised in a germ-free environment have impaired immune system development including small Peyer's patches, fewer mesenteric lymph nodes, fewer CD4+ T cells and greater susceptibility to infection (Hamada et al. 2002; Macpherson et al. 2001; Shi et al. 2017; Smith et al. 2007; Talham et al. 1999). Interestingly, if these germ-free mice receive a microbiota transplantation from other mice, their immune maturation commences (Round and Mazmanian 2009).

In the healthy state, the immune system maintains a symbiotic relationship with the gut microbiota. This provides protection against pathogens and cancers, and tolerance to innocuous antigens. This is partially achieved through the 'mucosal firewall', which refers to the combined role of mucosal endothelial cells, IgA, antimicrobial peptides, immune cells and mucus to minimise excessive contact between gut microbiota and endothelial cells (Macpherson et al. 2009). The microbiota can stimulate multiple different aspects of the immune system, including the adaptive inflammatory response, the adaptive immunoregulatory response or generic stimulation of innate immunity (Palm et al. 2015). By tempering the interaction between the gut microbiota and endothelium, this prevents untoward microbial translocation, immune activation and tissue inflammation. Conversely, failure to regulate the interaction between luminal antigens and the immune system, including regulating misdirected immune responses against microbiota-derived antigens, can provoke the development of allergic, inflammatory or autoimmune diseases (Belkaid and Hand 2014) (Fig. 11.1). This delicate balance of immune stimulation and inhibition can be disturbed by external factors manipulating the microbiota such as antibiotics, dietary changes and parasitic infections (Blaser and Falkow 2009; Johnston et al. 2014). For example, gut dysbiosis is thought to be one of the key drivers in the development of IBD, along with genetic, immune and environmental factors (Maloy and Powrie 2011). Furthermore, gut microbiota are also implicated in the development of malignancies, due to mechanisms such as overactive immune responses to dysbiotic states (Grivennikov and Karin 2010). The most recognised example is *Helicobacter pylori* causing gastric cancer, due to chronic inflammation and dysregulation of the host immune response (Marshall and Warren 1984). Microbial

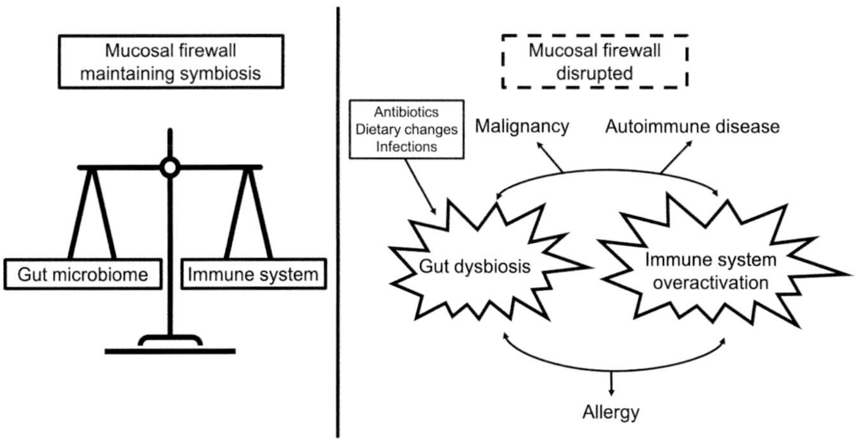

Fig. 11.1 Microbiota-immune system homeostasis

dysbiosis can also dysregulate bile acid synthesis, which can invoke development of HCC via inflammatory cytokine production, increased activation of mTOR and FXR signalling and accelerated fat synthesis (Wu et al. 2021; Yoshimoto et al. 2013). CRC is also associated with gut dysbiosis, characterised by an overall reduction in bacterial diversity including a reduction in *Clostridium, Blautia, Bifidobacterium* and *Faecalibacterium*, and an increase in *Bacteroides fragilis, Fusobacterium nucleatum, Enterococcaceae, Escherichia coli* and *Prevotella* (Sanchez-Alcoholado et al. 2020; Sobhani et al. 2011). This is highlighted by the ability to transfer CRC-susceptibility from mice affected by CRC to healthy mice after microbial transplantation (Chen et al. 2019). These microbial changes can promote tumourigenesis via reduced production of butyrate, increased pro-inflammatory cytokines and increased proliferation of endothelial cells (Sanchez-Alcoholado et al. 2020; Rubinstein et al. 2013; Kostic et al. 2012). Butyrate, a short-chain fatty acid produced from fermentation of dietary fibre, is essential for maintaining healthy colonic mucosa and suppressing local inflammation and carcinogenesis via expansion of regulatory T cells and IL-18 production (Salcedo et al. 2010; Singh et al. 2014).

Recent evidence has also implicated microbial dysbiosis and immune changes in the development of HCC (Ponziani et al. 2019). Behary et al. (2021) demonstrated that microbial dysbiosis and progressive changes in functional pathways precede the development of HCC. Microbial changes were shown to parallel changes in both the systemic and intrahepatic immune profiles, with the latter shifting from a pro-inflammatory to an immunosuppressed state as HCC developed (Behary et al. 2021).

11.3.2 Influence of the Immune System on the Microbiome

As well as being influenced by the microbiota, the immune system is also able to substantially affect the composition and development of the microbiota. Toll-like and Nod-like receptors of the innate immune system have a role in recognising foreign antigens, therefore contributing to the maintenance of host-gut homeostasis (Palm et al. 2015). Inexpression of these receptors has been associated with intestinal microbiota alterations in animal studies, as well as increased susceptibility to noncommunicable diseases associated with dysbiosis such as obesity, metabolic syndrome and colitis (Carvalho et al. 2012; Chassaing et al. 2014; Vijay-Kumar et al. 2010). In the adaptive immune system, B-lymphocytes produce secretory IgA which acts within the gut lumen to restrict the growth and function of gut commensals, and to maintain a diverse microbial composition (Palm et al. 2015). The necessity of IgA in shaping the microbial composition is well established, and many studies have noted adverse patterns of gut dysbiosis if IgA is lacking (Kawamoto et al. 2014; Kubinak et al. 2015; Mirpuri et al. 2014). T-lymphocytes, particularly T-regulatory and Th-17 cells, are credited with supporting microbial homeostasis through their role in helping B-lymphocytes to produce secretory IgA (Kato et al. 2014). Consequently, gut dysbiosis has also been identified in T cell deficient mice (Kawamoto et al. 2014; Kato et al. 2014).

11.4 Gut Microbiome and Immune Responses During Anti-cancer Therapy

11.4.1 Impact on Response to Therapy

Gut microbiota are able to modulate the response to cancer therapies, including both immunotherapies and some non-immunotherapies. This idea has gained significant traction in recent years, although it can originally be traced back to the 1800s when injections of *Streptococcus* and *Serratia* bacteria were noted to induce regression of sarcoma tumours (Coley 1891). Cyclophosphamide is a traditional chemotherapy agent able to alter the gut microbiota and allow selective bacterial translocation to stimulate production of Th1 and Th17 cells in the tumour microenvironment, subsequently optimising the anti-tumour response (Viaud et al. 2013). Gut microbiota can also modulate the effect of oxaliplatin, a platinum-based agent used for CRC, via their effect on myeloid cells within the tumour microenvironment (Iida et al. 2013). Tumour responses to both of these chemotherapeutic agents are lower in germ-free and antibiotic-treated mice which do not benefit from this microbiome effect (Viaud et al. 2013; Iida et al. 2013).

Checkpoint inhibitors such as PD-1/PD-L1 and CTLA4 agents are the most widely used immunotherapies in oncology, including in CRC, HCC, gastric and oesophageal cancers (Xu et al. 2019). Although their therapeutic effect is exerted at the interface between the cancer cells and immune cells, many studies have now proven that it is influenced by the gut microbiota. *Akkermansia muciniphila* and *E. coli* have been associated with augmented responses to anti PD-1/PD-L1 therapy, thought to be due to increased recruitment of CD4+ T-lymphocytes and enhanced Th1 response (Anker et al. 2018; Routy et al. 2018). *Bifidobacterium* is also associated with an augmented response to anti-PD-1/PD-L1 therapy, attributed to increased recruitment of dendritic cells and subsequent promotion of CD8+ T cell activity in the tumour microenvironment (Sivan et al. 2015). In CRC, *Bacteroides acidifaciens* was associated with improved responses to PD-1 therapy, attributed to increased expression of interferon-gamma and interleukin-2 (Lv et al. 2019). Additionally, *firmicutes* and *lachnospiraceae* enhanced the effect of PD-L1 inhibitors on CRC, attributed to increased CD8+ T-lymphocyte infiltration into the tumour microenvironment (Liu et al. 2020). In HCC, *Bifidobacterium dentium, Lactobacillus, Ruminococcaceae* and *Akkermansia muciniphila* are associated with improved response rates to PD-1 inhibitors, due to mechanisms including reduced inflammation and oxidative stress (Routy et al. 2018; Gopalakrishnan et al. 2018). *Faecalibacterium* and *bacteroides* have also been associated with improved responses to CTLA-4 inhibitors, due to increased induction of CD4+ T-lymphocytes and increased dendritic cells enhancing the Th1 response in the tumour microenvironment, respectively (Chaput et al. 2017; Vetizou et al. 2015). These microbial findings have therapeutic potential, with both animal and human studies confirming a clinical benefit from microbial transplantation from immunotherapy responders to non-responders (Routy et al. 2018; Gopalakrishnan et al. 2018; Davar et al. 2021). Furthermore, multiple studies have demonstrated shorter survival outcomes in patients exposed to antibiotic therapy prior to initiation of immunotherapy, regardless of cancer type (Derosa et al. 2018; Huang et al. 2019; Sen et al. 2018).

11.4.2 Impact on Immune-Mediated Toxicity

Immunotherapy agents not infrequently cause immune-mediated toxicity, such as colitis, hepatitis, pneumonitis and thyroiditis (Remash et al. 2021). The development of these toxicities is thought to correlate with tumour response, hence identifying effective ways to treat or prevent them is an important therapeutic goal (Michot et al. 2016). Certain microbial patterns have been associated with likelihood of developing immune-mediated toxicities, with the *Bacteroidetes* families of *Bacteroidaceae, Barnesiellaceae, Rikenellaceae and Tannerellaceae* found to be protective against immunotherapy-induced colitis (Chaput et al. 2017; Ding et al. 2018; Dubin et al. 2016; Liu et al. 2019). Conversely, an increased baseline prevalence of the *Firmicutes* species, including *Clostridiales bacterium* and *Faecalibacterium prausnitzii*, is associated with an increased likelihood of developing immunotherapy-induced colitis (Chaput et al. 2017). Patients with microbiota rich in *Faecalibacterium* who sustained good tumour responses yet high rates of immunotherapy-induced colitis have been found to have low levels of both CD4+ and CD8+ T-lymphocytes at baseline, yet high levels of CD4+ T-lymphocytes after therapy initiation (Chaput et al. 2017). Conversely, patients with microbiota rich in *Bacteroides* who had lower rates of immunotherapy-induced colitis had higher levels of CD4+ T-lymphocytes at baseline with no subsequent increase after therapy initiation (Chaput et al. 2017). These trends also have therapeutic potential, with bacterial supplementation and faecal microbiota transplantation (FMT) both able to improve immunotherapy-induced colitis in mice and humans with cancer, attributed to the reduced levels of CD8+ T-lymphocytes and increased FoxP3+ regulatory T cells within colonic mucosa (Vetizou et al. 2015; Wang et al. 2018). Furthermore, the increased microbial diversity conferred by FMT may also be protective, as low baseline diversity is associated with an increased risk of severe immune-mediated toxicities (Batten et al. 2019). In addition to influencing the development of immune-mediated toxicities, gut microbiota can also influence their severity, with microbial depletion due to antibiotic exposure associated with an increased requirement for hospitalisation and immunosuppressive treatment, particularly if antibiotics were commenced at the onset of the toxicity (Abu-Sbeih et al. 2019). Therefore, gut microbiota can provide useful information for predicting response, toxicity and severity of immunotherapy-induced toxicities, and can consequently provide an effective therapeutic avenue.

11.5 Modulating the Gut Microbiome and its Effect on Immune Responses in Gastrointestinal Cancer

Gut microbiota can be modulated via dietary changes, antibiotics, probiotics or FMT to affect the anti-cancer immune response and the response to immunotherapy as described above. This section will focus on the immune responses, as the other aspects of microbial modulation in gastrointestinal malignancies are covered elsewhere in this book.

11.5.1 Diet

Multiple studies have investigated the role of certain foods in boosting the immune system to combat infections and reduce neoplasia. For example, dietary fibres are prebiotic substances which undergo fermentation by the gut microbiota to produce short-chain fatty acids (SCFA), such as butyrate. Higher levels of SCFA have been associated with increased production and function of dendritic cells (Tan et al. 2016; Trompette et al. 2014) and improved response to PD-1 inhibitors in patients with cancer (Nomura et al. 2020). High fibre intake is also associated with increased levels of *Firmicutes*, which possesses anti-inflammatory and immunomodulatory effects (Fung et al. 2012). Multiple studies have demonstrated an inverse relationship between dietary fibre intake and butyrate production with the development of colon polyps and CRC (Bingham et al. 2003; Bishehsari et al. 2018; Deehan et al. 2020; O'Keefe et al. 2015).

11.5.2 Antibiotics

Antibiotics can be used to deplete and modulate microbial composition, subsequently affecting the immune response and tumourigenesis. The most well-known example is *Helicobacter pylori*, antibiotic-induced eradication of which can substantially reduce the risk of developing gastric adenocarcinoma and mucosa-associated lymphoid tissue (MALT) lymphoma, and can also induce regression of the latter (Choi et al. 2018; Roggero et al. 1995). Antibiotics have been demonstrated to correct the microbial dysbiosis which causes abnormal bile acid signalling and subsequent inflammation contributing to HCC development. By reducing bile acid generating bacteria, such as *Clostridium*, antibiotics are able to alter bile acid composition, increase recruitment of natural killer T-lymphocytes and reduce inflammation (Wu et al. 2021).

11.5.3 Probiotics

Studying the effects of probiotics is challenging as their ability to colonise and affect the host is influenced by multiple exogenous factors including baseline microflora and gene-expression profile (Cheng et al. 2020). Probiotics are postulated to improve the diversity and richness of gut microbiota, downgrade inflammation and reduce the production of carcinogenic compounds (Drago 2019; Ohara et al. 2011). Some strains, such as *Bifidobacterium animalis* subsp. *Lactis*, can also contribute to maintenance of immune-vigilance via activating phagocytes to eliminate early cancer cells (Bozkurt et al. 2019; Galdeano and Perdigón 2006). Preclinical mice models have identified the beneficial effect of *Lactobacillus rhamnosus* GG in reducing CRC growth, which is attributed to inhibition of inflammatory protein expression including NF-κB-p65, COX-2, and TNF-alpha (Banna et al. 2017; Gamallat et al. 2016). *Lactobacillus casei* BL23 has been shown to enhance the immune response in mice with colitis-associated CRC via reducing levels of regulatory T-lymphocytes (Jacouton et al. 2017). Mice models have also identified positive effects of probiotics in HCC, with the probiotic mixtures VSL#3 and Prohep both exhibiting anti-inflammatory effects and reducing HCC growth (Li et al. 2016; Zhang et al. 2012).

In humans, a randomised-controlled trial in people with colorectal adenomas and carcinomas demonstrated that a probiotic mixture of *Lactobacillus rhamnosus* and *Bifidobacterium Breve* induced microbial changes and reduced markers of CRC proliferation (Rafter et al. 2007). Another prospective study, in which probiotics containing *Lactobacillus acidophilus* NCFM and *Bifidobacterium lactis* BI-04 were administered to patients with CRC, identified advantageous microbiota changes including increased levels of butyrate-producing bacteria and reduced CRC-associated bacteria in both tumour and non-tumour colonic tissue (Hibberd et al. 2017). *Bifidobacteria* have also been shown to offer a synergistic benefit on reducing CRC tumour size when used concurrently with PD-L1 inhibitors (Routy et al. 2018; Ding et al. 2018). Similarly, an enhanced effect of CTLA-4 inhibitors against CRC with the addition of *Bacteroides fragilis* has been demonstrated in preclinical studies, associated with increased maturation and function of dendritic cells and memory T-lymphocytes (Vetizou et al. 2015).

11.5.4 Faecal Microbiota Transplantation

There are emerging data for the use of FMT in both benign and malignant diseases (Gough et al. 2011). In the oncology literature, a prospective study identified that FMT taken from patients with CRC increased the risk of CRC development in mice, and was associated with reduced microbial richness and increased levels of pro-inflammatory cytokines, Th-1 and Th-17 lymphocytes in the colon (Wong et al. 2017). Future studies are required to determine whether the reverse is true, if FMT from healthy donors could reduce CRC growth in affected patients. For pancreatic cancer, faecal samples taken from humans with prolonged pancreatic cancer survival conferred advantageous tumour outcomes compared to samples taken from humans with short pancreatic cancer survival when transplanted into mice (Riquelme et al. 2019). This includes improved microbial diversity and increased recruitment and activation of immune cells including CD8+ T-lymphocytes (Riquelme et al. 2019).

Akin to probiotics, the synergistic use of FMT with immunotherapy has been supported by preclinical studies. Faecal samples transplanted from patients responsive to immunotherapy into mice conferred increased efficacy of both CTLA-4 and PD-1/PD-L1 inhibitors compared to faecal samples taken from immunotherapy non-responders (Routy et al. 2018; Gopalakrishnan et al. 2018; Vetizou et al. 2015; Matson et al. 2018). These improved responses can likely be attributed to increased recruitment of CXCR3+ CD4+ and CD8+ T-lymphocytes and lower levels of Th-17 lymphocytes in the tumour microenvironment (Routy et al. 2018; Gopalakrishnan et al. 2018; Vetizou et al. 2015; Matson et al. 2018) (Table 11.2).

Table 11.2 Gut microbiome modulation to affect immune responses to gastrointestinal cancer

Method of modulation	Element modulated	Immune component affected
Diet	Dietary fibre and SCFAs	Dendritic cells Response to PD-1 inhibitors
Antibiotics	Helicobacter pylori	Gastric adenocarcinoma MALT lymphoma
	Bile acid generating bacteria	Natural killer T-lymphocytes
Probiotics	*Bifidobacterium animalis* subsp. *Lactis*	Phagocytes
	Lactobacillus rhamnosus GG	Inflammatory protein expression
	Lactobacillus casei BL23	Regulatory T-lymphocytes
	Bifidobacteria	Synergism with PD-L1 inhibitors
	Bacteroides fragilis	Synergism with CTLA-4 inhibitors Dendritic cells and memory T-lymphocytes
FMT	FMT from patients with CRC	Pro-inflammatory cytokines, Th-1 and Th-17 lymphocytes
	FMT from patients with pancreatic cancer	CD8+ T-lymphocytes
	FMT from patients responsive to immunotherapy	Synergism with CLTA-4 and PD-1/PD-L1 inhibitors Tumour microenvironment modulation

SCFA short-chain fatty acids, *MALT* mucosa-associated lymphoid tissue, *FMT* faecal microbiota transplantation, *CRC* colorectal cancer

11.6 Future Perspectives and Conclusions

The gut microbiota and host immune response play an integral role in influencing the initiation and development of gastrointestinal malignancies. This provides opportunities for prognostication and manipulation of the course of the malignancy, and is therefore an eminent focus of current medical research. Over the past decade, many associations have been made between certain bacterial species and their relationship with tumours and the immune system. The focus has subsequently shifted towards developing a further understanding of causal relationships (as opposed to associations) and mechanisms by which certain bacteria influence the development of and immune response to cancers. These questions will continue to dominant the research field moving forwards, with preliminary knowledge gained from preclinical mice studies being examined in human cohorts to ascertain whether similar associations exist in both species.

In addition to identifying associations and mechanistic relationships, human interventional studies are greatly needed. Further data are required on the efficacy and safety of microbial interventions, including diet, probiotics and FMT for prevention and treatment of cancers. Certain bacterial species have already been identified which can enhance the immune response to tumours and augment the immunotherapy response, as well as other strains with the opposing effects. Analysis should also focus on patients who are non-responsive to immunotherapy, to identify whether selective microbial manipulation can improve their therapeutic response. Large-scale prospective trials need to be designed to investigate the effects of these preliminary findings and to gain a better understanding of the clinical effects of therapeutic interventions. The eventual goal is to develop personalised medicine whereby patient microbiome analysis can inform treatment selection or methods of microbial manipulation to enhance the host immune response to the tumour and augment the effect of anti-cancer therapies. Other areas of uncertainty which require additional future research include the relationship between non-bacterial (viral and fungal) microbiota and the immune system in gastrointestinal malignancies, as well as the influence of metabolites on cancer development and response to immunotherapy.

References

Abu-Sbeih H, Herrera LN, Tang T, Altan M, Chaftari AP, Okhuysen PC, et al. Impact of antibiotic therapy on the development and response to treatment of immune checkpoint inhibitor-mediated diarrhea and colitis. J Immunother Cancer. 2019;7:242.

Anker JF, Naseem A, Mok H, Schaeffer AJ, Abdulkadir SA, Thumbikat P. Multi-faceted immunomodulatory and tissue-tropic clinical bacterial isolate potentiates prostate cancer immunotherapy. Nat Commun. 2018;9:1–14.

Banna G, Torino F, Marletta F, Santagati M, Salemi R, Cannarozzo E, et al. Lactobacillus rhamnosus GG: an overview to explore the rationale of its use in cancer. Front Pharmacol. 2017;8:603.

Batten M, Shanahan E, Silva IP, Adhikari C, Conway J, Tasker A. Low intestinal microbial diversity is associated with severe immune-related adverse events and lack of response to neoadjuvant combination antiPD1, anti- CTLA4 immunotherapy. Cancer Res. 2019;79:2822.

Behary J, Raposo AE, Amorim NML, Zheng H, Gong L, McGovern E, et al. Defining the temporal evolution of gut dysbiosis and inflammatory responses leading to hepatocellular carcinoma in Mdr2 −/− mouse model. BMC Microbiol. 2021;21:113.

Belkaid Y, Hand TW. Role of the microbiota in immunity and inflammation. Cell. 2014;157:121–41.

Bingham S, Day N, Luben RN, Ferrari P, Slimani N, Norat T, et al. Dietary fibre in food and protection against colorectal cancer in the European prospective investigation into cancer and nutrition (EPIC): an observational study. Lancet. 2003;361:1496–501.

Bishehsari F, Engen P, Preite NZ, Tuncil Y, Naqib A, Shaikh M, et al. Dietary fiber treatment corrects the composition of gut microbiota, promotes SCFA production, and suppresses colon carcinogenesis. Genes. 2018;9:102.

Blaser MJ, Falkow S. What are the consequences of the disappearing human microbiota? Nat Rev Microbiol. 2009;7:887–94.

Bozkurt H, Quigley E, Kara B. Bifidobacterium animalis subspecies lactis engineered to produce mycosporin-like amino acids in colorectal cancer prevention. SAGE Open Med. 2019;7:2050312119825784. https://doi.org/10.1177/2050312119825784.

Carvalho FA, Koren O, Goodrich JK, Johansson ME, Nalbantoglu I, Aitken JD, et al. Transient inability to manage proteobacteria promotes chronic gut inflammation in TLR5-deficient mice. Cell Host Microbe. 2012;12:139–52.

Chaput N, Lepage P, Coutzac C, Soularue E, Le Roux K, Monot C, et al. Baseline gut microbiota predicts clinical response and colitis in metastatic melanoma patients treated with ipilimumab. Ann Oncol. 2017;28:1368–79.

Chassaing B, Koren O, Carvalho F, Ley R, Gewirtz A. AIEC pathobiont instigates chronic colitis in susceptible hosts by altering microbiota composition. Gut. 2014;63:1069–80.

Chen D, Wu J, Jin D, Wang B, Cao H. Fecal microbiota transplantation in cancer management: current status and perspectives. Int J Cancer. 2019;145:2021–31.

Cheng W, Wu CY, Yu J. The role of gut microbiota in cancer treatment: friend or foe? Gut. 2020;69:1867–76.

Choi I, Kook M, Kim Y, Cho SJ, Lee JY, Kim CG, et al. Helicobacter pylori therapy for the prevention of metachronous gastric cancer. N Engl J Med. 2018;378:1085–95.

Coley W. Contribution to the knowledge of sarcoma. Am Surg. 1891;14:190.

Coppola A, Arriga R, Lauro D, Del Principe MI, Buccisano F, Maurillo L, et al. NK cell inflammation in the clinical outcome of colorectal carcinoma. Front Med. 2015;2:33.

Davar D, Dzutsev A, McCulloch JA, Rodrigues RR, Chauvin JM, Morrison RM, et al. Fecal microbiota transplant overcomes resistance to anti-PD-1 therapy in melanoma patients. Science. 2021;371:595–602.

Deehan E, Yang C, Perez-Muñoz M, Nguyen N, Cheng C, Triador L, et al. Precision microbiome modulation with discrete dietary fiber structures directs short-chain fatty acid production. Cell Host Microbe. 2020;27:389–404.

Derosa L, Hellmann M, Spaziano M, Halpenny D, Fidelle M, Rizvi H, et al. Negative association of antibiotics on clinical activity of immune checkpoint inhibitors in patients with advanced renal cell and non-small-cell lung cancer. Ann Oncol. 2018;29:1437–44.

Dienstmann R, Mason M, Sinicrope FA, Phipps AI, Tejpar S, Nesbakken A, et al. Prediction of overall survival in stage II and III colon cancer beyond TNM system: a retrospective, pooled biomarker study. Ann Oncol. 2017;28:1023–31.

Ding C, Tang W, Fan X, Wu G. Intestinal microbiota: a novel perspective in colorectal cancer biotherapeutics. Onco Targets Ther. 2018;11:4797–810.

Drago L. Probiotics and colon cancer. Microorganisms. 2019;7:66.

Dubin K, Callahan M, Ren B, Khanin R, Viale A, Ling L, et al. Intestinal microbiome analyses identify melanoma patients at risk for checkpoint-blockade-induced colitis. Nat Commun. 2016;7:10391.

Erreni M, Mantovani A, Allavena P. Tumor-associated macrophages (TAM) and inflammation in colorectal cancer. Cancer Microenviron. 2011;4:141–54.

Francescone R, Hou V, Grivennikov S. Microbiome, inflammation, and cancer. Cancer. 2014;20:181–9.

Fung T, Hu F, Schulze M, Pollak M, Wu T, Fuchs C, et al. A dietary pattern that is associated with C-peptide and risk of colorectal cancer in women. Cancer Causes Control. 2012;23:959–65.

Galdeano CM, Perdigón G. The probiotic bacterium Lactobacillus casei induces activation of the gut mucosal immune system through innate immunity. Clin Vaccine Immunol. 2006;13:219–26.

Gamallat Y, Meyiah A, Kuugbee ED, Hago AM, Chiwala G, Awadasseid A, et al. Lactobacillus rhamnosus induced epithelial cell apoptosis, ameliorates inflammation and prevents colon cancer development in an animal model. Biomed Pharmacother. 2016;83:536–41.

Gopalakrishnan V, Spencer C, Nezi L, Reuben A, Andrews MC, Karpinets TV, et al. Gut microbiome modulates response to anti-PD-1 immunotherapy in melanoma patients. Science. 2018;359:97–103.

Gough E, Shaikh H, Manges AR. Systematic review of intestinal microbiota transplantation (fecal bacteriotherapy) for recurrent Clostridium difficile infection. Clin Infect Dis. 2011;53:994–1002.

Greten F, Grivennikov S. Inflammation and cancer: triggers, mechanisms, and consequences. Immunity. 2019;51:27–41.

Grivennikov S. Inflammation and colorectal cancer: colitis-associated neoplasia. Semin Immunopathol. 2012;35:229–44.

Grivennikov SI, Karin M. Dangerous liaisons: STAT3 and NF-kappaB collaboration and crosstalk in cancer. Cytokine Growth Factor Rev. 2010;21:11–9.

Hamada H, Hiroi T, Nishiyama Y, Takahashi H, Masunaga Y, Hachimura S, et al. Identification of multiple isolated lymphoid follicles on the antimesenteric wall of the mouse small intestine. J Immunol. 2002;168:57–64.

Hibberd A, Lyra A, Ouwehand A, Rolny P, Lindegren H, Cedgård L, et al. Intestinal microbiota is altered in patients with colon cancer and modified by probiotic intervention. BMJ Open Gastroenterol. 2017;4:e000145.

Huang XZ, Gao P, Song YX, Xu Y, Sun JX, Chen XW, et al. Antibiotic use and the efficacy of immune checkpoint inhibitors in cancer patients: a pooled analysis of 2740 cancer patients. Oncoimmunology. 2019;8:e1665973.

Iida N, Dzutsev A, Stewart CA, Smith L, Bouladoux N, Weingarten RA, et al. Commensal bacteria control cancer response to therapy by modulating the tumor microenvironment. Science. 2013;342:967–70.

Jacouton E, Chain F, Sokol H, Langella P, Bermúdez-Humarán LG. Probiotic strain lactobacillus casei BL23 prevents colitis-associated colorectal cancer. Front Immunol. 2017;8:1553.

Johnston CJ, McSorley HJ, Anderton SM, Wigmore SJ, Maizels RM. Helminths and immunological tolerance. Transplantation. 2014;97:127–32.

Kato L, Kawamoto S, Maruya M, Fagarasan S. The role of the adaptive immune system in regulation of gut microbiota. Immunol Rev. 2014;260:67–75.

Kawamoto S, Maruya M, Kato LM, Suda W, Atarashi K, Doi Y, et al. Foxp3(+) T cells regulate immunoglobulin a selection and facilitate diversification of bacterial species responsible for immune homeostasis. Immunity. 2014;41:152–65.

Kostic AD, Gevers D, Pedamallu CS, Michaud M, Duke F, Earl AM, et al. Genomic analysis identifies association of Fusobacterium with colorectal carcinoma. Genome Res. 2012;22:292–8.

Kubinak JL, Petersen C, Stephens WZ, Soto R, Bake E, O'Connell R, et al. MyD88 signaling in T cells directs IgA-mediated control of the microbiota to promote health. Cell Host Microbe. 2015;17:153–63.

Li J, Sung C, Lee N, Ni Y, Pihlajamäki J, Panagiotou G, et al. Probiotics modulated gut microbiota suppresses hepatocellular carcinoma growth in mice. Proc Natl Acad Sci U S A. 2016;113:E1306–15.

Liu JZN, Li Q, Zhang W, Ke F, Leng Q, Wang H, Chen J, Wang H. Tumor-associated macrophages recruit CCR6+ regulatory T cells and promote the development of colorectal cancer via enhancing CCL20 production in mice. PLoS One. 2011;6:e19495.

Liu T, Xiong Q, Li L, Hu Y. Intestinal microbiota predicts lung cancer patients at risk of immune-related diarrhea. Immunotherapy. 2019;11:385–96.

Liu X, Wang L, Jing N, Jiang G, Liu Z. Biostimulating gut microbiome with bilberry anthocyanin combo to enhance anti-PD-L1 efficiency against murine colon cancer. Microorganisms. 2020;8:175.

Lv J, Li J, Kuai W, Li Y, Guo F, Xu X, et al. Gegen Qinlian decoction enhances the effect of PD-1 blockade in colorectal cancer with microsatellite stability by remodelling the gut microbiota and the tumour microenvironment. Cell Death Dis. 2019;10:415.

Macpherson AJ, Hunziker L, McCoy K, Lamarre A. IgA responses in the intestinal mucosa against pathogenic and non-pathogenic microorganisms. Microbes Infect. 2001;3:1021–35.

Macpherson AJ, Slack E, Geuking MB, McCoy KD. The mucosal firewalls against commensal intestinal microbes. Semin Immunopathol. 2009;31:145–9.

Maloy KJ, Powrie F. Intestinal homeostasis and its breakdown in inflammatory bowel disease. Nature. 2011;474:298–306.

Marcobal A, Barboza M, Froehlich JW, Block DE, German JB, Lebrilla CB, et al. Consumption of human milk oligosaccharides by gut-related microbes. J Agric Food Chem. 2010;58:5334–40.

Marshall BJ, Warren JR. Unidentified curved bacilli in the stomach of patients with gastritis and peptic ulceration. Lancet. 1984;1:1311–5.

Matson V, Fessler J, Bao R, Chongsuwat T, Zha Y, Alegre ML, et al. The commensal microbiome is associated with anti-PD-1 efficacy in metastatic melanoma patients. Science. 2018;359:104–8.

Michot JM, Bigenwald C, Champiat S, Collins M, Carbonnel F, Postel-Vinay S, et al. Immune-related adverse events with immune checkpoint blockade: a comprehensive review. Eur J Cancer. 2016;54:139–48.

Mirpuri J, Raetz M, Sturge CR, Wilhelm CL, Benson A, Savani RC, et al. Proteobacteria-specific IgA regulates maturation of the intestinal microbiota. Gut Microbes. 2014;5:28–39.

Nomura M, Nagatomo R, Doi K, Shimizu J, Baba K, Saito T, et al. Association of short-chain fatty acids in the gut microbiome with clinical response to treatment with nivolumab or pembrolizumab in patients with solid cancer tumors. JAMA Netw Open. 2020;3:e202895.

O'Donnell JS, Teng M, Smyth MJ. Cancer immunoediting and resistance to T cell-based immunotherapy. Nat Rev Clin Oncol. 2019;16:151–67.

O'Keefe S, Li J, Lahti L, Ou J, Carbonero F, Mohammed K, et al. Fat, fibre and cancer risk in African Americans and rural Africans. Nat Commun. 2015;6:6342.

Ohara T, Yoshino K, Kitajima M. Possibility of preventing colorectal carcinogenesis with probiotics. Hepatogastroenterology. 2011;57:1411–5.

Ormandy LA, Hilleman T, Wedemeyer H, Manns MP, Greten TF, Korangy F. Increased populations of regulatory T cells in peripheral blood of patients with hepatocellular carcinoma. Cancer Res. 2005;65:2457–64.

Palm NW, de Zoete MR, Flavell RA. Immune-microbiota interactions in health and disease. Clin Immunol. 2015;159:122–7.

Ponziani F, Bhoori S, Castelli C, Putignani L, Rivoltini L, Del Chierico F, et al. Hepatocellular carcinoma is associated with gut microbiota profile and inflammation in nonalcoholic fatty liver disease. Hepatology. 2019;69:107–20.

Rafter J, Bennett M, Caderni G, Clune Y, Hughes R, Karlsson P, et al. Dietary synbiotics reduce cancer risk factors in polypectomized and colon cancer patients. Am J Clin Nutr. 2007;85:488–96.

Remash D, Prince DS, McKenzie C, Strasser SI, Kao S, Liu K. Immune checkpoint inhibitor-related hepatotoxicity: a review. World J Gastroenterol. 2021;27:5376–91.

Riquelme E, Zhang Y, Zhang L, Montiel M, Zoltan M, Dong W, et al. Tumor microbiome diversity and composition influence pancreatic cancer outcomes. Cell. 2019;178:795–806.

Roggero E, Zucca E, Pinotti G, Pascarella A, Capella C, Savio A, et al. Eradication of Helicobacter pylori infection in primary low-grade gastric lymphoma of mucosa-associated lymphoid tissue. Ann Intern Med. 1995;122:767–9.

Round JL, Mazmanian S. The gut microbiota shapes intestinal immune responses during health and disease. Nat Rev Immunol. 2009;9:313–23.

Routy B, Derosa L, Duong CPM, Alou MT, Daillère R, Fluckiger A, et al. Gut microbiome influences efficacy of PD-1–based immunotherapy against epithelial tumors. Science. 2018;359:91–7.

Rubinstein MR, Wang X, Liu W, Hao Y, Cai G, Han YW. Fusobacterium nucleatum promotes colorectal carcinogenesis by modulating E-cadherin/b-catenin signaling via its FadA adhesin. Cell Host Microbe. 2013;14:195–206.

Salcedo R, Worschech A, Cardone M, Jones Y, Gyulai Z, Dai RM, Wang E, et al. MyD88-mediated signaling prevents development of adenocarcinomas of the colon: role of interleukin 18. J Exp Med. 2010;207:1625–36.

Sanchez-Alcoholado L, Ramos-Molina B, Otero A, Laborda-Illanes A, Ordonez R, Medina JA, et al. The role of the gut microbiome in colorectal cancer development and therapy response. Cancers (Basel). 2020;12:1406.

Santhakumar C, Gane EJ, Liu K, McCaughan GW. Current perspectives on the tumor microenvironment in hepatocellular carcinoma. Hepatol Int. 2020;14:947–57.

Sen S, Hess K, Viola GM, Subbiah V. Impact of antibiotic use on survival in patients with advanced cancers treated on immune checkpoint inhibitor phase I clinical trials. Ann Oncol. 2018;29:2396–8.

Shi NLN, Duan X, Niu H. Interaction between the gut microbiome and mucosal immune system. Military Med Res. 2017;4:14.

Singh N, Gurav A, Sivaprakasam S, Brady E, Padia R, Shi H, Thangaraju M, et al. Activation of Gpr109a, receptor for niacin and the commensal metabolite butyrate, suppresses colonic inflammation and carcinogenesis. Immunity. 2014;40:128–39.

Sinicrope F, Smyrk T, Foster N, Meyers J, Thibodeau S, Goldberg RM, et al. Association of tumor infiltrating lymphocytes (TILs) with molecular subtype and prognosis in stage III colon cancers (CC) from a FOLFOX-based adjuvant chemotherapy trial. J Clin Oncol. 2016;34:3518.

Sivan A, Corrales L, Hubert N, Williams JB, Aquino-Michaels K, Earley ZM, et al. Commensal Bifidobacterium promotes antitumor immunity and facilitates anti–PD-L1 efficacy. Science. 2015;350:1084–9.

Smith K, McCoy KD, Macpherson AJ. Use of axenic animals in studying the adaptation of mammals to their commensal intestinal microbiota. Semin Immunol. 2007;19:59–69.

Sobhani I, Tap J, Roudot-Thoraval F, Roperch JP, Letulle S, Langella P, et al. Microbial dysbiosis in colorectal cancer (CRC) patients. PLoS One. 2011;6:e16393.

Talham GL, Jiang HQ, Bos NA, Cebra JJ. Segmented filamentous bacteria are potent stimuli of a physiologically normal state of the murine gut mucosal immune system. Infect Immun. 1999;67:1992–2000.

Tan J, McKenzie C, Vuillermin PJ, Goverse G, Vinuesa CG, Mebius RE, et al. Dietary fiber and bacterial SCFA enhance oral tolerance and protect against food allergy through diverse cellular pathways. Cell Rep. 2016;15:2809–24.

Trompette A, Gollwitzer E, Yadava K, Sichelstiel AK, Sprenger N, Ngom-Bru C. Gut microbiota metabolism of dietary fiber influences allergic airway disease and hematopoiesis. Nat Med. 2014;20:159–66.

Vetizou M, Pitt J, Daillère R, Lepage P, Waldschmitt N, Flament C, et al. Anticancer immunotherapy by CTLA-4 blockade relies on the gut microbiota. Science. 2015;350:1079–84.

Viaud S, Saccheri F, Mignot G, Yamazaki T, Daillère R, Hannani D, et al. The intestinal microbiota modulates the anticancer immune effects of cyclophosphamide. Science. 2013;342:971–6.

Vijay-Kumar M, Aitken J, Carvalho FA, Cullender TC, Mwangi S, Srinivasan S, et al. Metabolic syndrome and altered gut microbiota in mice lacking Toll-like receptor 5. Science. 2010;328:228–31.

Waldman AD, Fritz JM, Lenardo MJ. A guide to cancer immunotherapy: from T cell basic science to clinical practice. Nat Rev Immunol. 2020;20:651–68.

Wang Y, Wiesnoski D, Helmink BA, Gopalakrishnan V, Choi K, DuPont HL, et al. Fecal microbiota transplantation for refractory immune checkpoint inhibitor-associated colitis. Nat Med. 2018;24:1804–8.

Wilkinson K, Ng W, Roberts T, Becker T, Lim S, Chua W, et al. Tumour immune microenvironment biomarkers predicting cytotoxic chemotherapy efficacy in colorectal cancer. J Clin Pathol. 2021;74:625–34.

Wong S, Zhao L, Zhang X, Nakatsu G, Han J, Xu W, et al. Gavage of fecal samples from patients with colorectal cancer promotes intestinal carcinogenesis in germ-free and conventional mice. Gastroenterology. 2017;153:1621–33.

Wu L, Feng J, Li J, Yu Q, Ji J, Wu J, et al. The gut microbiome-bile acid axis in hepatocarcinogenesis. Biomed Pharmacother. 2021;133:111036.

Xu W, Liu K, Chen M, Sun JY, McCaughan GW, Lu XJ, et al. Immunotherapy for hepatocellular carcinoma: recent advances and future perspectives. Ther Adv Med Oncol. 2019;11:1758835919862692.

Yoshimoto S, Loo TM, Atarashi K, Kanda H, Sato S, Oyadomari S, et al. Obesity-induced gut microbial metabolite promotes liver cancer through senescence secretome. Nature. 2013;499:97–101.

Zhang H, Yu L, Yang W, Tang L, Lin Y, Wu H, et al. Profound impact of gut homeostasis on chemically- induced pro-tumorigenic inflammation and hepatocarcinogenesis in rats. J Hepatol. 2012;57:803–12.

Zhang Y, Jin N, Wang J. Mechanisms of immunosuppression in colorectal cancer. Cancers (Basel). 2020;12:3850.

Chapter 12
Animal Models in the Study of Microbiome in Gastrointestinal Cancer

Xinning Wang and Hong Wei

Abstract The high incidence and mortality of gastrointestinal (GI) cancer always attracted a great deal of attention from academia and industry. Efforts have been made to clarify the pathogenesis of GI cancer and identify therapeutic targets, which led to profound progress in the establishment and application of animal models. Currently, the study of cancer microbiome marks one of the most important trends in this field, putting forward demands that animal models be more elaborate. In this chapter, we have profiled representative animal models used in major types of GI cancer to support the study of corresponding microbiome, along with the findings obtained based on them. Looking to the future, animal models need to be further upgraded to conform to academic and industrial demands for establishing causality and developing microbiome therapeutics.

Keywords Animal models · GI cancer · Microbiome · Germ-free · Causal relationship

12.1 Introduction

The human gastrointestinal (GI) tract is the passageway that extends from the mouth to the anus, which contains the main digestive organs including the esophagus, stomach, and intestines. The GI tract is critical to human health since it is responsible for the digestion of food and absorption of nutrients. Unfortunately, it is also responsible for more incidence and mortality rates of cancer than any other parts of human body. In 2020, major types of GI cancer (cancers of colorectum, stomach, liver, esophagus, pancreas) account for 26% of new cancer cases and 35.6% of cancer deaths worldwide, which have posed huge burden on human health (Sung et al. 2021).

X. Wang · H. Wei (✉)
Precision Medicine Institute, The First Affiliated Hospital, Sun Yat-Sen University, Guangzhou, China

J. Yu (ed.), *Microbiome in Gastrointestinal Cancer*,
https://doi.org/10.1007/978-981-19-4492-5_12

Generally speaking, the pathogenesis of GI cancer is closely related to inherited genetic factors, latent conditions, and modifiable lifestyles (Arnold et al. 2020). Notably, a growing body of evidence has demonstrated that host microbiome plays critical roles in GI cancer. Given that the GI tract harbors most of the commensal microbes in human body, discovering and developing microbiome-related diagnostic and prognostic biomarkers, novel drugs, and clinical strategies are considered to have broad prospect of fighting against GI cancer.

In order to better understand the pathogenesis and develop effective intervention methods, animal models are indispensable tools to mimic human conditions and receive various in vivo tests without causing potential harm to human. In the study of microbiome in GI cancers, animal models are constructed using various approaches including tumor xenograft, genetic engineering, chemical induction, and sterilization. Currently, cancer microbiome study has covered all major organs of the GI tract and the digestive system, namely the esophagus, stomach, intestines, liver, and pancreas. The following content of this chapter will describe the typical animal models used in microbiome study according to GI cancer types.

12.2 Animal Models

12.2.1 Esophageal Cancer

The esophagus is an organ which connects the pharynx with the stomach, which is responsible for delivering food down to the stomach. In recent years, esophageal cancer has been occupying the seventh place in the ranking of new cancer cases and the sixth in cancer mortality globally (Sung et al. 2021). The two main histologic subtypes of esophageal cancer are esophageal squamous cell carcinoma (ESCC) and esophageal adenocarcinoma (EAC). Usually occurs in the upper or middle part of the esophagus, ESCC is more common in developing countries. EAC occurs in the lower part of the esophagus, and it accounts for the majority of esophageal cancer cases in developed countries. Increasing evidence have suggested that the microbiome could be related to the occurrence and development of esophageal cancer and the corresponding animal models are essential to elucidating the intricate relationships.

Recently, the cross-talk between the gut microbiome and ESCC has been found. In one study, the composition of gut and esophageal microbiota of nude mice were found altered after implantation with human ESCC cells (EC-109) (Cheung et al. 2020). Further, nude mice were administered antibiotics (ABX) to deplete the native gut microbiota. These ABX-treated mice were then xenografted with EC-109 cells to establish ESCC models. Afterwards, fecal microbiota transplantation (FMT) experiments were carried out on these models and the gut microbiota from healthy mice led to attenuated tumor metastasis. These animal model-based results indicate that an intact gut microbiota could be beneficial to ESCC treatment. In another study, a similar ESCC cell line-derived xenograft (CDX) mouse model was constructed. Through characterizing the gut microbiota of ESCC mice and implementing chemotherapy to treat them, the adjuvant role of natural product cepharanthine hydrochloride in chemotherapy by regulating host microbiome was revealed (Zhou et al. 2019). Considering the rising need for more translatable results into clinical gains and precision medicine, patient-derived xenograft (PDX) models based on immunodeficient mice are due to replace the CDX models gradually (Ledford 2016; Byrne et al. 2017; Risbridger et al. 2020).

Barrett's esophagus (BE), caused by gastroesophageal reflux disease, is considered as a premalignant condition of EAC (Gatenby et al. 2014; Peters et al. 2019). Animal model-based studies on the pathogenesis of BE and the development process from BE to EAC have revealed the potential diagnostic, prognostic, therapeutic roles of microbiome. In an attempt to investigate underlying factors that influencing tumorigenesis of BE, a transgenic mouse model expressing human interleukin-1β in the esophagus epithelium called L2-IL1B mouse (a model of BE) was used (Munch et al. 2019). In this study, the L2-IL1B mice fed a high-fat diet (HFD) exhibited acceleration of the inflammatory and tumor development in contrast to mice treated with control diet. The accelerated dysplasia phenotype in mouse models was found associated with altered composition of host microbiota. 16S rRNA gene sequencing of fecal samples showed an increased Firmicutes/Bacteroidetes ratio in HFD-treated L2-IL1B mice. Bedding transfer from HFD group to control diet group led to tumor phenotype transmission. Next, germ-free (GF) L2-IL1B mice were generated via embryo transfer into GF mothers. The depletion of microbes under GF conditions led to suppressed oncogenesis.

12.2.2 Gastric Cancer

Gastric cancer (GC) is the fourth most commonly diagnosed cancer and the fourth leading cause of cancer death in 2020 with an estimated 1.1 million new cases and 0.77 million deaths (Sung et al. 2021). The relationship between GC and microbiome is very close. Firstly, the primary cause of most GC cases is *Helicobacter pylori* infection (Plummer et al. 2015). *H. pylori* is associated with chronic atrophic gastritis at the beginning of GC development and is the most recognized bacterial carcinogen to date. More than half of the world's population is infected with *H. pylori*, in which only a small percentage of people will eventually develop GC (Hooi et al. 2017). Noticeably, although only a smaller number of bacteria live in the acidic environment of the stomach, microbes other than *H. pylori* have also been revealed to be involved in gastric cancer (Noto and Peek Jr. 2017; Ferreira et al. 2018).

Transgenic insulin-gastrin mouse (INS-GAS) model on an FVB/N background overexpresses human gastrin by an insulin promoter. It has high circulating levels of gastrin and is capable of developing atrophic gastritis spontaneously. After being infected with *H. pylori*, the INS-GAS mice will further develop gastrointestinal intraepithelial neoplasia, making them useful tools for studying relationship between microbiome and the development of gastric cancer (Stewart et al. 2020). In a typical study to investigate the role of microbiota in gastric cancer, *H. pylori*-infected, GF, and specific pathogen free (SPF) INS-GAS mice were used. The results showed that it took GF INS-GAS mice much longer time to develop gastric lesions when compared with the SPF control. Colonization of *H. pylori* in INS-GAS mice significantly promoted progressive gastric pathology. And 16s rRNA gene sequencing of microbiome composition in the stomach indicated that the relative number of Bacteroidetes was reduced in *H. pylori*-infected male mice while Firmicutes was increased in contrast to uninfected controls. As for the gut microbiome, no significant difference was detected (Lofgren et al. 2011).

Myeloid differentiation primary response gene 88 (MyD88) is a key regulator in several inflammatory pathways and the protective role of MyD88 in *H. felis*-induced GC was previously demonstrated in a *Myd88*-deficient mouse model (Banerjee et al. 2014). The *H. felis*-infected *Myd88*$^{-/-}$ model shows a rapid progression to cancerous lesions and recapitulates the process of human GC. Thus, the microbiome signature changes in GC progression after *Helicobacter* infection were studied in mice with different genotypic background including *Myd88*$^{-/-}$ mice. Analysis of stomach mucosal tissue showed an overall reduction in microbial diversity after infection with *H. felis*. Significant reduction of Campylobacterales was found in infected models while the abundance of Lactobacillales increased dramatically after infection. Further histological data from mouse models also confirmed Lactobacillales are closely related to GC development upon *Helicobacter* infection (Bali et al. 2021).

To verify the causal relationship between human gastric microbiome and GC, GF mice can serve as an effective model. For example, gastric microbiota profiles in patients with gastric dysplasia or GC were found similar. On the basis of correlation, gastric microbiota transplantation (GMT) from patients in different disease stages to GF mice was performed. Inoculation of microbiota from intestinal metaplasia and GC mucosal showed elevated inflammation and metaplasia in the stomachs of GF mouse recipients compared with that of chronic superficial gastritis mucosal-inoculated mice. On the other hand, GMT using gastric fluid samples from corresponding patients resulted in similar premalignant lesions to recipient GF mice (Kwon et al. 2021). This example fully demonstrated the unique role of GF animal models in reproducing premalignant changes and establishing causality in the study of microbiome in gastric cancer.

12.2.3 Colorectal Cancer

As the one with the largest number of patients and deaths among GI cancers, colorectal cancer (CRC) is one of the key targets for global cancer prevention and treatment (Keum and Giovannucci 2019). In many developing countries, the incidence of colorectal cancer has been steadily increasing with economic development and lifestyle changes. Many CRC risk factors such as alcohol consumption, smoking, and high intake of red or processed meat profoundly modulate the microbiome. And given that most of the commensal microbes reside within the gut, studies on the relationship between CRC and gut microbiome have been more common and in-depth, and the demand for appropriate animal models is continuing to rise.

One of the most widely used animal model in CRC research is *Apc*$^{min/+}$ mouse model. The heterozygous *Apc* gene mutation can trigger multiple intestinal neoplasia (Min) in the intestine while homozygous ApcMin/+ mice are not viable (Moser et al. 1990, 1995). The genetic feature and phenotype of *Apc*$^{min/+}$ mice resemble human familial adenomatous polyposis (FAP), which is an important precancerous lesion of CRC (Madhu et al. 2020). When it comes to CRC microbiome research, this model and its derivatives also play an indispensable role. It has long been recognized that the gut microbiome as a whole could be important for the development of intestinal adenomas (Dove et al. 1997). *Apc*$^{min/+}$ mice have been utilized to validate the functional role of certain gut microbiota in CRC tumorigenesis. Enterotoxigenic *Bacteroides fragilis* colonized *Apc*$^{min/+}$ mice can develop colonic colitis and accelerated tumorigenesis (Wu et al. 2009). By introducing *Fusobacterium nucleatum* into *Apc*$^{min/+}$ mice, colonic tumorigenesis was also accelerated but without causing colitis. *F. nucleatum* in *Apc*$^{min/+}$ mice was enriched in tumor tissues compared with adjacent tissues, which is consistent with human CRC (Kostic et al. 2013). Analysis on the intestinal tumors of *Fusobacterium*-treated Apc$^{min/+}$ mice revealed that *F. nucleatum* induced tumor-promoting microenvironment through recruitment of myeloid-derived immune cells (Kostic et al. 2013). The carcinogenic mechanism of *F. nucleatum* involving a TLR4/p-PAK1/p-β-catenin S675 cascade was also discovered with the help of *Apc*$^{min/+}$ mice (Wu et al. 2018). In a study to dissect the relationship among microbiome, inflammation, and colon tumorigenesis, *Apc*$^{Min/+}$*;Il10*$^{-/-}$ mice were generated from crossbreeding between *Apc*$^{min/+}$ mice and *Il10*$^{-/-}$ colitis mouse models. Inflammatory cytokine expression was decreased and colon tumorigenesis completely disappeared in GF *Apc*$^{Min/+}$*;Il10*$^{-/-}$ mice as compared with SPF mice, implying that microbiome is essential for promoting inflammation and initiating CRC (Tomkovich et al. 2017). The same study further proved that *Apc*$^{Min/+}$*;Il10*$^{-/-}$ mice were sensitive to specific microbial profiles and colibactin produced by *Escherichia coli* was a driver of colon tumor development in *Apc*$^{Min/+}$*;Il10*$^{-/-}$ mice (Tomkovich et al. 2017).

In addition to genetically engineered models, chemically induced models are also used in the study of microbiome in CRC because of convenient modeling process and affordable cost. Azoxymethane (AOM) is a carcinogen that causes colon tumors in mice through inducing DNA alkylation and base mismatches. Routinely, intraperitoneal injection of AOM in mice is either implemented alone or in conjunction with administration of dextran sulfate sodium (DSS), a colitogenic agent, to generate chemically induced CRC mouse models (De Robertis et al. 2011). Transfer of fecal microbiota from patients with CRC into antibiotic-treated AOM mice as well as GF mice successfully recapitulated the human phenotypes, suggesting a potential deleterious composition of the microbiome in CRC patients (Wong et al. 2017). A recent study saw the depletion of aerobic gut microbe *Lysinibacillus sphaericus* in AOM/DSS mice enhanced the efficacy of aspirin-mediated CRC prevention. Further metagenomics analysis of fecal microbiota from both AOM/DSS and $Apc^{Min/+}$ mice revealed that the administration of aspirin elevated the abundance of some probiotics (Zhao et al. 2020). Besides, it is reasonable to integrate chemical induction with gene editing in a CRC model for the purpose of studying the intricate mechanism of tumorigenesis involving the microbiome (Arthur et al. 2012).

Human tumor xenograft models are also used in the study of CRC microbiome (Cougnoux et al. 2014; Bullman et al. 2017; Chen et al. 2020). Immunodeficient mice transplanted with human-derived CRC cells or tissues replicate more biological characteristics of the primary tumor in histopathology, oncogene expression, and drug response than do the mouse CRC cell line-derived xenograft models.

12.2.4 Liver Cancer

Among all GI cancers, the mortality rate of primary liver cancer is second only to CRC. As the most important type of liver cancer, hepatocellular carcinoma (HCC) accounts for 80% of cases (Sung et al. 2021). The risk factors vary in different regions of the world, and the potential role of gut–liver axis (Wahlstrom et al. 2016; Gruner and Mattner 2021) in the development of liver cancer has been underlined in recent years through experiments based on animal models.

Obesity is one of the main risk factors for HCC. To elucidate the mechanism of obesity-induced dysbacteriosis participating in the development of HCC, mice were treated with carcinogenic chemical dimethylbenz[a]anthracene (DMBA) and fed HFD diet to establish HCC models (Yoshimoto et al. 2013). Interestingly, transgenic p21-*p*-luc mice featuring with noninvasively detectable $p21^{Waf1/Cip1}$ gene expression (a senescence marker) (Ohtani et al. 2007) were deployed in this study to facilitate the monitoring of HCC development. In another study investigating the role of microbiota in non-alcoholic steatohepatitis (NASH)-associated HCC development, C57BL/6J mice were fed a steatohepatitis-inducing HFD with or without antibiotics, which induced NASH pathology in a relatively short time. The following HCC development was achieved without carcinogenic chemicals (Yamada et al. 2018).

Bile acid metabolism mediated by gut microbiome can promote accumulation of hepatic CXCR6^{+} natural killer T (NKT) cells and production of interferon-γ (IFN-γ) production, reinforcing immune response against primary and metastatic liver tumors. The underlying mechanism was well illustrated mainly by a series of in vivo experiments implemented in liver-specific MYC mice (Ma et al. 2018). As a conditional transgenic model constructed by using Tet system, expression of human MYC proto-oncogene can be regulated in liver cells of MYC mice (Xu et al. 2004). To induce spontaneous HCC, MYC transgenic mice were fed a methionine–choline-deficient diet (Ma et al. 2016).

12.2.5 *Pancreatic Cancer*

Generally speaking, pancreatic cancer is more prevalent in developed countries but incidence rates in many other countries of the world are gradually increasing in these years. Because pancreatic ductal adenocarcinoma (PDAC) accounts for over 90% of pancreatic cancer diagnoses, most animal models and microbiome studies have aimed at PDAC diagnosis, pathogenesis, and treatment. Given that activating mutations in the KRAS proto-oncogene are observed in most PDAC cases (Hashimoto et al. 2016), genetically engineered mouse models featuring mutant *Kras* are intensively used in this field.

KC mouse model, expressing oncogenic *Kras* in the pancreas, can spontaneously develop slowly progressive pancreatic neoplasia. It has been a popular tool for PDAC study since it was first established by Tuveson's group (Hingorani et al. 2003). They first inserted a Lox-STOP-Lox (LSL) construct into the mouse KRAS locus upstream of modified exon 1 containing a G12D mutation to give *LSL-Kras*^{G12D} strain. Next, by crossing *LSL-Kras*^{G12D} mice with pancreatic-specific Cre strains such as *Pdx-1-Cre* and *p48-Cre* mice, the resulting KC mice were established. By incorporating mutant tumor suppressor genes (e.g., *Trp53*, *Smad4*, *Pten*, and *Cdkn2a*) and *Kras*, variants of KC mice were constructed by many groups (Lee et al. 2016). These genetically engineered models have played important roles in the study of microbiome in PDAC.

Gut bacteria from PDAC mice showed higher ability for translocation to the pancreas compared with wild-type gut bacteria in a study using KC and *Pdx1*^{Cre}*;LSL-Kras*^{G12D}*;Trp53*^{R172H} (KPC) mice (Pushalkar et al. 2018). With the help of these models, it was further demonstrated that bacteria accelerated the progression of pancreatic oncogenesis through dampening immunosuppression characteristic of PDAC. The fungal mycobiome is also an important player in PDAC although most studies so far have focused on bacteria. A typical study revealed fungal dysbiosis during tumorigenesis by using KC mice. Ablation of the mycobiome was protective against the growth of both tumors in KC mice and orthotopic tumors derived from KPC mice (Aykut et al. 2019). A separate study sequencing the gut microbiota from KPC mice showed significantly changing bacterial species over time. Proteobacterial and Firmicutes were found to be the dominant bacteria at the early stages of PDAC. The metabolic landscape of the microbiota showed elevated polyamine metabolism in the progression of PDAC, which could be exploited as biomarker in early detection of this disease (Mendez et al. 2020).

12.3 Conclusions and Future Perspectives

Animal models in the study of microbiome in GI cancer have seen significant advances in recent years. It is noteworthy that the integrated use of multiple types of models such as xenograft models, genetically engineered models, diet induced models, and chemically induced models has made great contributions to our understanding of the role of microbiome in GI cancer. Indeed, the correlation between host microbiome and cancer development has been proposed in all major GI cancer types by numerous studies as mentioned above. However, validation of causality and clinical translation are still difficult. From the perspective of animal models, some inherent limitations of current GI cancer models need to be addressed urgently and models conforming to the development trends of microbiome research shall be constructed.

Firstly, the existence of commensal microbiota of SPF models could mislead our understanding of the functional role of specific bacteria in GI cancer although it is generally sufficient for discovering a correlation. A conventional and economical practice is to treat models with ABX cocktail for the purpose of eliminating possible background interference caused by commensal bacteria. But complete depletion of bacteria is impossible to achieve in this way let alone maintain a sterile state. Hence, in order to establish explicit cause-and-effect relationship or mechanistic link between defined microbiome and a phenotype, the usage of GF mice is rapidly growing in recent years (Uzbay 2019; Kamareddine et al. 2020). Theoretically, most SPF mouse strain can be converted into its GF counterpart via either cesarean birth or embryo transfer. In addition to conventional C57BL/6 and BALB/c strains, those genetically engineered mouse models described above are worthy of being developed into corresponding GF strains to facilitate precise study of microbiome in GI cancer. Secondly, tissue-specific and tumorigenesis controllable models need to be further exploited so as to yield mechanistic insights into the role of microbiome under conditions that better mimic human pathological characteristics of GI cancer. For example, most tumor lesions in conventional $Apc^{min/+}$ mouse model occur in the small intestine (Moser et al. 1995; Ren et al. 2019), which is divergent from human CRC. Conditional gene targeting approaches can provide feasible solutions to support establishment of more accurate and controllable models (Shibata et al. 1997; Barker et al. 2009) and it would be significant to microbiome research if the GF feature should be integrated. Last but not least, more efforts from academia and industry should now focus on constructing dependable animal models to support preclinical evaluations of novel microbiome-targeted therapies for GI cancer. As an innovative approach to alter host microbiome, FMT has already exerted striking efficacy in cancer management although its safety is still controversial (Baruch et al. 2021; Davar et al. 2021; Elkrief and Routy 2021). Additionally, commensal bacteria strains with therapeutic potential in cancer immunotherapy are being continually identified (Routy et al. 2018; Tanoue et al. 2019; Hou et al. 2021). One foreseeable picture is the ascent of live biotherapeutic products (LBPs) for cancer treatment based on specific functional strains (Laute-Caly et al. 2019; Lythgoe et al. 2020). The close relationship between microbiome and GI cancer will spur attempts to expend indications for microbiome therapeutics to GI cancer in the near term. The development of animal models is largely demand-driven and we anticipate it being in a new window of opportunity given the soaring enthusiasm for microbiome study in GI cancer (Fig. 12.1).

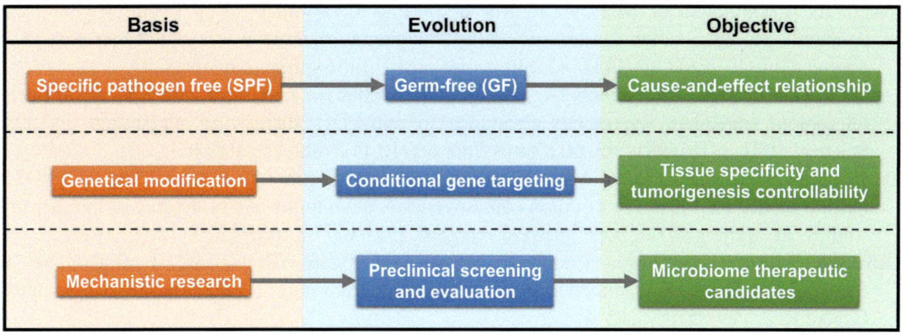

Fig. 12.1 Future perspectives on animal models in the study of microbiome in GI cancer

References

Arnold M, Abnet CC, Neale RE, Vignat J, Giovannucci EL, McGlynn KA, et al. Global burden of 5 major types of gastrointestinal cancer. Gastroenterology. 2020;159(1):335–349.e15. https://doi.org/10.1053/j.gastro.2020.02.068.

Arthur JC, Perez-Chanona E, Mühlbauer M, Tomkovich S, Uronis JM, Fan T-J, et al. Intestinal inflammation targets cancer-inducing activity of the microbiota. Science. 2012;338(6103):120–3. https://doi.org/10.1126/science.1224820.

Aykut B, Pushalkar S, Chen R, Li Q, Abengozar R, Kim JI, et al. The fungal mycobiome promotes pancreatic oncogenesis via activation of MBL. Nature. 2019;574(7777):264–7. https://doi.org/10.1038/s41586-019-1608-2.

Bali P, Coker J, Lozano-Pope I, Zengler K, Obonyo M. Microbiome signatures in a fast- and slow-progressing gastric cancer murine model and their contribution to gastric carcinogenesis. Microorganisms. 2021;9(1):189. https://doi.org/10.3390/microorganisms9010189.

Banerjee A, Thamphiwatana S, Carmona EM, Rickman B, Doran KS, Obonyo M. Deficiency of the myeloid differentiation primary response molecule MyD88 leads to an early and rapid development of Helicobacter-induced gastric malignancy. Infect Immun. 2014;82(1):356–63. https://doi.org/10.1128/IAI.01344-13.

Barker N, Ridgway RA, van Es JH, van de Wetering M, Begthel H, van den Born M, et al. Crypt stem cells as the cells-of-origin of intestinal cancer. Nature. 2009;457(7229):608–11. https://doi.org/10.1038/nature07602.

Baruch EN, Youngster I, Ben-Betzalel G, Ortenberg R, Lahat A, Katz L, et al. Fecal microbiota transplant promotes response in immunotherapy-refractory melanoma patients. Science. 2021;371(6529):602–9. https://doi.org/10.1126/science.abb5920.

Bullman S, Pedamallu CS, Sicinska E, Clancy TE, Zhang X, Cai D, et al. Analysis of *Fusobacterium* persistence and antibiotic response in colorectal cancer. Science. 2017;358(6369):1443–8. https://doi.org/10.1126/science.aal5240.

Byrne AT, Alferez DG, Amant F, Annibali D, Arribas J, Biankin AV, et al. Interrogating open issues in cancer precision medicine with patient-derived xenografts. Nat Rev Cancer. 2017;17(4):254–68. https://doi.org/10.1038/nrc.2016.140.

Chen YC, Miao ZF, Yip KL, Cheng YA, Liu CJ, Li LH, et al. Gut fecal microbiota transplant in a mouse model of orthotopic rectal cancer. Front Oncol. 2020;10:568012. https://doi.org/10.3389/fonc.2020.568012.

Cheung MK, Yue GGL, Tsui KY, Gomes AJ, Kwan HS, Chiu PWY, et al. Discovery of an interplay between the gut microbiota and esophageal squamous cell carcinoma in mice. Am J Cancer Res. 2020;10(8):2409–27.

Cougnoux A, Dalmasso G, Martinez R, Buc E, Delmas J, Gibold L, et al. Bacterial genotoxin colibactin promotes colon tumour growth by inducing a senescence-associated secretory phenotype. Gut. 2014;63(12):1932–42. https://doi.org/10.1136/gutjnl-2013-305257.

Davar D, Dzutsev AK, McCulloch JA, Rodrigues RR, Chauvin J-M, Morrison RM, et al. Fecal microbiota transplant overcomes resistance to anti-PD-1 therapy in melanoma patients. Science. 2021;371(6529):595–602. https://doi.org/10.1126/science.abf3363.

De Robertis M, Massi E, Poeta ML, Carotti S, Morini S, Cecchetelli L, et al. The AOM/DSS murine model for the study of colon carcinogenesis: from pathways to diagnosis and therapy studies. J Carcinog. 2011;10:9. https://doi.org/10.4103/1477-3163.78279.

Dove WF, Clipson L, Gould KA, Luongo C, Marshall DJ, Moser AR, et al. Intestinal neoplasia in the ApcMin mouse: independence from the microbial and natural killer (beige locus) status. Cancer Res. 1997;57(5):812–4.

Elkrief A, Routy B. First clinical proof-of-concept that FMT can overcome resistance to ICIs. Nat Rev Clin Oncol. 2021;18(6):325–6. https://doi.org/10.1038/s41571-021-00502-3.

Ferreira RM, Pereira-Marques J, Pinto-Ribeiro I, Costa JL, Carneiro F, Machado JC, et al. Gastric microbial community profiling reveals a dysbiotic cancer-associated microbiota. Gut. 2018;67(2):226–36. https://doi.org/10.1136/gutjnl-2017-314205.

Gatenby P, Caygill C, Wall C, Bhatacharjee S, Ramus J, Watson A, et al. Lifetime risk of esophageal adenocarcinoma in patients with Barrett's esophagus. World J Gastroenterol. 2014;20(28):9611–7. https://doi.org/10.3748/wjg.v20.i28.9611.

Gruner N, Mattner J. Bile acids and microbiota: multifaceted and versatile regulators of the liver-gut axis. Int J Mol Sci. 2021;22(3):1397. https://doi.org/10.3390/ijms22031397.

Hashimoto D, Arima K, Yokoyama N, Chikamoto A, Taki K, Inoue R, et al. Heterogeneity of KRAS mutations in pancreatic ductal adenocarcinoma. Pancreas. 2016;45(8):1111–4. https://doi.org/10.1097/mpa.0000000000000624.

Hingorani SR, Petricoin EF III, Maitra A, Rajapakse V, King C, Jacobetz MA, et al. Preinvasive and invasive ductal pancreatic cancer and its early detection in the mouse. Cancer Cell. 2003;4(6):437–50. https://doi.org/10.1016/S1535-6108(03)00309-X.

Hooi JKY, Lai WY, Ng WK, Suen MMY, Underwood FE, Tanyingoh D, et al. Global prevalence of Helicobacter pylori infection: systematic review and meta-analysis. Gastroenterology. 2017;153(2):420–9. https://doi.org/10.1053/j.gastro.2017.04.022.

Hou F, Pan Z, Yang R, Zhi F, Bi Y. Gold digging: searching for gut microbiota that enhances antitumor immunity. J Cell Physiol. 2021;236(8):5495–511. https://doi.org/10.1002/jcp.30272.

Kamareddine L, Najjar H, Sohail MU, Abdulkader H, Al-Asmakh M. The microbiota and gut-related disorders: insights from animal models. Cell. 2020;9(11):2401. https://doi.org/10.3390/cells9112401.

Keum N, Giovannucci E. Global burden of colorectal cancer: emerging trends, risk factors and prevention strategies. Nat Rev Gastroenterol Hepatol. 2019;16(12):713–32. https://doi.org/10.1038/s41575-019-0189-8.

Kostic AD, Chun E, Robertson L, Glickman JN, Gallini CA, Michaud M, et al. Fusobacterium nucleatum potentiates intestinal tumorigenesis and modulates the tumor-immune microenvironment. Cell Host Microbe. 2013;14(2):207–15. https://doi.org/10.1016/j.chom.2013.07.007.

Kwon SK, Park JC, Kim KH, Yoon J, Cho Y, Lee B, et al. Human gastric microbiota transplantation recapitulates premalignant lesions in germ-free mice. Gut. 2021;71(7):1266–76. https://doi.org/10.1136/gutjnl-2021-324489.

Laute-Caly DL, Raftis EJ, Cowie P, Hennessy E, Holt A, Panzica DA, et al. The flagellin of candidate live biotherapeutic Enterococcus gallinarum MRx0518 is a potent immunostimulant. Sci Rep. 2019;9(1):801. https://doi.org/10.1038/s41598-018-36926-8.

Ledford H. US cancer institute to overhaul tumour cell lines. Nature. 2016;530(7591):391. https://doi.org/10.1038/nature.2016.19364.

Lee JW, Komar CA, Bengsch F, Graham K, Beatty GL. Genetically engineered mouse models of pancreatic cancer: the KPC model (LSL-Kras(G12D/+) ;LSL-Trp53(R172H/+) ;Pdx-1-Cre), its variants, and their application in immuno-oncology drug discovery. Curr Protoc Pharmacol. 2016;73:14.39.1–14.39.20. https://doi.org/10.1002/cpph.2.

Lofgren JL, Whary MT, Ge Z, Muthupalani S, Taylor NS, Mobley M, et al. Lack of commensal flora in Helicobacter pylori-infected INS-GAS mice reduces gastritis and delays intraepithelial neoplasia. Gastroenterology. 2011;140(1):210–20. https://doi.org/10.1053/j.gastro.2010.09.048.

Lythgoe M, Stebbing J, Pickford E, Glasmacher A, Adriani M, Fyvie G, et al. 805 Safety and emerging evidence of immune modulation of the live biotherapeutic MRx0518 in the neoadjuvant setting for patients awaiting surgical removal of solid tumours. J Immunother Cancer. 2020;8(Suppl 3):A481–2. https://doi.org/10.1136/jitc-2020-SITC2020.0805.

Ma C, Kesarwala AH, Eggert T, Medina-Echeverz J, Kleiner DE, Jin P, et al. NAFLD causes selective CD4(+) T lymphocyte loss and promotes hepatocarcinogenesis. Nature. 2016;531(7593):253–7. https://doi.org/10.1038/nature16969.

Ma C, Han M, Heinrich B, Fu Q, Zhang Q, Sandhu M, et al. Gut microbiome-mediated bile acid metabolism regulates liver cancer via NKT cells. Science. 2018;360(6391):eaan5931. https://doi.org/10.1126/science.aan5931.

Madhu B, Uribe-Lewis S, Bachman M, Murrell A, Griffiths JR. Apc(Min/+) tumours and normal mouse small intestines show linear metabolite concentration and DNA cytosine hydroxymethylation gradients from pylorus to colon. Sci Rep. 2020;10(1):13616. https://doi.org/10.1038/s41598-020-70579-w.

Mendez R, Kesh K, Arora N, Di Martino L, McAllister F, Merchant N, et al. Microbial dysbiosis and polyamine metabolism as predictive markers for early detection of pancreatic cancer. Carcinogenesis. 2020;41(5):561–70. https://doi.org/10.1093/carcin/bgz116.

Moser AR, Pitot HC, Dove WF. A dominant mutation that predisposes to multiple intestinal neoplasia in the mouse. Science. 1990;247(4940):322–4. https://doi.org/10.1126/science.2296722.

Moser AR, Luongo C, Gould KA, McNeley MK, Shoemaker AR, Dove WF. ApcMin: a mouse model for intestinal and mammary tumorigenesis. Eur J Cancer. 1995;31A(7–8):1061–4. https://doi.org/10.1016/0959-8049(95)00181-h.

Munch NS, Fang HY, Ingermann J, Maurer HC, Anand A, Kellner V, et al. High-fat diet accelerates carcinogenesis in a mouse model of Barrett's esophagus via interleukin 8 and alterations to the gut microbiome. Gastroenterology. 2019;157(2):492–506.e2. https://doi.org/10.1053/j.gastro.2019.04.013.

Noto JM, Peek RM Jr. The gastric microbiome, its interaction with Helicobacter pylori, and its potential role in the progression to stomach cancer. PLoS Pathog. 2017;13(10):e1006573. https://doi.org/10.1371/journal.ppat.1006573.

Ohtani N, Imamura Y, Yamakoshi K, Hirota F, Nakayama R, Kubo Y, et al. Visualizing the dynamics of p21(Waf1/Cip1) cyclin-dependent kinase inhibitor expression in living animals. Proc Natl Acad Sci U S A. 2007;104(38):15034–9. https://doi.org/10.1073/pnas.0706949104.

Peters Y, Al-Kaabi A, Shaheen NJ, Chak A, Blum A, Souza RF, et al. Barrett oesophagus. Nat Rev Dis Primers. 2019;5(1):35. https://doi.org/10.1038/s41572-019-0086-z.

Plummer M, Franceschi S, Vignat J, Forman D, de Martel C. Global burden of gastric cancer attributable to Helicobacter pylori. Int J Cancer. 2015;136(2):487–90. https://doi.org/10.1002/ijc.28999.

Pushalkar S, Hundeyin M, Daley D, Zambirinis CP, Kurz E, Mishra A, et al. The pancreatic cancer microbiome promotes oncogenesis by induction of innate and adaptive immune suppression. Cancer Discov. 2018;8(4):403–16. https://doi.org/10.1158/2159-8290.CD-17-1134.

Ren J, Sui H, Fang F, Li Q, Li B. The application of Apc(Min/+) mouse model in colorectal tumor researches. J Cancer Res Clin Oncol. 2019;145(5):1111–22. https://doi.org/10.1007/s00432-019-02883-6.

Risbridger GP, Lawrence MG, Taylor RA. PDX: moving beyond drug screening to versatile models for research discovery. J Endocr Soc. 2020;4(11):bvaa132. https://doi.org/10.1210/jendso/bvaa132.

Routy B, Chatelier EL, Derosa L, Duong CPM, Alou MT, Daillère R, et al. Gut microbiome influences efficacy of PD-1-based immunotherapy against epithelial tumors. Science. 2018;359(6371):91–7. https://doi.org/10.1126/science.aan3706.

Shibata H, Toyama K, Shioya H, Ito M, Hirota M, Hasegawa S, et al. Rapid colorectal adenoma formation initiated by conditional targeting of the *Apc* gene. Science. 1997;278(5335):120–3. https://doi.org/10.1126/science.278.5335.120.

Stewart OA, Wu F, Chen Y. The role of gastric microbiota in gastric cancer. Gut Microbes. 2020;11(5):1220–30. https://doi.org/10.1080/19490976.2020.1762520.

Sung H, Ferlay J, Siegel RL, Laversanne M, Soerjomataram I, Jemal A, et al. Global cancer statistics 2020: GLOBOCAN estimates of incidence and mortality worldwide for 36 cancers in 185 countries. CA Cancer J Clin. 2021;71(3):209–49. https://doi.org/10.3322/caac.21660.

Tanoue T, Morita S, Plichta DR, Skelly AN, Suda W, Sugiura Y, et al. A defined commensal consortium elicits CD8 T cells and anti-cancer immunity. Nature. 2019;565(7741):600–5. https://doi.org/10.1038/s41586-019-0878-z.

Tomkovich S, Yang Y, Winglee K, Gauthier J, Muhlbauer M, Sun X, et al. Locoregional effects of microbiota in a preclinical model of colon carcinogenesis. Cancer Res. 2017;77(10):2620–32. https://doi.org/10.1158/0008-5472.CAN-16-3472.

Uzbay T. Germ-free animal experiments in the gut microbiota studies. Curr Opin Pharmacol. 2019;49:6–10. https://doi.org/10.1016/j.coph.2019.03.016.

Wahlstrom A, Sayin SI, Marschall HU, Backhed F. Intestinal crosstalk between bile acids and microbiota and its impact on host metabolism. Cell Metab. 2016;24(1):41–50. https://doi.org/10.1016/j.cmet.2016.05.005.

Wong SH, Zhao L, Zhang X, Nakatsu G, Han J, Xu W, et al. Gavage of fecal samples from patients with colorectal cancer promotes intestinal carcinogenesis in germ-free and conventional mice. Gastroenterology. 2017;153(6):1621–33.e6. https://doi.org/10.1053/j.gastro.2017.08.022.

Wu S, Rhee KJ, Albesiano E, Rabizadeh S, Wu X, Yen HR, et al. A human colonic commensal promotes colon tumorigenesis via activation of T helper type 17 T cell responses. Nat Med. 2009;15(9):1016–22. https://doi.org/10.1038/nm.2015.

Wu Y, Wu J, Chen T, Li Q, Peng W, Li H, et al. Fusobacterium nucleatum potentiates intestinal tumorigenesis in mice via a toll-like receptor 4/p21-activated kinase 1 Cascade. Dig Dis Sci. 2018;63(5):1210–8. https://doi.org/10.1007/s10620-018-4999-2.

Xu P, Widmer G, Wang Y, Ozaki LS, Alves JM, Serrano MG, et al. The genome of Cryptosporidium hominis. Nature. 2004;431(7012):1107–12. https://doi.org/10.1038/nature02977.

Yamada S, Takashina Y, Watanabe M, Nagamine R, Saito Y, Kamada N, et al. Bile acid metabolism regulated by the gut microbiota promotes non-alcoholic steatohepatitis-associated hepatocellular carcinoma in mice. Oncotarget. 2018;9(11):9925–39.

Yoshimoto S, Loo TM, Atarashi K, Kanda H, Sato S, Oyadomari S, et al. Obesity-induced gut microbial metabolite promotes liver cancer through senescence secretome. Nature. 2013;499(7456):97–101. https://doi.org/10.1038/nature12347.

Zhao R, Coker OO, Wu J, Zhou Y, Zhao L, Nakatsu G, et al. Aspirin reduces colorectal tumor development in mice and gut microbes reduce its bioavailability and chemopreventive effects. Gastroenterology. 2020;159(3):969–83.e4. https://doi.org/10.1053/j.gastro.2020.05.004.

Zhou P, Li Z, Xu D, Wang Y, Bai Q, Feng Y, et al. Cepharanthine hydrochloride improves cisplatin chemotherapy and enhances immunity by regulating intestinal microbes in mice. Front Cell Infect Microbiol. 2019;9:225. https://doi.org/10.3389/fcimb.2019.00225.

Chapter 13
Machine Learning on Microbiome Research in Gastrointestinal Cancer

Henley Cheung and Yufeng Lin

Abstract Gastrointestinal cancers remain a major threat to the global community. In recent years, the multifaceted effect of the microbiome in cancer development modulation and its potential therapeutic role are gaining well-deserved recognition. Artificial intelligence has been put to test in assisting clinicians with excellent performance. With the influx of data generated from sequencings in microbiome studies, there is an uprising application of artificial intelligence in microbiome data analysis. In this article, we discuss the pivotal role of the microbiome in gastrointestinal cancers, current approaches for microbiome research, and the potential applications of artificial intelligence in microbiome data analysis.

Keywords Artificial intelligence · Deep learning · Data analysis · Gut microbiome · Gastrointestinal cancers · Machine learning

13.1 Introduction

Gastrointestinal cancers are one of the major cancer incidents and leading causes of cancer death worldwide. Colorectal, esophageal, gastric, liver, and pancreas cancers are accountable for 26.1% of all new cases and 35.6% of all cancer deaths globally in 2020 (Sung et al. 2021). Multiple risk factors contribute to gastrointestinal cancer, such as genetics, diet, alcohol consumption, smoking, and infection (Arnold et al. 2020). Over the past decades, with the advancement of next-generation sequencing, the understanding of the role of the gut microbiome and its influences on human health is advancing progressively. The Human Microbiome Project was initiated in 2007 aiming to explore the fundamental roles of the microbiome in

H. Cheung (✉) · Y. Lin (✉)
Institute of Digestive Disease and the Department of Medicine and Therapeutics, State Key Laboratory of Digestive Disease, Li Ka Shing Institute of Health Sciences, The Chinese University of Hong Kong, Hong Kong, China
e-mail: henleycheung@link.cuhk.edu.hk; yufenglin@link.cuhk.edu.hk

J. Yu (ed.), *Microbiome in Gastrointestinal Cancer*,
https://doi.org/10.1007/978-981-19-4492-5_13

human health (Turnbaugh et al. 2007). In the following decades, researchers around the globe participated in the same pursuit and generated an enormous amount of sequencing data. The difficulties in accurate and efficient data analysis have become an immediate challenge that must be tackled. The recently proliferated field of machine learning shed new light on such tasks.

13.2 What Do We Know About the Gut Microbiome?

Microbiomes coexist with humans in many habitats, such as the gut, skin as well as oral, nasal, and vaginal cavities. A previous estimation suggested that the number of bacteria inhabiting the human body largely outnumber human cells by 10-folds (Hsiao et al. 2008), yet a recent study suggests that the ratio is around 1:1 (Sender et al. 2016). Our understanding of microbiomes is still progressing, but microbiome certainly exerts extensive biological significance to human health.

The establishment of the microbiome begins at the moment of birth: the sterile infant would be colonized immediately by the surrounding microbes and shape the microbiome composition in early childhood (Bokulich et al. 2016). Notably, the composition differs between vaginally and cesarean section delivered newborns (Peroni et al. 2020). The microbe composition would be further shaped by environmental factors such as geographical location, diet, and antibiotic usage until it reaches maximum diversity in adolescence (Gorkiewicz and Moschen 2018). In healthy individuals, the human gut microbiome co-exists commensally and aids functionally in nearly all physiological processes such as digestion, immunity, and metabolism (Belkaid and Hand 2014; Guinane and Cotter 2013).

Currently, the major research focuses on the gut microbiome due to the greatest abundance and compositional variety of microbes observed on this site. The standard practice to initiate a study begins with the collection of fecal samples. Fecal sample collection is considered advantageous due to its noninvasive nature and ease of preservation, which also provide a detailed representation of the gut microbiome with minimal host genome contamination. Another less common sampling method is mucosal biopsy. Although biopsy could reflect the microbiome composition at precise locations before passing through the low gastrointestinal tract, its invasion nature deems it more difficult and costly to obtain.

To explore the fundamental roles of the human microbiome, several large-scale projects were carried out in the past decades, such as the Human Microbiome Project with 4788 specimens collected from up to 18 body sites from 242 individuals for an extensive overview of the microbiome (Turnbaugh et al. 2007). Based on these studies, the microbiome compositions are broadly similar in population but different in detail among individuals. For example, the *Firmicutes* and *Bacteroidetes* are the two predominant phyla inhabiting the gut in healthy adults, and yet the ratio between them is not the same in all individuals.

Recent studies have linked or confirmed the effect of the gut microbiome on human health, especially in multiple cancers development and progression. In gastric cancer, the diversity and richness of the gastric microbiome are found to be high in tumor tissues. A higher proportion of ten genera, including *Bacteroides, Lactobacillus,* and *Streptococcus,* was found in gastric cancer patients compared to healthy individuals. These microbes may promote gastric tumor growth through metabolites and modulation of oncogenic signaling pathways (Dai et al. 2021). Furthermore, *Bacteroides* and *Ruminococcaceae* members, which are correlated with inflammation and immunity markers are enriched in patients with nonalcoholic fatty liver disease-related hepatocellular carcinoma (NAFLD-HCC). The bacterial extracts from the NAFLD-HCC microbiota also have an immunomodulatory effect of inducing Tregs and resulted in immunotolerance by attenuation of cytotoxic CD8+ T cell function (Behary et al. 2021). In colorectal cancer (CRC), a high abundance of *Fusobacterium nucleatum* was found in CRC tissue and promoted metastasis by inducing a decline of the m^6A writer, METTL3, by inhibition of Hippo pathway, followed by activation of YAP signaling and reduction of FOXD3 expression (Chen et al. 2022). The gut microbiome could be beneficial to human health. For example, *Lactobacillus gallinarum* was found to increase the probiotics abundance and inhibit CRC through metabolite production (Sugimura et al. 2021).

Another research direction focuses on developing noninvasive diagnostic tools and improving treatment efficacy for GI cancers. A 2018 study demonstrated that hepatocellular carcinoma (HCC) patients have a lower abundance of butyrate-producing bacterial families decreased and a higher abundance of lipopolysaccharide-producing bacterial families. The authors also identified 30 microbial markers that predict the probability of disease with an area under the curve (AUC) of 80.64% between 75 early HCC and 105 non-HCC samples (Ren et al. 2019). Furthermore, *F. nucleatum* was found to improve therapeutic responses to PD-1 blockade in CRC patients by activating STING signaling and increasing the accumulation of interferon-gamma CD8+ tumor-infiltrating lymphocytes (Gao et al. 2021).

13.3 The Current Approaches for Studying the Gut Microbiome

The advancement of high-throughput sequencing (HTS) technology has led to the blooming accumulating microbiome data and the rising need for follow-up analysis. Several HTS methods are routinely applied in the study of the gut microbiome, namely amplicon, shotgun metagenomic, metatranscriptomics, metaproteomics, and metabolomics sequencings.

Amplicon sequencing is a widely used HTS method to profile microbial communities by targeting the 16s ribosomal RNA housekeeping marker gene. Shotgun metagenomic sequencing is another common HTS tool to simultaneously examine all genes contained in a sample by shearing the extracted DNA into small fragments followed by sequencing (Sharpton 2014). To capture the real-time functional activities of the microbiome, metatranscriptomics and metaproteomics sequencing assess the microbial RNA and protein, respectively, to extract information on gene expression (Li et al. 2019; Verberkmoes et al. 2009). Metabolites secreted by the microbiome could be profiled by metabolomics sequencing (Clish 2015).

Massive amounts of sequencing data are generated with the wide applications of multi-omics tools. For example, the Human Microbiome Project produced 2.3 terabytes of 16s ribosomal RNA data by amplicon sequencing and metagenomic sequencing could generate 6 to 300 gigabytes of data for each human stool sample (Liu et al. 2021). These data could lay the foundation for further investigation of the roles of the microbiome in human health, but the influx of data imposes a rising challenge for effective interpretation and analysis.

13.4 Artificial Intelligence, Machine Learning, and Deep Learning

In addition to microbiome research, another beneficiary of technological advancement is the field of artificial intelligence (AI). AI is the programming of a machine to learn and perform tasks associated with intelligent beings (Goldenberg et al. 2019). It is regarded as the new frontier across different fields and is no exception to the scientific research and medical fields. By 2022, there are already 71 FDA-approved AI-related devices (Luchini et al. 2022). The progression of AI encountered many doubts. It was not until the exponential growth of available training data, graphical processing units designed to make parallel data processing possible, and the development of machine learning (ML) algorithms that allowed AI flourished. The recent advancement of AI has achieved great success and even surpassed human abilities in certain tasks, such as AlphaGo defeating human champions in the game of Go (Silver et al. 2016).

ML is the cornerstone of the current AI studies. It is the application of carefully designed algorithms for the machine to extract, learn, and conclude from the input data. ML can be further divided into two main approaches, supervised learning and unsupervised learning. In supervised learning, a large training data set of manually labeled input and output data is prepared and fed to the machine for training. The machine would extrapolate the labeled features and generate a score for each of the samples. Initially, there will likely be discrepancies between the machine-generated score and the manually labeled score. The goal of the machine is to reduce the discrepancies by applying optimization algorithms such as gradient descent to adjust its internal parameters. The training is considered completed once the minimum average of discrepancies is achieved. Another manually prepared data set is fed to the machine for scoring to verify the machine's learned ability. Unsupervised learning is considered an imitation of the learning habit of intellectual beings. The data is processed in the same fashion but with higher independency for the machine to extract and determine features of the input data without manual labeling. The algorithm may explore the intrinsic properties of the input data beyond human observations (Eraslan et al. 2019).

Deep learning is another maturing application of machine learning with the construction of multi-layer neural networks. The method is inspired by the brain structure, and the data processing units are named neurons. Raw data are fed into the input layer, multiple hidden layers, and eventually the output layer. Data without manually defined features are extracted and recomposed into higher and more complex features recognized by the machine between the hidden layers. For example, in the case of facial recognition, the machine would first extract each pixel in the image, followed by composing the edges and shapes, and finally the facial feature (Obermeyer and Emanuel 2016). The convolutional neural network (CNN) is an example of deep learning that has been recognized for its performance on object and facial recognition tasks (LeCun et al. 2015). CNN is constructed with three main layers: convolutional, pooling, and fully connected layers. The input data, such as an image, is captured in portions by the feature detector of the convolutional layer. Next, similar features are merged in the pooling layers for higher feature extraction. After multiple rounds of convolutional and pooling layers, the data would reach the fully connected layers for the machine to output its classification.

As the magnitudes of multi-omics data accumulate, the need of deploying ML to interpret and analysis handle these data are increasing. In a 2022 study, a supervised learning method was applied to data generated from metagenomic and metabolomic sequencing, as well as in the KEGG orthology database to predict early and late-onset CRC. Although each of the markers reached high predictive power with an AUC of about 85%, the combination of these three markers generated the highest AUC of 92.34% in the testing phase (Kong et al. 2022). Moreover, another study also used supervised learning and found that the fecal microbiome signatures generated from shotgun and amplicon sequencing are associated with clinical outcomes in patients with melanoma treated with anti-PD-1 (McCulloch et al. 2022). Machine learning also has great potential to improve the quality and cost of patient care as well. With supervised learning, the diagnosis computer-aided diagnosis (CADx) of colorectal polyps removal reached a negative predictive value of 97.6% and CADx-assisted endoscopists provided a high-confidence diagnosis of 94.6% (Hassan et al. 2022). Careful sample labeling and data management are always essential. However, mislabeled data are inevitable during the processing and pooling of many samples. Supervised classifiers are shown to be able to reliably detect and correct mislabeled data on 16s RNA sequencing until 30–40% of the samples are mislabeled (Knights et al. 2011). This application could be potentially applied to all microbiome research as a safety net practice as mistakes occur.

13.5 Challenges

Multi-omics tools and machine learning are showing great prospects to assist and improve microbiome research. One important note is that the data analysis and output are only as good as the input. Limited data may result in cohort heterogeneity. Therefore, it is essential to expand the sample size to properly represent the general demographic. Furthermore, the current standard practice for microbiome research relies heavily on stool samples. However, data extracted from stool samples are mostly a representation of the microbial composition of the lower GI tract. The current approach may not fully cover the microbiome features of the upper GI tract such as the esophagus (Vuik et al. 2019). Collaboration and data sharing between multiple institutes could be the solution but patient privacy and other legality must be respected.

Supervised learning is the leading machine learning method in microbiome research. With the proper input of training data, the machine can perform as well as or even surpass human experts. However, the current clinical studies are often retrospective studies using previously known datasets and may not guarantee a smooth translation in real-world settings. Another concern is that the input and output are being processed by the machine in a "black box" which is unknown or uninterpretable to humans. The reproducibility and reliability of such results would be questionable without thoroughly understanding the entirety of the process.

13.6 Conclusion

The gut microbiome is a significant physiological factor that influences human health in all aspects. It has been shown to affect tumor progression, treatment efficacy, and could serve as a noninvasive diagnostic tool for GI cancers. Initiated by the Human Microbiome Project and multi-omics technological advancement, emerging evidence is elucidating the role of the gut microbiome and the underlying relationship with GI cancer. Machine learning is a promising tool to provide efficient and accurate analysis or even prediction based on the data generated from the multi-omics sequencings. Such tools could also be used in clinical settings to assist physicians in better patient care. To realize these potentials, a global effort is required to foster a higher sample number and maintain sample quality for the continuous improvement of data integration (Fig. 13.1).

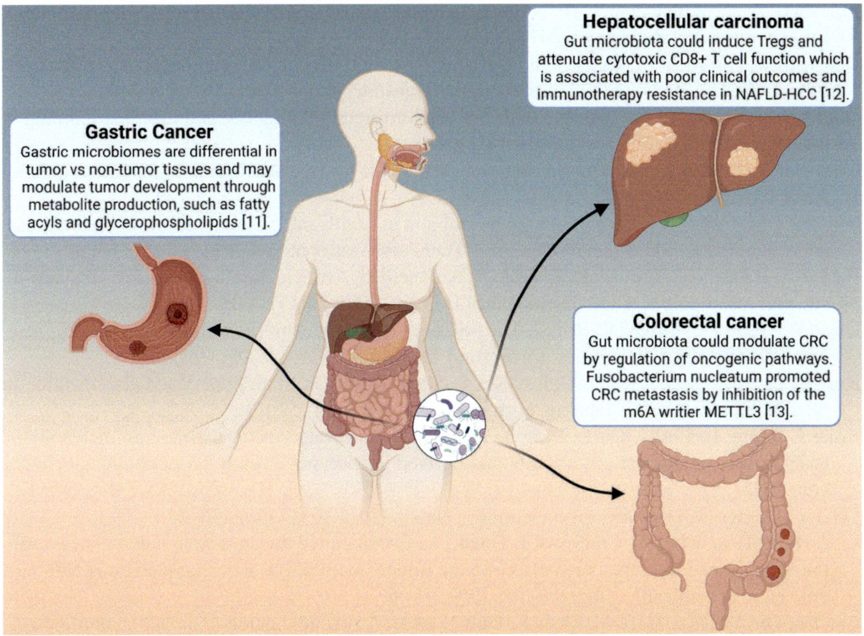

Fig. 13.1 Microbiome exerts its influence on cancer progression in multiple ways. In gastric cancer, the gastric microbiomes of tumor and non-tumor tissues are found to be different. Further investigation revealed that gastric microbiomes may modulate tumor development through metabolite production. Microbiome could also affect the cancer immune environment by Tregs induction and cytotoxic CD8+ T cell attenuation in NAFLD-HCC, which lead to poor clinical outcomes and immunotherapy. Besides, the m6A writer, METTL3, is downregulated by *Fusobacterium nucleatum* and promoted CRC metastasis

References

Arnold M, Abnet CC, Neale RE, Vignat J, Giovannucci EL, McGlynn KA, et al. Global burden of 5 major types of gastrointestinal cancer. Gastroenterology. 2020;159(1):335–349.e15.

Behary J, Amorim N, Jiang XT, Raposo A, Gong L, McGovern E, et al. Gut microbiota impact on the peripheral immune response in non-alcoholic fatty liver disease related hepatocellular carcinoma. Nat Commun. 2021;12(1):187.

Belkaid Y, Hand TW. Role of the microbiota in immunity and inflammation. Cell. 2014;157(1):121–41.

Bokulich NA, Chung J, Battaglia T, Henderson N, Jay M, Li H, et al. Antibiotics, birth mode, and diet shape microbiome maturation during early life. Sci Transl Med. 2016;8(343):343ra82.

Chen S, Zhang L, Li M, Zhang Y, Sun M, Wang L, et al. Fusobacterium nucleatum reduces METTL3-mediated m(6)A modification and contributes to colorectal cancer metastasis. Nat Commun. 2022;13(1):1248.

Clish CB. Metabolomics: an emerging but powerful tool for precision medicine. Cold Spring Harb Mol Case Stud. 2015;1(1):a000588.

Dai D, Yang Y, Yu J, Dang T, Qin W, Teng L, et al. Interactions between gastric microbiota and metabolites in gastric cancer. Cell Death Dis. 2021;12(12):1104.

Eraslan G, Avsec Z, Gagneur J, Theis FJ. Deep learning: new computational modelling techniques for genomics. Nat Rev Genet. 2019;20(7):389–403.

Gao Y, Bi D, Xie R, Li M, Guo J, Liu H, et al. Fusobacterium nucleatum enhances the efficacy of PD-L1 blockade in colorectal cancer. Signal Transduct Target Ther. 2021;6(1):398.

Goldenberg SL, Nir G, Salcudean SE. A new era: artificial intelligence and machine learning in prostate cancer. Nat Rev Urol. 2019;16(7):391–403.

Gorkiewicz G, Moschen A. Gut microbiome: a new player in gastrointestinal disease. Virchows Arch. 2018;472(1):159–72.

Guinane CM, Cotter PD. Role of the gut microbiota in health and chronic gastrointestinal disease: understanding a hidden metabolic organ. Ther Adv Gastroenterol. 2013;6(4):295–308.

Hassan C, Balsamo G, Lorenzetti R, Zullo A, Antonelli G. Artificial intelligence allows leaving-in-situ colorectal polyps. Clin Gastroenterol Hepatol. 2022;20(11):2505–2513.e4.

Hsiao WW, Metz C, Singh DP, Roth J. The microbes of the intestine: an introduction to their metabolic and signaling capabilities. Endocrinol Metab Clin N Am. 2008;37(4):857–71.

Knights D, Kuczynski J, Koren O, Ley RE, Field D, Knight R, et al. Supervised classification of microbiota mitigates mislabeling errors. ISME J. 2011;5(4):570–3.

Kong C, Liang L, Liu G, Du L, Yang Y, Liu J, et al. Integrated metagenomic and metabolomic analysis reveals distinct gut-microbiome-derived phenotypes in early-onset colorectal cancer. Gut. 2022.

LeCun Y, Bengio Y, Hinton G. Deep learning. Nature. 2015;521(7553):436–44.

Li F, Hitch TCA, Chen Y, Creevey CJ, Guan LL. Comparative metagenomic and metatranscriptomic analyses reveal the breed effect on the rumen microbiome and its associations with feed efficiency in beef cattle. Microbiome. 2019;7(1):6.

Liu YX, Qin Y, Chen T, Lu M, Qian X, Guo X, et al. A practical guide to amplicon and metagenomic analysis of microbiome data. Protein Cell. 2021;12(5):315–30.

Luchini C, Pea A, Scarpa A. Artificial intelligence in oncology: current applications and future perspectives. Br J Cancer. 2022;126(1):4–9.

McCulloch JA, Davar D, Rodrigues RR, Badger JH, Fang JR, Cole AM, et al. Intestinal microbiota signatures of clinical response and immune-related adverse events in melanoma patients treated with anti-PD-1. Nat Med. 2022;28(3):545–56.

Obermeyer Z, Emanuel EJ. Predicting the future—big data, machine learning, and clinical medicine. N Engl J Med. 2016;375(13):1216–9.

Peroni DG, Nuzzi G, Trambusti I, Di Cicco ME, Comberiati P. Microbiome composition and its impact on the development of allergic diseases. Front Immunol. 2020;11:700.

Ren Z, Li A, Jiang J, Zhou L, Yu Z, Lu H, et al. Gut microbiome analysis as a tool towards targeted non-invasive biomarkers for early hepatocellular carcinoma. Gut. 2019;68(6):1014–23.

Sender R, Fuchs S, Milo R. Are we really vastly outnumbered? Revisiting the ratio of bacterial to host cells in humans. Cell. 2016;164(3):337–40.

Sharpton TJ. An introduction to the analysis of shotgun metagenomic data. Front Plant Sci. 2014;5:209.

Silver D, Huang A, Maddison CJ, Guez A, Sifre L, van den Driessche G, et al. Mastering the game of go with deep neural networks and tree search. Nature. 2016;529(7587):484–9.

Sugimura N, Li Q, Chu ESH, Lau HCH, Fong W, Liu W, et al. Lactobacillus gallinarum modulates the gut microbiota and produces anti-cancer metabolites to protect against colorectal tumourigenesis. Gut. 2021;71(10):2011–21.

Sung H, Ferlay J, Siegel RL, Laversanne M, Soerjomataram I, Jemal A, et al. Global cancer statistics 2020: GLOBOCAN estimates of incidence and mortality worldwide for 36 cancers in 185 countries. CA Cancer J Clin. 2021;71(3):209–49.

Turnbaugh PJ, Ley RE, Hamady M, Fraser-Liggett CM, Knight R, Gordon JI. The human microbiome project. Nature. 2007;449(7164):804–10.

Verberkmoes NC, Russell AL, Shah M, Godzik A, Rosenquist M, Halfvarson J, et al. Shotgun metaproteomics of the human distal gut microbiota. ISME J. 2009;3(2):179–89.

Vuik F, Dicksved J, Lam SY, Fuhler GM, van der Laan L, van de Winkel A, et al. Composition of the mucosa-associated microbiota along the entire gastrointestinal tract of human individuals. United European Gastroenterol J. 2019;7(7):897–907.

Chapter 14
Gut Microbiota Modulation: Probiotics and Prebiotics in GI Cancer

Phillip Lung Wai Au-Doung, Ryan Hei Chan, William Ka Kei Wu, and Qing Li

Abstract Gastrointestinal (GI) cancers are major public health problems as they are one of the most common types of cancer worldwide. Despite recent treatment advancements due to a better understanding of the molecular mechanisms of GI cancer tumorigenesis, a high mortality rate still occurs, especially in the metastatic stage of GI cancers. Modulating intestinal microbiota with probiotics and prebiotics becomes a novel strategy for the prevention and treatment of GI cancers as intestinal microbiota has been shown to play a key role in GI cancer development. The literature has provided ample evidence that probiotics could help to prevent or treat GI cancers by slowing down the progression or acting as adjunctive therapy to cancer treatment. In this chapter, we summarize the involvement of intestinal microbiota in GI cancer development, the potential mechanism of actions of probiotics/prebiotics, and related preclinical and clinical studies in the prevention and treatment of GI cancers to highlight their potential therapeutic values.

Keywords Probiotics · Prebiotics · Gastrointestinal cancer · Gut microbiota Gastric microbiome

---

Phillip Lung Wai Au-Doung and Ryan Hei Chan are co-first authors.

P. L. W. Au-Doung · R. H. Chan
Department of Anaesthesia and Intensive Care and Peter Hung Pain Research Institute, The Chinese University of Hong Kong, Hong Kong, China

School of Pharmacy, The Chinese University of Hong Kong, Hong Kong, China

W. K. K. Wu (✉) · Q. Li (✉)
Department of Anaesthesia and Intensive Care and Peter Hung Pain Research Institute, The Chinese University of Hong Kong, Hong Kong, China

State Key Laboratory of Digestive Disease, LKS Institute of Health Science, The Chinese University of Hong Kong, Hong Kong, China
e-mail: wukakei@cuhk.edu.hk; qingli@cuhk.edu.hk

J. Yu (ed.), *Microbiome in Gastrointestinal Cancer*,
https://doi.org/10.1007/978-981-19-4492-5_14

14.1 Introduction

Gastrointestinal (GI) cancers are a major public health problem, accounting for 26% of the incidence rate and 35% of all cancer-related deaths globally (Arnold et al. 2020). In 2018, there were estimated 4.8 million new cases and 3.4 million cancer-related deaths in the world (Arnold et al. 2020). Esophageal cancer, gastric cancer (GC), and liver cancer were more common in Asia. Meanwhile, colorectal cancer (CRC) and pancreatic cancer were more common in Europe and North America (Bray et al. 2018). Interestingly, the intestinal microbiota has been shown to play a pivotal role in GI cancer development (Cheng et al. 2020). Therefore, modulating intestinal microbiota with probiotics and prebiotics becomes a novel strategy for the prevention and treatment of GI cancer (Lebeer et al. 2008; Kumar et al. 2010), particularly CRC, GC, liver cancer, and pancreatic cancer (Javanmard et al. 2018). This chapter aims to summarize (1) the mechanism on how the intestinal microbiota is involved in GI cancer development, (2) the potential mechanism of probiotics/prebiotics in the prevention and treatment of GI cancer and (3) the preclinical and clinical studies to highlight their potential therapeutic values.

14.1.1 Probiotics and Prebiotics

Probiotics are living microorganisms that are beneficial to the host when ingested an adequate amount (Hill et al. 2014). *Lactobacillus*, *Bifidobacterium,* and *Saccharomyces* are the most common types of marketed probiotics (Lebeer et al. 2010). Other probiotics include *Clostridiales*, *Bacteroidales*, and *Bacillus spp.*, (O'Toole et al. 2017). Prebiotics are compounds that induce the growth of beneficial bacteria in the gut (Gibson et al. 2017).

14.2 Colorectal Cancer and Intestinal Microbiota

CRC is the third most lethal cancer among all cancer types. Nearly two million people were diagnosed in 2018 globally (Rawla et al. 2019a). Red meat consumption, alcohol intake, and cigarette smoking are associated with increased risk for CRC (Rawla et al. 2019a). Intestinal microbiota also plays a crucial role in CRC tumorigenesis (Tlaskalova-Hogenova et al. 2014). A systematic review found that microbial dysbiosis is associated with CRC development (Borges-Canha et al. 2015). Compared to healthy individuals, patients with CRC usually had an abnormal composition and low diversity of the intestinal flora (Fong et al. 2020; Chen et al. 2012), containing a greater proportion of bacteria that cause inflammation and produce carcinogenic metabolites (Yang et al. 2017). The microbiota adhered to the intestinal mucosa are different from those in the intestinal lumen although both can contribute to CRC development (Eckburg et al. 2005; Flemer et al. 2017). Among the mucosa-adherent microbiota, *Bifidobacterium*, *Faecalibacterium*, and *Blautia* were reduced in patients with CRC, whereas *Fusobacterium*, *Porphyromonas*, and *Peptostreptococcus* were enriched. In the lumen, *Erysipelotrichaceae*, *Prevotellaceae*, and *Coriobacteriaceae* were increased in patients with CRC (Chen et al. 2012). The gut luminal microflora promotes CRC development via co-metabolism or metabolic exchange with the host. Meanwhile, the mucosa-associated microbiota promotes CRC development through direct interaction with the host (Chen et al. 2012). For instance, *Fusobacterium nucleatum* is associated with a worsened prognosis (Castellarin et al. 2012; Mima et al. 2016). It causes mutations in the tumor suppressor *APC* and alters the intestinal epithelial barrier by causing the loss of tight junctions, affecting epithelial polarity, and mitigating the mucus layer (Grivennikov et al. 2012). This promotes further infiltration of *Fusobacteria* and other bacteria to accumulate in the intestinal barrier (Kostic et al. 2013). *Fusobacteria* can utilize amino acids and peptides as nutrient sources to generate formyl-methionyl-leucyl-phenylalanine, which is a myeloid cell chemoattractant and contributes to tumorigenesis (Kostic et al. 2013). *Streptococcus bovis*, a bacterium involved in bacteremia and endocarditis, was reported as a risk factor for CRC (Gupta et al. 2010; Abdulamir et al. 2011). Statistically, between 25 and 80% of patients with *S. bovis* infection were diagnosed with CRC (Abdulamir et al. 2011). In vivo study showed that *S. bovis* promotes the tumor cell proliferation and induces the level of interleukin-8 (IL-8) in the gut mucosa by inducing oxidative stress (Xie 2001). *Clostridium spp.* was found to attach to colon cells under the mucus layer (Molska and Reguła 2019). The activated inflammation-related genes and proteins, such as COX-2, NF-kB, TNF-a, IL-6, IL-8, and IL-12, were also associated with CRC tumorigenesis (Reis et al. 2019). In contrast, the number of potentially beneficial bacteria species, including the well-known probiotics and some promising next-generation probiotics, which can produce beneficial metabolites [short-chain fatty acids (SCFAs), small molecules, enzymes, bacteriocins] were reduced (Reis et al. 2019).

14.2.1 Probiotic and Prebiotic in the Treatment and Prevention of CRC

Probiotics may be able to restore the microbial balance and produce anti-inflammatory, antiproliferative effects, and promote apoptosis in colon cancer cells (Fong et al. 2020). The mechanisms on how probiotics induce the inhibitory effect in CRC are still under investigation (Górska et al. 2019). Table 14.1 shows the current progress of in vitro and in vivo studies.

Lowering the colonization of pathobionts is one of the strategies to inhibit CRC development, as these carcinogenic microbes can cause inflammation (Fong et al. 2020). Probiotics reduce the bacterial colonization by (1) adhering to the surface of gut epithelial cells (Tuomola et al. 1999), (2) competing nutrients (Kamada et al. 2012), and (3) co-aggregating with the pathogenic bacteria (Campana et al. 2017).

Alterations in intestinal microbiota will increase intestinal permeability and therefore lead to gut barrier dysfunction and cause inflammation (Alvarez et al. 2016; Martín et al. 2019). The tight junction proteins such as claudin-1, occludin, ZO-1, ZO-2 are responsible for the organization of the tight junction structure (Shen et al. 2011). Loss of tight junction proteins will induce epithelial-mesenchymal transition (EMT) and metastasis

Table 14.1 Summary of the in vitro and in vivo studies related to probiotics and CRC

Probiotics	Cell line/ Animals	Findings	References
In vitro			
Bacillus polyfermenticus KU3	HT-29, LoVo	Inhibited the proliferation of colon cancer cells	Lee et al. (2015)
Bacillus polyfermenticus	HT-29, DLD-1 and Caco-2	Inhibited tumor growth through suppressing ErbB2 and ErbB3	Ma et al. (2010a)
Bifidobacterium adolescentis SPM0212	Caco-2, HT-29, and SW480	Decreased tumor cell proliferation by increasing the secretion of TNF-α and NO from macrophages	Lee et al. (2008)
Clostridium butyricum	HCT116, Caco-2, and HCT8	Decreased proliferation by GPR43 gene silencing and increased apoptosis	Chen et al. (2020a)
Clostridium butyricum and dextran	Murine subcutaneous and orthotopic tumor models of colon cancers	Inhibited tumor growth up to 89% and 65% in subcutaneous and orthotopic tumor models, respectively	Zheng et al. (2020)
Clostridium butyricum ATCC and *Bacillus subtilis* ATCC 9398	HCT116 and SW1116	Promoted antiproliferative effect, apoptosis, and anti-inflammatory effects by reducing mRNA and protein levels of NF-κB in SW1116 cells	Chen et al. (2015)
Enterococcus faecium FP51, Pediococcus pentosaceus FP3 and Lactobacillus salivarius FP25/FP35	Caco-2	Adhered to cancer cells and triggered the bioproduction of short-chain fatty acids	Thirabunyanon and Hongwittayakorn (2013)
Enterococcus faecium RM11 and *Lactobacillus fermentum* RM28	Caco-2	Adhered to epithelial cells to trigger antiproliferative effects on colon cancer cells	Thirabunyanon et al. (2009)
Exopolysaccharides (EPSs) obtained from *Lactobacillus* spp	HT-29	Induced apoptosis	Tukenmez et al. (2019)
EPSs obtained from *Lactobacillus casei* 01	HT-29	Induced antiproliferative effects	Liu et al. (2011)
EPSs obtained from *Lactobacillus acidophilus* 606	HT-29	Inhibited the proliferation by directly affecting cell morphology; Activated autophagic cell death by the induction of Beclin-1 and GRP78, as well as indirectly through the induction of Bcl-2 and Bak	Kim et al. (2010)

Table 14.1 (continued)

Probiotics	Cell line/ Animals	Findings	References
Lactobacillus casei ATCC 393	HT-29 and CT-26	Induced antiproliferative effect	Tiptiri-Kourpeti et al. (2016)
Lactobacillus casei and *Lactobacillus rhamnosus* GG	HCT-116	Inhibited colon cancer cell invasion by influencing matrix metalloproteinase-9 (MMP-9) activity and levels of the tight junction protein zona occludens-1 (ZO-1)	Escamilla et al. (2012)
Lactobacillus gallinarum	HCT116, Lovo	Decreased the cell proliferation; induced cell apoptosis	Sugimura et al. (2022)
Lactococcus lactis NK34	DLD-1, HT-29	Inhibited the proliferation of cancer cells and production of pro-inflammatory cytokines	Han et al. (2015)
Lactobacillus paracasei IMPC2.1 and *Lactobacillus rhamnosus* GG	DLD-1	Induced antiproliferative effect and apoptosis; Reduced the inflammation effect on the host gastric mucosa	Orlando et al. (2012)
Lactobacillus pentosus B281 and *Lactobacillus plantarum* B282	Caco-2. HT-29	Induced antiproliferative effect; produced cytotoxic effect; alter the cell-cycle distribution	Saxami et al. (2016)
Lactobacillus plantarum A7 and *Lactobacillus rhamnosus* GG	Caco-2 and HT-29	Induced antiproliferative effect	Sadeghi-Aliabadi et al. (2014)
Lactobacillus rhamnosus GG *Bifidobacterium lactis* Bb12	Caco-2	Induced apoptosis through the mitochondrial pathway by inducing BAX translocation, cytochrome c release, caspase-9 and -3 cleavage	Altonsy et al. (2010)
Lactobacillus rhamnosus GG	Caco-2, HT29, SW480	Induced antiproliferative effect; induced apoptosis	Orlando et al. (2016)
Streptococcus thermophilus	HCT116, HT29, and Caco-2,	Decreased the cell proliferation by secretion of β-galactosidase and promoted cell apoptosis	Li et al. (2021)
In vivo			
Bifidobacterium species	AOM/DSS induced CRC mice	Reduced tumor size BC-treated mice than those observed in untreated CRC mice	Parisa et al. (2020)

(continued)

Table 14.1 (continued)

Probiotics	Cell line/ Animals	Findings	References
Clostridium butyricum	*Apc*$^{min/+}$ mice	Suppressed the Wnt/β-catenin signaling pathway and modulated the gut microbiota composition	Chen et al. (2020a)
Clostridium butyricum ATCC and *Bacillus subtilis* ATCC 9398	DMH induced CRC mice	Inhibited the development of DMH induced CRC; the mechanism involved reduced inflammation and improved immune homeostasis	Chen et al. (2015)
Enterococcus faecalis (heat killed)	DSS induced CRC mice	Reduced the severity of intestinal inflammation and the formation of CRC in wild-type mice	Chung et al. (2019)
Enterococcus faecium CRL 183	DMH induced CRC mice	Produced antitumor effect by increasing IL-4, IFN-γ, and TNF-α to stimulate the immune response	Sivieri et al. (2008)
Lactobacillus acidophilus	DMH/DSS induced CRC mice	Enhanced the colonic expression of p53 and Bax; Increased the ratio of Bax/Bcl-2	Lin et al. (2019)
Lactobacillus acidophilus	Xenograft CRC mice model (CT26)	Enhanced apoptosis of CT-26 cells in mouse model; Downregulated expression of CXCR4 mRNA and MHC class I	Chen et al. (2012)
Lactobacillus casei ATCC334	Xenograft CRC mice model (SW620)	Initiated a tumor-suppressive effect by the activation of the JNK signaling pathway	Konishi et al. (2016)
Lactobacillus casei ATCC393	Xenograft CRC mice model (CT26)	Induced apoptosis by upregulating TRAIL and downregulating survivin	Tiptiri-Kourpeti et al. (2016)
Lactobacillus casei BL23	AOM/DSS induced CRC mice	Produced an immunomodulatory effect by downregulating the IL-22; Produced an antiproliferative effect by upregulating *caspase-7, caspase-9, and Bik*	Jacouton et al. (2017)
Lactobacillus gasseri and *Cudrania tricuspidata* leaf extract	AOM/DSS induced CRC mice	Suppressed pro-inflammatory cytokines (TNF-α, IFN-γ, IL-1β, and IL-6); Enhanced the production of anti-inflammatory cytokines (IL-4 and IL-10)	Oh et al. (2020)

Table 14.1 (continued)

Probiotics	Cell line/ Animals	Findings	References
Lactobacillus gallinarum	*Apc*$^{min/+}$ mice AOM/DSS induced CRC mice	Produced a visually smaller colon tumor in *L. gallinarum* group (*Apc*$^{min/+}$ mice); Reduced colorectal tumor number and size in *L. gallinarum* group (AOM/DSS induced CRC mice)	Sugimura et al. (2022)
Lactobacillus GG	DMH induced CRC mice	Produced antiproliferative effects	Goldin et al. (1996)
Lactobacillus plantarum AS1	DMH induced CRC mice	Produced antitumor effect through its antioxidant properties	Kumar et al. (2012)
Lactobacillus plantarum YYC-3	*Apc*$^{min/+}$ mice	Suppressed the expression of the inflammatory cytokines IL-6, IL-17 F, and IL-22; Suppressed the activation of the NF-κB and Wnt signaling pathways	Yue et al. (2020)
Lactobacillus rhamnosus GG	DMH induced CRC mice	Induced apoptosis and anti-inflammatory effect by reducing the expression of β-catenin, the anti-apoptotic protein Bcl-2, the inflammatory proteins NFκB-p65, COX-2, and TNFα, and increased the expression of the pro-apoptotic proteins Bax, casp3, and p53	Gamallat et al. (2016)
Lactobacillus reuteri	AOM/DSS induced CRC mice	Decreased tumor growth and prolonged survival in mice	Bell et al. (2022)
Streptococcus thermophilus	AOM induced CRC mice	Reduced tumor formation through secreting β-galactosidase	Li et al. (2021)
VSL#3 (A commercial probiotic composed of eight bacterial species)	DMH induced CRC mice	Showed antioxidant activity; Protected the mucosa from damage caused by chemical carcinogen and increased SCFA concentrations therefore resulted in reduced intestinal permeability	Cruz et al. (2021)
VSL#3	AOM/DSS induced CRC mice	Reduced the tumor load; Decreased the level of TNF-α and IL-6 in colon tissue	Wang et al. (2018)
VSL#3 and metformin	AOM/DSS induced CRC mice	Reduced colitis and tumor growth by inhibiting macrophage infiltration and maintaining epithelial integrity	Chung et al. (2017)

(Ahmad et al. 2017). Probiotics Lactobacillus rhamnosus, Lactobacillus plantarum, and Escherichia coli Nissle 1917 have been shown to improve gut barrier function by upregulating or normalizing expression of tight junction proteins (claudin-1, occludin, ZO-1, ZO-2) (Alvarez et al. 2016; Escamilla et al. 2012), stimulate mucus production, and suppress inflammation (Martín et al. 2019). This is possibly due to the upregulated colonic expression of the TRAF-interaction protein with a forkhead-associated domain (TIFA), which further activates TRAF2 which can enhance the survival of colonic epithelial cells and reduce inflammation (Lin et al. 2011).

Adhesion of probiotic bacteria to colon cancer cells was shown to induce apoptosis. They can also produce SCFAs and thereby exerting an antitumor effect (Thirabunyanon et al. 2009; Thirabunyanon and Hongwittayakorn 2013; Saxami et al. 2016; Banna et al. 2017). *Lactobacillus casei* adhered to colon cancer cells to reduce cell viability and induce apoptotic cell death (Tiptiri-Kourpeti et al. 2016). SCFAs, including acetate, propionate, and butyrate, are produced by the fermentation of prebiotics (Fong et al. 2020). They can interact with the bacteria receptor and prevent pathogens attaching to the epithelial cells and therefore inhibit colonization (Monteagudo-Mera et al. 2019). It can also be directly absorbed into intestinal cells and induce an immune response by altering the intestinal gene expression (Fong et al. 2020). SCFAs are the energy source for colon cells and maintain the acidic environment of the intestine (Floch 2010). Butyrate is a histone deacetylase inhibitor and has been suggested to promote apoptosis of CRC cells (Canani et al. 2011). In patients with CRC, there is an obvious reduction of SCFAs when compared to healthy individuals (Macfarlane and Macfarlane 2003). Therefore, the consumption of probiotics can help to increase the daily production of SCFAs (Lu et al. 2021). SCFAs can induce intestinal epithelial cells to produce antibacterial peptides and enhance the expression of tight junctions to strengthen intestinal barrier function (Kahouli et al. 2013). Furthermore, exopolysaccharides (EPSs) isolated from *Lactobacillus* had cytotoxicity effects on colon cancer cells in vitro due to the activation of cell death pathway (Kim et al. 2010; Liu et al. 2011; Tukenmez et al. 2019). Some harmful bacteria can activate Wnt/β-catenin through bacterial effectors and toxins, such as *Helicobacter pylori* and *Salmonella enterica* (Gagnaire et al. 2017). *Clostridium butyricum* was found to modulate the gut microbiota composition by suppressing the Wnt/β-catenin signaling pathway and therefore inhibit tumor growth (Chen et al. 2020a). A more recent study demonstrated that *Streptococcus thermophilus* suppressed intestinal tumorigenesis in mice models by downregulation of the Hippo pathway kinases and decreased the proliferation by secretion of β-galactosidase (Li et al. 2021). Other possible mechanisms include downregulation of inflammation mediators such as IL-22 (Jacouton et al. 2017), activation of apoptosis (Tiptiri-Kourpeti et al. 2016; Gamallat et al. 2016), and antioxidant effects (Kumar et al. 2012; Cruz et al. 2021).

14.2.2 Clinical Studies of Probiotics Related to CRC

Few clinical studies have explored the potential effects of probiotics in CRC (Table 14.2). Two of them were conducted in Asia while the other were conducted in Europe. Long-term consumption of yogurt could lower the risk of CRC (adjusted

Table 14.2 Summary of clinical studies of probiotics related to CRC

Types of probiotics or probiotics containing product	Country	Number of participants	Study design	Study duration	Findings	References
Bifidobacterium lactis Bl-04 and *Lactobacillus acidophilus* NCFM	Sweden	15	A randomized intervention with probiotics in patients with colon cancer Biopsy samples were obtained from the normal mucosa and tumor vs biopsies from non-cancer controls	Probiotics intake ranged from 8 to78 days	Probiotics increased abundance of butyrate-producing bacteria, e.g., *Faecalibacterium* and *Clostridiales sp* and decreased abundances of CRC-associated bacteria such as *Fusobacterium* and *Peptostreptococcus*	Hibberd et al. (2017)
Lactobacillus casei	Japan	380	Randomized trial recruited participants who had at least 2 colorectal tumors removed	4 years	More tumor occurred in the wheat bran group after 4 years (adjusted OR 1.31 vs control group) Less tumor occurred in the *Lactobacillus casei* group (adjusted OR 0.76 vs control group)	Ishikawa et al. (2005)
Lactobacillus gasseri	Japan	10	Analysis of stool specimen and peripheral blood specimen from healthy participants and patients with CRC	12 weeks	A deterioration of the intestinal environment was observed in the CRC patients when compared to the healthy controls; patients with CRC after intake of probiotics; decreased total amount of *Clostridium perfringens and* increased in the short-chain fatty acid Blood IL-1 beta and NK cell activity values were significantly higher before taking probiotics	Ohara et al. (2010)

(continued)

Table 14.2 (continued)

Types of probiotics or probiotics containing product	Country	Number of participants	Study design	Study duration	Findings	References
Lactobacillus rhamnosus LC705 and *Propionibacterium freudenreichii* ssp. shermanii JS	Finland	38	Randomized, double-blind, placebo-controlled, two-period crossover study recruited non-CRC patients	Two period with 4 weeks treatment	Increased in the fecal counts of *lactobacilli* and *propionibacteria;* decrease in the activity of β-glucosidase	Hatakka et al. (2008)
Synbiotic preparation with probiotics components—*Lactobacillus rhamnosus* GG and *Bifidobacterium lactis* Bb12	Ireland	37	Randomized, double-blind, placebo-controlled trial recruited participants with colon cancer	12 weeks	Synbiotic intervention resulted in significant changes in fecal flora: *Bifidobacterium* and *Lactobacillus* increased and *Clostridium perfringens* decreased Increased IFN-γ production in patients with CRC A significant 20% reduction in proliferative activity compared with control subjects	Rafter et al. (2007)
Yogurt	Italy	45,241	Prospective study recruited volunteers	Follow-up 12 years	Yogurt consumption was inversely associated with CRC risk (adjusted HR: 0.65 higher intake versus lower intake)	Pala et al. (2011)

HR: 0.65) (Pala et al. 2011). This may be due to the *Streptococcus thermophilus* and *Lactobacillus delbrueckii* in yogurt have anti-inflammatory properties (Perdigón et al. 2002). The other studies also showed that patients with CRC who consumed probiotics can change the intestinal flora composition such as increased abundance of butyrate-producing bacteria and decreased CRC-associated bacteria (Rafter et al. 2007; Hibberd et al. 2017) and reduced the inflammatory mediators such as IL-1 beta and NK cell activity (Ohara et al. 2010). Another study recruited healthy volunteers and confirmed that probiotics were able to decrease the activity of CRC carcinogenic substances such as the bacterial β-glucosidase (Hatakka et al. 2008).

14.3 Gastric Cancer (GC)

The mortality rate of GC came after CRC and caused nearly 770,000 deaths globally in 2020 (Sung et al. 2021). The early stage of GC is often asymptomatic until it develops to a late-stage tumor (Luan et al. 2020; Yang et al. 2021). The most common type of GC is gastric adenocarcinoma and is classified histologically into "diffuse" and "intestinal" types. In some cases, the tumor can exhibit both "diffuse" and "intestinal" properties (Lauren 1965). The signaling pathways underlying the pathogenesis of these two GC subtypes are different. Intestinal GC is associated with substantial inflammation and goes through various pre-malignant stages, such as atrophic gastritis and intestinal metaplasia. While diffuse GC lacks differentiated cell morphology and is associated with poor survival compared to the intestinal type (Kunz et al. 2012). Intestinal GC exhibits higher genetic and chromosomal instability than the diffuse adenocarcinoma (Vauhkonen et al. 2005), which is associated with small-sized amplifications and mutations in E-cadherin gene (The Cancer Genome Atlas Research Network 2014). Apart from adenocarcinoma, there is a relatively rare subtype, namely gastrointestinal stromal tumors (GIST), which originate from the interstitial cells of Cajal and have *KIT* or *PDGRA* mutations (Oppelt et al. 2017).

14.3.1 Gastric Carcinogenesis and **Helicobacter pylori (H. pylori)** *Infection*

H. pylori is more frequently found in patients with intestinal GC (Wang et al. 2014). Chronic *H. pylori* infection is considered a major risk factor for GC development (Sarhadi et al. 2021). As it can cause chronic gastritis which is the early manifestation of tenacious inflammation and proceeds to damage the endothelial cell (Kidane 2018). *H. pylori* infection stimulates immune responses via the regulation of various signaling pathways and results in achlorhydria, epithelial atrophy, and dysplasia (Toh and Wilson 2020).

Oncoproteins cytotoxin-associated gene A (CagA) and vacuolating toxin A (VacA) produced by *H. pylori* drastically increase the risk of GC by upregulation of mitogen-activated protein (MAP) kinase and ERK1/2 expression and increasing vascular endothelial growth factor to angiogenesis (Backert et al. 2000; Khatoon et al. 2016). They can also promote the release of cytokines and inflammatory factors including interferon-γ, TNF-α, IL-1, IL1β, IL-6, IL-7, IL-8, IL-10, and IL-18 (Backert et al. 2000). Eventually signaling pathways such as ERK/MAPK, NF-κB, Ras, as well as STAT3 are triggered and upregulated upon the infection of Cag^+ *H. pylori* strains (Meng et al. 2018). The tumor-suppressing mechanisms (e.g., p53) can be disarmed by *H. pylori* by causing mutation (Yong et al. 2015). *H. pylori* can also cause DNA hypermethylation on tumor suppressor genes, including trefoil factor 2 (TFF2), which increases the risk of carcinogenesis (Sitaraman 2014).

14.3.2 Gastric Cancer and Gastric Microbiome

The microbial diversity is markedly reduced in GC patients when compared to healthy individuals (Iizasa et al. 2015; Ferreira et al. 2018; Liu et al. 2019). *Prevotella copri* and *Bacteroides uniformis* were reduced, whereas *Prevotella melaninogenica*, *Streptococcus anginosus*, and *Propionibacterium acnes* were enriched in tumor tissue (Liu et al. 2019). *Novosphingobium*, *Ralstonia*, *Ochrobactrum*, *Anoxybacillus*, and *Pseudoxanthomonas* were increased in the early stage of GC, whereas *Burkholderia*, *Tsukamurella*, *Uruburuella*, and *Salinivibrio* were more populated in late-stage GC (Wang et al. 2020). Interestingly, lactic acid-producing bacteria also play a role in gastric carcinogenesis (Vinasco et al. 2019). A recent in vivo study revealed that the enrichment of *Lactobacillales* in the stomach could accelerate the development of GC although the exact mechanism is still under investigation (Bali et al. 2021).

Little is known about the microbiome environment among GC subtypes (Sarhadi et al. 2021). Recent research compared two subtypes of GC and showed that *Fusobacteria*, *Bacteroidetes*, *Patescibacteria* were more frequently observed in gastric signet-ring cell carcinoma (a rare but highly malignant form of GC), while *Proteobacteria* and *Acidobacteria were observed* in gastric adenocarcinoma (Ravegnini et al. 2020). Another research showed that a lower abundance of *Lachnoclostridium*, *Bifidobacterium*, *Parabacteroides,* and *Barnesiella* was only seen in the adenocarcinoma patients when compared to GIST patients (Sarhadi et al. 2021).

14.3.3 Probiotic in the Treatment and Prevention of GC

As GC is mainly associated with *H. pylori* infection, many researchers investigated if the combination of probiotics with *H. pylori* eradiation therapy can enhance the eradication rate and reduce adverse effects (Table 14.3). The Toronto Consensus

Table 14.3 Summary of clinical studies of probiotics related to *H. pylori* eradication

Types of probiotics or probiotics containing product	Country	Study design and interventions	Number of participants	Treatment duration	Findings	References
Lactobacillus casei supplementation	Italy	A prospective, randomized study to divide participants into group A (with supplementation) & group B (without supplementation)	70 patients with resistant *H. pylori infection* and dyspepsia symptoms	10 days	Probiotic supplementation improved the eradication rate slightly and reduced side effects of the quadruple therapy	Tursi et al. (2004)
Lactobacillus acidophilus La5 *Bifidobacterium lactis* Bb12	Taiwan	Randomized study Intervention group: triple therapy + yogurt control group: triple therapy only	160 patients with *H. pylori* infection	4 weeks	Eradication rate increased in the intervention group	Sheu et al. (2002)
Lactobacillus acidophilus La5 *Bifidobacterium lactis* Bb12	Taiwan	Participants were randomly assigned to either yogurt + quadruple therapy group or a quadruple therapy only group	138 patients with resistant *H. pylori* infection and dyspepsia symptoms	4 weeks	Yogurt + quadruple therapy group had an increase in the eradication rate	Sheu et al. (2006)
Lactobacillus acidophilus LB	Italy	Single center, randomized trial	120 patients with *H. pylori* infection with dyspepsia symptoms	10 days	Eradication rate increased; no significant difference in the reduction of triple therapy's side effects	Canducci et al. (2000)
Lactobacillus reuteri	Italy	A prospective, single-center, randomized study. Patients divided into two groups: with/without receiving probiotics along with 7-day course triple therapy for 14 days	90 patients with *H. pylori* infection	14 days	Significantly increased the eradication rate in the probiotic group	Ojetti et al. (2012)

(continued)

Table 14.3 (continued)

Types of probiotics or probiotics containing product	Country	Study design and interventions	Number of participants	Treatment duration	Findings	References
Lactobacillus rhamnosus LC *Propionibacterium freudenreichii* *Bifidobacterium breve*	Finland	Randomized double-blinded with patients for receiving either probiotics or placebo treatment	47 patients with *H. pylori* infection	3 weeks	Eradication rate similar in both groups; reduced urease activity, gastritis, and *H. pylori* colonization in probiotic group	Myllyluoma et al. (2005)
Lactobacillus rhamnosus GG	Italy	Open, randomized study	120 healthy adults with no symptoms	2 weeks	Side effects of the eradication therapy were significantly reduced in the probiotic group	Armuzzi et al. (2001)
Lactobacillus rhamnosus GG *Saccharomyces boulardii* *Lactobacillus* spp. *bifidobacteria*	US	Randomized into 4 groups Group 1: *Lactobacillus* GG Group 2: *Saccharomyces boulardii* Group 3: *Lactobacillus* spp. and *bifidobacteria* Group 4: Placebo	85 patients with *H. pylori* infection but asymptomatic	2 weeks	Probiotics groups were superior to placebo for side effect prevention but no significant difference in eradication rate between the probiotic group and the placebo group	Cremonini et al. (2002)

established in 2016 strongly recommends adding probiotics to the eradication therapy (Fallone et al. 2016). Notably, they can be only used as supplements to antibiotic therapy to decrease *H. pylori*-induced inflammatory response and achieve a gastric mucosa protective effect (Zhu and Liu 2017).

14.4 Liver Cancer

Liver cancer is the fourth most prominent cause of cancer death and caused approximately 830,000 deaths and 906,000 new cases globally in 2018 (Bray et al. 2018). Hepatocellular carcinoma (HCC) is the most common type of primary liver cancer (Balogh et al. 2016). Various chronic liver diseases can progress to HCC, including alcoholic liver disease (ALD), non-alcoholic fatty liver disease (NAFLD), as well as hepatitis B or C (Forner et al. 2018). The majority of patients with HCC have underlying chronic liver disease and/or liver cirrhosis (Sherman 2010).

14.4.1 Gut Microbiota and HCC

The leaky gut and dysbiosis are the prominent features of liver cirrhosis and hepatocarcinogenesis (Yu and Schwabe 2017). This is caused by an increase in exposure to a wide range of toll-like receptor (TLR) ligands as well as other bacterial products and metabolites (Schwabe and Greten 2020). The leaky gut triggered by gram-negative bacteria lipopolysaccharide (LPS)-mediated inflammation via TLR4 results in the translocation the dysbiotic microbiota to the liver (Lin et al. 1995). TLR4 also promotes the development of liver fibrosis and upregulates the expression of epiregulin, a potent HCC-promoting hepatomitogen (Dapito et al. 2012; Bultman 2014). Furthermore, a high-fat diet can enhance bacteria to generate more secondary bile acid (deoxycholic acid, DCA) (Schwabe and Greten 2020). DCA increases TLR2 expression on hepatic stellate cells and activates prostaglandin E_2 (PGE_2) to suppress the antitumor immunity, resulting in HCC carcinogenesis (Loo et al. 2017).

Dysbiosis alters the metabolic pathways in the gut microbiota and leads to HCC progression (Yu and Schwabe 2017; Schwabe and Greten 2020). The microbiota composition in patients with HCC was not consistent between studies. This is possibly due to different etiologies, geographical areas, and underlying causes of cirrhosis (Schwabe and Greten 2020). Patients with HCC progressed from NASH-induced cirrhosis had a higher amount of *Bacteroides* and *Ruminococcaceae* compared to patients with NASH-induced cirrhosis only (Ponziani et al. 2019). Patients with ALD were found to have a higher amount of *Enterobacteriaceae* and *Proteobacteria* and a lesser amount of *Bacteroidetes* and *Firmicutes* when compared to healthy individuals (Mutlu et al. 2012).

14.4.2 Probiotics in the Treatment and Prevention of HCC

Probiotics have been studied in a few in vitro and in vivo studies on their potential HCC-suppressing effects (Table 14.4). An in vivo study discovered that probiotics composed of *Lactobacillus rhamnosus* GG, *Escherichia coli* Nissle 1917, and heat-inactivated VSL#3 (1:1:1) increased the amount of beneficial bacteria such as *Prevotella* and *Oscillibacter*, and therefore reduced the growth of HCC and Th17 cell differentiation (Li et al. 2016). Selenium-glutathione-enriched probiotic mixture *S. cerevisiae* and *L. acidophilus* activate silent information regulator 1 (SIRT1) to relieve hepatic oxidative stress (Liu et al. 2018). It predominantly prevented CCl4-induced hepatic inflammation in rat livers as indicated by the reduced serum level of alanine aminotransferase (ALT) and aspartate transaminase (AST) (Liu et al. 2018). Probiotics can regulate the host gene expression to alleviate the pathogenesis of HCC through modulating DNA methylation and histone modification (Miro-Blanch and Yanes 2019; Heydari et al. 2019). *Paraplantarum* decreased the rate of hepatic inflammation and fibrosis significantly by downregulating the transcription of the CCAAT enhancer-binding protein β (C/EBP/β) and α-2 macroglobulin (A2MG) expression (Mihailović et al. 2017).

14.4.3 Clinical Studies on Probiotics Related to HCV Infection and NAFLD

Although the mechanisms of action of probiotics at the molecular level are largely unknown, studies demonstrated that they can moderate liver inflammatory response and immunity to improve non-alcoholic steatohepatitis (NASH) and virus-induced HCC progression (Schwabe and Greten 2020). HCV and NAFLD are risk factors for HCC (Forner et al. 2018; Than and Newsome 2015). There are 4 randomized controlled studies and 2 single-center studies that explored the effects of probiotic administration in patients with NAFLD and HCV, respectively (Table 14.5). Results showed that the serum level of ALT and AST were decreased and the HCV treatment response was enhanced (Oo et al. 2016; Nanis et al. 2019). For the patients with NAFLD, probiotics can decrease serum ALT and AST levels, and no adverse effects were observed in the studies (Nabavi et al. 2014; Ahn et al. 2019; Duseja et al. 2019) . In addition, probiotics can provide additional benefits such as reducing the risk of hepatic inflammation and fibrosis and downregulating TNF-α expression (Ahn et al. 2019; Duseja et al. 2019).

Table 14.4 Summary of the in vitro and in vivo studies related to probiotics in preventing of HCC development

Probiotics	Cell line/Animals	Findings	References
In vitro			
Bifidobacterium adolescentis SPM0212	24 h incubation of HepG2.2.15 cells along with probiotic cell extracts	The probiotic cell extract activated MxA protein by upregulating STAT1, therefore inhibited HBV replication	Lee et al. (2013)
Cranberry proanthocyanidin extract biotransformed by *Lactobacillus rhamnosus*	48 h incubation of HepG2 cells with biotransformed cranberry proanthocyanidins extract (10–500 μg/mL)	Depleted mitochondria in HepG2 cells	Rupasinghe et al. (2019)
Lactobacillus bulgaricus 761N	96 h incubation of HepG2 cells with extracellular probiotic microbes and HCV virus	HCV count was reduced	Adawi et al. (2015)
In vivo			
Bifidobacterium infantis, *Lactobacillus acidophilus*, and *Bacillus cereus*	Male SPF SD rats on a HSHF (high-fat high sucrose) diet were supplemented with the probiotic mixture for 12 weeks	The probiotic mixture restored the loss of GM richness, and gut barrier function in rats fed with HSHF diet, which in turn reduced the serum LPS level and TLR4 induced immune response	Xue et al. (2017)
Lactobacillus acidophilus and *Bifidobacterium bifidum*	Male Balb/c mice (6 weeks) were treated with the two probiotics separately for 5 months. Ten days into the treatment the mice were injected with carcinogen, azoxymethane weekly for three weeks to result in colorectal cancer	Probiotic supplementation downregulated onco-miRNAs (miR-155 and miR-221) and oncogenes (Bcl-w and K-Ras) in liver tissue; Upregulated tumor suppressors miR-122 and PU.1	Heydari et al. (2019)
Lactobacillus paraplantarum BGCG11	Albino Wistar rats were treated intraperitoneal with streptozotocin for 5 days, then supplemented with probiotic bacteria for 4 weeks	Probiotic reduced inflammatory response and hepatic oxidative stress by restoring SOD activity	Mihailović et al. (2017)
Lactobacillus. plantarum EMCC-1039	Wistar rats with liver cirrhosis is cultivated with thioacetamide (200 mg/kg) three times a day, they they receive 1.2×10^9 cfu/mL of probiotic bacteria daily	Probiotics controlled thioacetamide-induced cirrhosis in Wistar rats by downregulating TLR4, CXCL9, and PREX-2	Elshaer et al. (2019)

(continued)

Table 14.4 (continued)

Probiotics	Cell line/Animals	Findings	References
Lactobacillus. rhamnosus, Escherichia E. coli Nissle 1917	Male C57BL6/N mice (5–6 weeks) were nourished with the probiotic mixture enriched with libitum and inject hepatoma cell subcutaneously	Repressed tumorigenesis by downregulation of IL-17 and upregulation of anti-inflammatory cytokines	Li et al. (2016)
Saccharomyces cerevisiae and *Lactobacillus acidophilus* enriched with selenium and glutathione	Liver fibrosis rats were cultivated with intraperitoneal CCl4 twice a week for 7 weeks, then supplemented with probiotic mixture for 7 weeks	Probiotics simultaneously reduced hepatic damage and fibrosis; Reduced CCl4-induced oxidative stress, ER stress, and serum level of AST and ALT in blood	Liu et al. (2018)

Table 14.5 Summary of clinical studies of probiotics related to HCV infection and NAFLD

Types of probiotics or probiotics containing product	Country	Study design	Number of participants	Interventions	Treatment duration	Findings	References
A mixture of *Lactobacillus acidophilus* and *Bifidobacteria* supplementation	Egypt	A prospective single-center study	20 patients with HCV	Participants treated with probiotic mixture daily, before initiating HCV treatment with pegylated IFN-α and ribavirin	1 month	Treatment response to pegylated IFN-α and ribavirin was enhanced by probiotics by 25%	Nanis et al. (2019)
Heat-treated *Enterococcus faecalis* FK-23	Japan	A single-arm, non-comparative clinical drug trial study	39 patients with HCV	HCV positive patients treated with heat-treated probiotics	A minimum 3 months to maximum 36 months	Serum level of alanine aminotransferase (ALT) and aspartate transaminase (AST) decreased during the treatment period	Oo et al. (2016)
A multi-strain probiotic mixture of *Lactobacillus paracasei* DSM 24733, *Lactobacillus plantarum* DSM 24730, *Lactobacillus acidophilus* DSM 24735 and *Lactobacillus delbrueckii* subsp. *bulgaricus* DSM 24734, *Bifidobacterium longum* DSM 24736, *Bifidobacterium infantis* DSM 24737, *Bifidobacterium breve* DSM 24732, and *Streptococcus thermophilus* DSM 24731	India	A double-blind randomized clinical trial	39 patients with NAFLD	Intervention group: exercising and healthy diet received multi-strain probiotic mixture for 12 months Placebo group: exercising and healthy diet received placebo (microcrystalline cellulose) for 12 months	12 months	Probiotic supplementation reduced hepatocyte ballooning and hepatic fibrosis; Reduced hepatic lobular inflammation and ALT serum level, adipocytokines, leptin, and endotoxins	Duseja et al. (2019)

(continued)

Table 14.5 (continued)

Types of probiotics or probiotics containing product	Country	Study design	Number of participants	Interventions	Treatment duration	Findings	References
A probiotic mixture of *Lactobacillus acidophilus* CBT LA1, *L. rhamnosus* CBT LR5, *L. paracasei* CBT LPC5, *Pediococcus pentosaceus* CBT SL4, *Bifidobacteria lactis* CBT BL3, and *Bifidobacteria breve* CBT BR3	Korea	A double-blind randomized clinical trial	68 patients with NAFLD	Intervention group: probiotic mixture daily for Placebo group: composed of dextran, maltodextrin, lemon flavor, and Mg stearate	3 months	Probiotic mixture significantly lowered participants' body weight, body cholesterol and fat levels; Downregulated TNF-α in NAFLD patients	Ahn et al. (2019)
A yogurt with *Lactobacillus acidophilus* La5 and *Bifidobacteria lactis* Bb12	Iran	A double-blind randomized clinical trial	72 patients with NAFLD	Intervention group: 300 g of the probiotic yogurt daily Placebo group: 300 g of conventional yogurt daily	2 months	Probiotic yogurt reduced AST (5.42%) and ALT (4.67%) serum level and total cholesterol level (4.1%)	Nabavi et al. (2014)
Lactobacillus bulgaricus and *Streptococcus thermophilus*	Spain	A double-blind randomized clinical trial	30 patients with NAFLD	Intervention group: treated with probiotics Placebo group: treated with placebo (starch)	3 months	Serum level of ALT and AST decreased significantly	Aller et al. (2011)

14.5 Pancreatic Cancer

Pancreatic cancer (PC) is one of the most fatal cancer types due to its high malignancy and poor prognosis (Rawla et al. 2019b). Although it is the seventh leading cause of cancer-related deaths worldwide (Rawla et al. 2019b), the 5-year overall survival rate of PC remains <10% (Bray et al. 2018). Lack of alarming symptoms and therefore delay in diagnosis contribute to the high mortality rate (Kamisawa et al. 2016).

14.5.1 Risk Factors of PC Development

Obesity significantly increases the risk of PC development (Li et al. 2009). In vivo study demonstrated that adipose tissue released pro-inflammatory cytokines such as IL-1, IL-6, and TNF-α to activate the innate immune system via abnormal regulation of the NF-kB signaling pathway (Creely et al. 2007; Hertzer et al. 2016). Further, obesity is associated with insulin resistance and the elevation in the insulin-like growth factor 1 (IGF-1) level (Xu et al. 2018). IGF-1 can in turn stimulate the phosphatidylinositol 3-kinase (PI3K)/AKT/mTOR pathway which induces proliferation and inhibits apoptosis in PC cells (Rozengurt 2014). The overactivation of IGF-1 can also downregulate tumor suppressors such as PTEN which contributes to PC development (Ma et al. 2010b).

Chronic heavy alcohol consumption is another risk factor for PC but the exact mechanism remains unclear (Rahman et al. 2015; Herreros-Villanueva et al. 2013). The alcohol metabolite acetaldehyde may damage the pancreatic cells (Duell 2012). It can also alter the DNA repair process (Garro et al. 1986). In addition, CYP enzymes (CYP2E1) are expressed in pancreatic tissues and may play a role in generating alcohol metabolites (Burim et al. 2004). These metabolites can damage the pancreatic tissues and stimulate the secretion of pro-inflammatory cytokines, eventually leading to pancreatitis and may progress to PC (Feingold et al. 1990).

A meta-analysis showed that dietary cholesterol may increase the risk of PC development (Wang et al. 2015). Although there are several potential mechanisms to explain the linkage of cholesterol to PC, the exact mechanism remains unclear (Wang et al. 2015). In addition, cholesterol level affects bile excretion and may cause bile reflux into the head of the pancreas via the common duct, where the PC most likely occurs anatomically (Baghurst et al. 1991).

Poor oral hygiene has been proposed to increase the risk of PC (Huang et al. 2016). The presence of dental plaque, oral mucosal lesions, or tongue lesions may promote the growth of bacteria such as nitrate-reducing bacteria to form nitrosamine (Nair et al. 1996). It is considered one of the potential pancreatic carcinogens (Risch 2003). Another hypothesis is that oral pathogens such as *Porphyromonas gingivalis* can impair innate immunity (Curtis 2014).

H. pylori may increase the risk of PC (Bao et al. 2010). A prospective cohort study showed that men with gastric ulcers had an increased risk of PC (RR, 1.83; 95% CI:1.13–2.97) (Bao et al. 2010). The bacterium might catalyze nitrosamines, which induce DNA damage in the pancreas could eventually cause pancreatic tumor development (Hecht 2003). Altered gut microbiota may also contribute to PC (Li et al. 2020). *Enterococcus and Enterobacter* species commonly found in bile can flow and penetrate to the pancreatic tissues (Maekawa et al. 2018). Penetrated bacterial metabolites such as LPS can also induce inflammation and immune responses by binding to TLR and Nod-like receptor (NLR) and activate NF-kB and mitogen-activated protein kinase (MAPK) signaling pathways (Li et al. 2020). NF-kB regulates the gene transcription to increase the expression of pro-inflammatory mediators (Zhang and Rigas 2006). Those inflammatory mediators will further attract immune cells and lead to inflammation and promote pancreatitis development (Zhang and Rigas 2006). Furthermore, lipoteichoic acid (LTA) is a surface component of gram-positive bacteria and can trigger the secretion of pro-inflammatory factors by binding to CD14 or TLR2 (Hermann et al. 2002). A recent in vivo study showed that the infection of *Enterococcus faecalis* may contribute to the progression of chronic pancreatitis and PC development (Maekawa et al. 2018).

However, only limited in vitro and in vivo studies were available (Singhal et al. 2016). But probiotics may have antitumor effects or be able to provide syngenetic effects to standard chemotherapy (Table 14.6). The possible mechanisms include reduced proliferation of tumor cells (Kuno et al. 2015) and induction of apoptosis by activating the p38 MAPK signaling pathway (Konishi et al. 2021). More clinical studies are warranted to further elucidate and confirm the potential role of probiotics in PC prevention and treatment.

Table 14.6 Summary of in vitro and in vivo studies of the effect of probiotics in PC

Probiotics	Cell line/Animals	Methods	Findings	References
Aspergillus oryzae (a fungus)	The human pancreatic cancer cell lines SUIT2 BALB/c nude mice and BALB/c mice	Probiotic was administered to pancreatic cancer cell lines Heptelidic acid (metabolite of *Aspergillus oryzae*) was directly injected into the transplanted tumor in mice	Tumor-suppressive effect was observed; *Aspergillus oryzae* released tumor-suppressive molecules (heptelidic acid)	Konishi et al. (2021)
Fermented brown rice *Aspergillus oryzae* (FBRA)	Male Syrian golden hamsters	The hamsters were divided into 7 groups Group 1: received basal diet during the experimental period Groups 2 and 3: received 5 and 10% FBRA in the diet, respectively, during and 1 week after BOP injection. Then changed to the control diet until they were 27 weeks of age Group 4 and 5: received basal diet during BOP injection, received 5% and 10% FBRA in the diet during and 1 week after BOP injection until 27 weeks of age Group 6: received 10% FBRA in the diet during the whole experimental period Group 7: non-treatment control *Group 1–5: with pancreatic cancer* *Group 6 to 7: without pancreatic cancer*	Intake of 10% FBRA during the post-initiation phase reduced the multiplicity and inhibited the progression of precancerous lesions of ductal adenocarcinoma	Kuno et al. (2015)

(continued)

Table 14.6 (continued)

Probiotics	Cell line/Animals	Methods	Findings	References
Lactobacillus paracasei GMNL-133 and *Lactobacillus reuteri* GMNL-89	LSL-K-ras$^{G12D/-}$-Pdx-1-Cre mouse model of pancreatic ductal adenocarcinoma (PDAC)	Mice with pancreatic cancer were treated with gemcitabine in combination with the oral administration of probiotics	A lower grade of pancreatic intraepithelial neoplasia (PanIN) was observed in the mice treated with gemcitabine and probiotics; An inhibitory effect on PanIN was observed in the mice treated with high-dose probiotics alone	Chen et al. (2020b)

14.6 Use of Probiotics to Increase the Efficacies of Anti-GI Cancer Therapy

There were few preclinical studies focusing on enhancing the efficacy of the chemotherapy agent 5- fluorouracil (5-FU) against CRC. The combination therapy of *Lactobacillus plantarum* (LP) supernatant (SN) and 5-FU inhibited the survival of CRC cells (HT-29 and HCT- 116) and led to cell death by inducing caspase-3 activity. The possible mechanism may be due to the inactivation of the Wnt/β-catenin signaling of chemoresistant CRC cells (JaeJin 2016). In vivo studies showed that the combination therapy of *L. rhamnosus* and 5-FU can reduce the inflammatory response in the colon by modulating K-ras and Treg/IL-10 transcription levels (Hadad et al. 2019). *L. rhamnosus* was also being tested in in vivo studies to combine with capecitabine for GC treatment. The results showed that the combination therapy increased apoptotic and necrotic responses in the grafted tumor and the size was reduced when compared with control group (Rahimi et al. 2021).

Furthermore, preclinical studies showed that gut microbiota can help to achieve an effective immune response in immunotherapy (Routy et al. 2018), such as enhancing the immune checkpoint inhibitors response to target the programmed death receptor 1 (PD-1)/programmed death-ligand 1 (PD-L1) axis (Sivan et al. 2015) and the cytotoxic T lymphocyte-associated antigen 4 (CTLA-4) axis (Vétizou et al. 2015). PD-L1 is associated with the inhibition of T cell activation (Salmaninejad et al. 2019) and expressed in various types of non-GI and GI cancers, especially in non-small cell lung cancer (NSCLC), melanoma, GC, and liver cancer (Chae et al. 2018). CTLA-4 recognizes B7 ligands on the surface of tumor cells and further inhibits T cell activation (Ganesan et al. 2018). Specific bacteria were positively correlated with immunotherapeutic response, including *Bifidobacterium* spp. (Sivan et al. 2015). Furthermore, a consortium published in 2019 identified 11 bacterial strains that could enhance the action of immune checkpoint inhibitors to inhibit tumor growth in a tumor model derived from a mouse colon adenocarcinoma cell line (Tanoue et al. 2019). Based on these findings, further research is needed to confirm the therapeutic responses of probiotics in immunotherapy in GI cancer and incorporate the preclinical studies' findings into clinical trials (Wong and Yu 2019).

Although there are limited clinical trials on probiotics for treating and preventing GI cancer, ample evidence supports the beneficial effects of probiotics in attenuating the anti-GI cancer therapy-related diarrhea and surgery-related complications (Lu et al. 2021). These complications negatively impact on patients' recovery and prolong the length of hospital stay (Lu et al. 2019). In such cases, probiotics such as *Bifidobacterium* and *Lactobacillus* have been shown to improve the gastrointestinal barrier function and normalize the gut microbiota environment (He et al. 2013; Zhao et al. 2017; Xu et al. 2019). Chemotherapy will damage the normal intestinal cells and cause the change of gut microbiota composition in patients (Lu et al. 2021; Touchefeu et al. 2014). Reduced *Bifidobacteria* and *Clostridium* genus and increased in *Enterobacter* and *Bacteroides* then in turn contribute to intestinal mucositis and cause chemotherapy-induced diarrhea (CID) (Touchefeu et al. 2014). In this connection, patients with CRC after surgery with adjuvant chemotherapy received *Lactobacillus rhamnosus* GG supplements daily had mild diarrhea and lower incidence of grade 3 or 4 diarrhea (experimental group vs control group: 22% vs 37%) (Osterlund et al. 2007). A meta-analysis also showed that patients with CRC using probiotics can reduce the frequency of CID (Lu et al. 2019). In addition, patients with CRC who used probiotics before and after colorectal surgery may help to reduce surgery-related complications, such as the superficial incisional surgical site infection (Aisu et al. 2015). Probiotics improved the intestinal microbial environment and activated host immune function, leading to the prevention of infectious complications (Aisu et al. 2015). Besides, post-surgical GC patients receiving fiber and probiotics for 7 consecutive days can reduce the frequency of enteral nutrition-related diarrhea (Zhao et al. 2017).

14.7 Future Probiotics Development

"Next-generation probiotics" is a relatively new approach for probiotics development (O'Toole et al. 2017). Researchers continue to identify different new probiotic strains in fermented food and human feces (Mejía-Caballero et al. 2021). This can help to evaluate the human microbiota distribution in different GI cancers and identify potential new probiotics that may help to treat or prevent GI cancers. Researchers also start to use engineering techniques to modify probiotic strains to exert different functions, such as transforming them into a vehicle for the delivery of drug molecules to the target site in GI cancer, producing anti-inflammatory effect alongside cancer immunotherapy (Mejía-Caballero et al. 2021). *Bifidobacterium bifidum* BGN4 has been genetically engineered to produce interleukin IL-10 to produce anti-inflammatory effects with cancer immunotherapy in human intestines (Hong et al. 2021). *E coli* Nissle has been engineered to release the lytic protein HlyE to induce tumor regression (Chiang and Huang 2021). Engineered probiotics could also be used as cancer diagnostic tools. For instance, the engineered probiotic *E. coli* Nissle 1917 specifically colonizing liver tumors in mice by carting specific gene circuits produced a detectable signal in urine (Danino et al. 2015). Furthermore, since probiotics are considered as dietary supplements, more future work such as establishing comprehensive guidance of probiotics' efficacy and safety in GI cancer is warranted (Lu et al. 2021).

14.8 Conclusions

Despite a better understanding of the molecular mechanisms of GI cancer tumorigenesis since the past decade and the advancement of treatment, a high mortality rate due to metastasis is still an issue worldwide. Abnormal gut microbiota composition has been shown to be causally linked to GI cancers. There is a need for the development of new therapeutic agents and new strategies, including prebiotics and probiotics, to target the gut microbiota. Literature demonstrated that probiotics could help to prevent or treat GI cancers by slowing down their progression or act as adjunctive therapy to cancer treatment. However, only limited clinical trials are available. More preclinical and clinical research are warranted to understand the complex mechanisms of GI cancer development and to identify the most suitable probiotic strains for the prevention and treatment.

References

Abdulamir AS, Hafidh RR, Abu Bakar F. The association of Streptococcus bovis/gallolyticus with colorectal tumors: the nature and the underlying mechanisms of its etiological role. J Exp Clin Cancer Res. 2011;30(1):11.

Adawi HE, Nour I, Fattouh F, Deeb NE. Investigation of the antiviral bioactivity of Lactobacillus bulgaricus 761N extracellular extract against hepatitis C virus (HCV). Int J Pharmacol. 2015;11(1):19–26.

Ahmad R, Kumar B, Chen Z, Chen X, Müller D, Lele SM, et al. Loss of claudin-3 expression induces IL6/gp130/Stat3 signaling to promote colon cancer malignancy by hyperactivating Wnt/β-catenin signaling. Oncogene. 2017;36(47):6592–604.

Ahn SB, Jun DW, Kang B-K, Lim JH, Lim S, Chung M-J. Randomized, double-blind, placebo-controlled study of a multispecies probiotic mixture in nonalcoholic fatty liver disease. Sci Rep. 2019;9(1):5688.

Aisu N, Tanimura S, Yamashita Y, Yamashita K, Maki K, Yoshida Y, et al. Impact of perioperative probiotic treatment for surgical site infections in patients with colorectal cancer. Exp Ther Med. 2015;10(3):966–72.

Aller R, De Luis DA, Izaola O, Conde R, Gonzalez Sagrado M, Primo D, et al. Effect of a probiotic on liver aminotransferases in nonalcoholic fatty liver disease patients: a double blind randomized clinical trial. Eur Rev Med Pharmacol Sci. 2011;15(9):1090–5.

Altonsy MO, Andrews SC, Tuohy KM. Differential induction of apoptosis in human colonic carcinoma cells (Caco-2) by Atopobium, and commensal, probiotic and enteropathogenic bacteria: mediation by the mitochondrial pathway. Int J Food Microbiol. 2010;137(2–3):190–203.

Alvarez C-S, Badia J, Bosch M, Giménez R, Baldomà L. Outer membrane vesicles and soluble factors released by probiotic Escherichia coli Nissle 1917 and commensal ECOR63 enhance barrier function by regulating expression of tight junction proteins in intestinal epithelial cells. Front Microbiol. 2016;7:1981.

Armuzzi A, Cremonini F, Ojetti V, Bartolozzi F, Canducci F, Candelli M, et al. Effect of Lactobacillus GG supplementation on antibiotic-associated gastrointestinal side effects during Helicobacter pylori eradication therapy: a pilot study. Digestion. 2001;63(1):1–7.

Arnold M, Abnet CC, Neale RE, Vignat J, Giovannucci EL, McGlynn KA, et al. Global burden of 5 major types of gastrointestinal cancer. Gastroenterology. 2020;159(1):335–49.e15.

Backert S, Ziska E, Brinkmann V, Zimny-Arndt U, Fauconnier A, Jungblut PR, et al. Translocation of the Helicobacter pylori CagA protein in gastric epithelial cells by a type IV secretion apparatus. Cell Microbiol. 2000;2(2):155–64.

Baghurst PA, McMichael AJ, Slavotinek AH, Baghurst KI, Boyle P, Walker AM. A case-control study of diet and cancer of the pancreas. Am J Epidemiol. 1991;134(2):167–79.

Bali P, Coker J, Lozano-Pope I, Zengler K, Obonyo M. Microbiome signatures in a fast- and slow-progressing gastric cancer murine model and their contribution to gastric carcinogenesis. Microorganisms. 2021;9(1):189.

Balogh J, Victor D 3rd, Asham EH, Burroughs SG, Boktour M, Saharia A, et al. Hepatocellular carcinoma: a review. J Hepatocell Carcinoma. 2016;3:41–53.

Banna GL, Torino F, Marletta F, Santagati M, Salemi R, Cannarozzo E, et al. Lactobacillus rhamnosus GG: an overview to explore the rationale of its use in cancer. Front Pharmacol. 2017;8:603.

Bao Y, Spiegelman D, Li R, Giovannucci E, Fuchs CS, Michaud DS. History of peptic ulcer disease and pancreatic cancer risk in men. Gastroenterology. 2010;138(2):541–9.

Bell HN, Rebernick RJ, Goyert J, Singhal R, Kuljanin M, Kerk SA, et al. Reuterin in the healthy gut microbiome suppresses colorectal cancer growth through altering redox balance. Cancer Cell. 2022;40(2):185–200.e6.

Borges-Canha M, Portela-Cidade JP, Dinis-Ribeiro M, Leite-Moreira AF, Pimentel-Nunes P. Role of colonic microbiota in colorectal carcinogenesis: a systematic review. Rev Esp Enferm Dig. 2015;107(11):659–71.

Bray F, Ferlay J, Soerjomataram I, Siegel RL, Torre LA, Jemal A. Global cancer statistics 2018: GLOBOCAN estimates of incidence and mortality worldwide for 36 cancers in 185 countries. CA Cancer J Clin. 2018;68(6):394–424.

Bultman SJ. Emerging roles of the microbiome in cancer. Carcinogenesis. 2014;35(2):249–55.

Burim RV, Canalle R, de Lôurdes Candolo Martinelli A, Takahashi CS. Polymorphisms in glutathione S-transferases GSTM1, GSTT1 and GSTP1 and cytochromes P450 CYP2E1 and CYP1A1 and susceptibility to cirrhosis or pancreatitis in alcoholics. Mutagenesis. 2004;19(4):291–8.

Campana R, van Hemert S, Baffone W. Strain-specific probiotic properties of lactic acid bacteria and their interference with human intestinal pathogens invasion. Gut Pathog. 2017;9:12.

Canani RB, Costanzo MD, Leone L, Pedata M, Meli R, Calignano A. Potential beneficial effects of butyrate in intestinal and extraintestinal diseases. World J Gastroenterol. 2011;17(12):1519–28.

Canducci F, Armuzzi A, Cremonini F, Cammarota G, Bartolozzi F, Pola P, et al. A lyophilized and inactivated culture of Lactobacillus acidophilus increases Helicobacter pylori eradication rates. Aliment Pharmacol Ther. 2000;14(12):1625–9.

Castellarin M, Warren RL, Freeman JD, Dreolini L, Krzywinski M, Strauss J, et al. Fusobacterium nucleatum infection is prevalent in human colorectal carcinoma. Genome Res. 2012;22(2):299–306.

Chae YK, Arya A, Iams W, Cruz MR, Chandra S, Choi J, et al. Current landscape and future of dual anti-CTLA4 and PD-1/PD-L1 blockade immunotherapy in cancer; lessons learned from clinical trials with melanoma and non-small cell lung cancer (NSCLC). J Immunother Cancer. 2018;6(1):39.

Chen W, Liu F, Ling Z, Tong X, Xiang C. Human intestinal lumen and mucosa-associated microbiota in patients with colorectal cancer. PLoS One. 2012;7(6):e39743.

Chen ZF, Ai LY, Wang JL, Ren LL, Yu YN, Xu J, et al. Probiotics Clostridium butyricum and Bacillus subtilis ameliorate intestinal tumorigenesis. Future Microbiol. 2015;10(9):1433–45.

Chen D, Jin D, Huang S, Wu J, Xu M, Liu T, et al. Clostridium butyricum, a butyrate-producing probiotic, inhibits intestinal tumor development through modulating Wnt signaling and gut microbiota. Cancer Lett. 2020a;469:456–67.

Chen SM, Chieng WW, Huang SW, Hsu LJ, Jan MS. The synergistic tumor growth-inhibitory effect of probiotic Lactobacillus on transgenic mouse model of pancreatic cancer treated with gemcitabine. Sci Rep. 2020b;10(1):20319.

Cheng Y, Ling Z, Li L. The intestinal microbiota and colorectal cancer. Front Immunol. 2020;11(3100):615056.

Chiang C-J, Huang P-H. Metabolic engineering of probiotic Escherichia coli for cytolytic therapy of tumors. Sci Rep. 2021;11(1):5853.

Chung EJ, Do EJ, Kim SY, Cho EA, Kim DH, Pak S, et al. Combination of metformin and VSL#3 additively suppresses western-style diet induced colon cancer in mice. Eur J Pharmacol. 2017;794:1–7.

Chung I-C, OuYang C-N, Yuan S-N, Lin H-C, Huang K-Y, Wu P-S, et al. Pretreatment with a heat-killed probiotic modulates the NLRP3 inflammasome and attenuates colitis-associated colorectal cancer in mice. Nutrients. 2019;11(3):516.

Creely SJ, McTernan PG, Kusminski CM, Fisher FM, Da Silva NF, Khanolkar M, et al. Lipopolysaccharide activates an innate immune system response in human adipose tissue in obesity and type 2 diabetes. Am J Physiol Endocrinol Metab. 2007;292(3):E740–7.

Cremonini F, Di Caro S, Covino M, Armuzzi A, Gabrielli M, Santarelli L, et al. Effect of different probiotic preparations on anti-helicobacter pylori therapy-related side effects: a parallel group, triple blind, placebo-controlled study. Am J Gastroenterol. 2002;97(11):2744–9.

Cruz B, de Sousa Moraes LF, De Nadai ML, Dias KA, Murad LB, Sarandy MM, et al. Evaluation of the efficacy of probiotic VSL#3 and synbiotic VSL#3 and yacon-based product in reducing oxidative stress and intestinal permeability in mice induced to colorectal carcinogenesis. J Food Sci. 2021;86(4):1448–62.

Curtis MA. Periodontal microbiology—the lid's off the box again. J Dent Res. 2014;93(9):840–2.

Danino T, Prindle A, Kwong GA, Skalak M, Li H, Allen K, et al. Programmable probiotics for detection of cancer in urine. Sci Transl Med. 2015;7(289):289ra84.

Dapito DH, Mencin A, Gwak GY, Pradere JP, Jang MK, Mederacke I, et al. Promotion of hepatocellular carcinoma by the intestinal microbiota and TLR4. Cancer Cell. 2012;21(4):504–16.

Duell EJ. Epidemiology and potential mechanisms of tobacco smoking and heavy alcohol consumption in pancreatic cancer. Mol Carcinog. 2012;51(1):40–52.

Duseja A, Acharya SK, Mehta M, Chhabra S, Rana S, Das A, et al. High potency multistrain probiotic improves liver histology in non-alcoholic fatty liver disease (NAFLD): a randomised, double-blind, proof of concept study. BMJ Open Gastroenterol. 2019;6(1):e000315.

Eckburg PB, Bik EM, Bernstein CN, Purdom E, Dethlefsen L, Sargent M, et al. Diversity of the human intestinal microbial flora. Science (New York, NY). 2005;308(5728):1635–8.

Elshaer AM, El-Kharashi OA, Hamam GG, Nabih ES, Magdy YM, Abd El Samad AA. Involvement of TLR4/CXCL9/PREX-2 pathway in the development of hepatocellular carcinoma (HCC) and the promising role of early administration of lactobacillus plantarum in Wistar rats. Tissue Cell. 2019;60:38–47.

Escamilla J, Lane MA, Maitin V. Cell-free supernatants from probiotic Lactobacillus casei and Lactobacillus rhamnosus GG decrease colon cancer cell invasion in vitro. Nutr Cancer. 2012;64(6):871–8.

Fallone CA, Chiba N, van Zanten SV, Fischbach L, Gisbert JP, Hunt RH, et al. The Toronto consensus for the treatment of Helicobacter pylori infection in adults. Gastroenterology. 2016;151(1):51–69.e14.

Feingold KR, Soued M, Adi S, Staprans I, Shigenaga J, Doerrler W, et al. Tumor necrosis factor–increased hepatic very-low-density lipoprotein production and increased serum triglyceride levels in diabetic rats. Diabetes. 1990;39(12):1569.

Ferreira RM, Pereira-Marques J, Pinto-Ribeiro I, Costa JL, Carneiro F, Machado JC, et al. Gastric microbial community profiling reveals a dysbiotic cancer-associated microbiota. Gut. 2018;67(2):226–36.
Flemer B, Lynch DB, Brown JMR, Jeffery IB, Ryan FJ, Claesson MJ, et al. Tumour-associated and non-tumour-associated microbiota in colorectal cancer. Gut. 2017;66(4):633.
Floch MH. The effect of probiotics on host metabolism: the microbiota and fermentation. J Clin Gastroenterol. 2010;44(Suppl 1):S19–21.
Fong W, Li Q, Yu J. Gut microbiota modulation: a novel strategy for prevention and treatment of colorectal cancer. Oncogene. 2020;39(26):4925–43.
Forner A, Reig M, Bruix J. Hepatocellular carcinoma. Lancet. 2018;391(10127):1301–14.
Gagnaire A, Nadel B, Raoult D, Neefjes J, Gorvel JP. Collateral damage: insights into bacterial mechanisms that predispose host cells to cancer. Nat Rev Microbiol. 2017;15(2):109–28.
Gamallat Y, Meyiah A, Kuugbee ED, Hago AM, Chiwala G, Awadasseid A, et al. Lactobacillus rhamnosus induced epithelial cell apoptosis, ameliorates inflammation and prevents colon cancer development in an animal model. Biomed Pharmacother. 2016;83:536–41.
Ganesan A, Moon TC, Barakat KH. Revealing the atomistic details behind the binding of B7-1 to CD28 and CTLA-4: a comprehensive protein-protein modelling study. Biochim Biophys Acta Gen Subj. 2018;1862(12):2764–78.
Garro AJ, Espina N, Farinati F, Salvagnini M. The effects of chronic ethanol consumption on carcinogen metabolism and on O6-methylguanine transferase-mediated repair of alkylated DNA. Alcohol Clin Exp Res. 1986;10(6 Suppl):73s–7s.
Gibson GR, Hutkins R, Sanders ME, Prescott SL, Reimer RA, Salminen SJ, et al. Expert consensus document: the International Scientific Association for Probiotics and Prebiotics (ISAPP) consensus statement on the definition and scope of prebiotics. Nat Rev Gastroenterol Hepatol. 2017;14(8):491–502.
Goldin BR, Gualtieri LJ, Moore RP. The effect of Lactobacillus GG on the initiation and promotion of DMH-induced intestinal tumors in the rat. Nutr Cancer. 1996;25(2):197–204.
Górska A, Przystupski D, Niemczura MJ, Kulbacka J. Probiotic bacteria: a promising tool in cancer prevention and therapy. Curr Microbiol. 2019;76(8):939–49.
Grivennikov SI, Wang K, Mucida D, Stewart CA, Schnabl B, Jauch D, et al. Adenoma-linked barrier defects and microbial products drive IL-23/IL-17-mediated tumour growth. Nature. 2012;491(7423):254–8.
Gupta A, Madani R, Mukhtar H. Streptococcus bovis endocarditis, a silent sign for colonic tumour. Color Dis. 2010;12(3):164–71.
Hadad SE, Hazmi BA, Alhebshi A, Aldahlawi AM, Bassam RA. *Lactobacillus rhamnosus* enhances the immunological antitumor effect of 5-fluorouracil against colon cancer. Pak J Biol Sci. 2019;22(12):597–606.
Han KJ, Lee NK, Park H, Paik HD. Anticancer and anti-inflammatory activity of probiotic Lactococcus lactis NK34. J Microbiol Biotechnol. 2015;25(10):1697–701.
Hatakka K, Holma R, El-Nezami H, Suomalainen T, Kuisma M, Saxelin M, et al. The influence of Lactobacillus rhamnosus LC705 together with Propionibacterium freudenreichii ssp. shermanii JS on potentially carcinogenic bacterial activity in human colon. Int J Food Microbiol. 2008;128(2):406–10.
He D, Wang HY, Feng JY, Zhang MM, Zhou Y, Wu XT. Use of pro-/synbiotics as prophylaxis in patients undergoing colorectal resection for cancer: a meta-analysis of randomized controlled trials. Clin Res Hepatol Gastroenterol. 2013;37(4):406–15.
Hecht SS. Tobacco carcinogens, their biomarkers and tobacco-induced cancer. Nat Rev Cancer. 2003;3(10):733–44.
Hermann C, Spreitzer I, Schröder NW, Morath S, Lehner MD, Fischer W, et al. Cytokine induction by purified lipoteichoic acids from various bacterial species—role of LBP, sCD14, CD14 and failure to induce IL-12 and subsequent IFN-gamma release. Eur J Immunol. 2002;32(2):541–51.
Herreros-Villanueva M, Hijona E, Bañales JM, Cosme A, Bujanda L. Alcohol consumption on pancreatic diseases. World J Gastroenterol. 2013;19(5):638–47.

Hertzer KM, Xu M, Moro A, Dawson DW, Du L, Li G, et al. Robust early inflammation of the peripancreatic visceral adipose tissue during diet-induced obesity in the KrasG12D model of pancreatic cancer. Pancreas. 2016;45(3):458–65.

Heydari Z, Rahaie M, Alizadeh AM. Different anti-inflammatory effects of Lactobacillus acidophilus and Bifidobacterium bifidum in hepatocellular carcinoma cancer mouse through impact on microRNAs and their target genes. J Nutr Intermed Metab. 2019;16:100096.

Hibberd AA, Lyra A, Ouwehand AC, Rolny P, Lindegren H, Cedgård L, et al. Intestinal microbiota is altered in patients with colon cancer and modified by probiotic intervention. BMJ Open Gastroenterol. 2017;4(1):e000145.

Hill C, Guarner F, Reid G, Gibson GR, Merenstein DJ, Pot B, et al. The International Scientific Association for Probiotics and Prebiotics consensus statement on the scope and appropriate use of the term probiotic. Nat Rev Gastroenterol Hepatol. 2014;11(8):506–14.

Hong N, Ku S, Yuk K, Johnston TV, Ji GE, Park MS. Production of biologically active human interleukin-10 by Bifidobacterium bifidum BGN4. Microb Cell Fact. 2021;20(1):16.

Huang J, Roosaar A, Axéll T, Ye W. A prospective cohort study on poor oral hygiene and pancreatic cancer risk. Int J Cancer. 2016;138(2):340–7.

Iizasa H, Ishihara S, Richardo T, Kanehiro Y, Yoshiyama H. Dysbiotic infection in the stomach. World J Gastroenterol. 2015;21(40):11450–7.

Ishikawa H, Akedo I, Otani T, Suzuki T, Nakamura T, Takeyama I, et al. Randomized trial of dietary fiber and Lactobacillus casei administration for prevention of colorectal tumors. Int J Cancer. 2005;116(5):762–7.

Jacouton E, Chain F, Sokol H, Langella P, Bermúdez-Humarán LG. Probiotic strain Lactobacillus casei BL23 prevents colitis-associated colorectal cancer. Front Immunol. 2017;8:1553.

JaeJin A. Combination therapy of Lactobacillus plantarum supernatant and 5-Fluouracil increases chemosensitivity in colorectal cancer cells. J Microbiol Biotechnol. 2016;26(8):1490–503.

Javanmard A, Ashtari S, Sabet B, Davoodi SH, Rostami-Nejad M, Esmaeil Akbari M, et al. Probiotics and their role in gastrointestinal cancers prevention and treatment; an overview. Gastroenterol Hepatol Bed Bench. 2018;11(4):284–95.

Kahouli I, Tomaro-Duchesneau C, Prakash S. Probiotics in colorectal cancer (CRC) with emphasis on mechanisms of action and current perspectives. J Med Microbiol. 2013;62(Pt 8):1107–23.

Kamada N, Kim YG, Sham HP, Vallance BA, Puente JL, Martens EC, et al. Regulated virulence controls the ability of a pathogen to compete with the gut microbiota. Science. 2012;336(6086):1325–9.

Kamisawa T, Wood LD, Itoi T, Takaori K. Pancreatic cancer. Lancet. 2016;388(10039):73–85.

Khatoon J, Rai RP, Prasad KN. Role of Helicobacter pylori in gastric cancer: updates. World J Gastrointest Oncol. 2016;8(2):147–58.

Kidane D. Molecular mechanisms of H. pylori-induced DNA double-strand breaks. Int J Mol Sci. 2018;19(10):2891.

Kim Y, Oh S, Yun HS, Oh S, Kim SH. Cell-bound exopolysaccharide from probiotic bacteria induces autophagic cell death of tumour cells. Lett Appl Microbiol. 2010;51(2):123–30.

Konishi H, Fujiya M, Tanaka H, Ueno N, Moriichi K, Sasajima J, et al. Probiotic-derived ferrichrome inhibits colon cancer progression via JNK-mediated apoptosis. Nat Commun. 2016;7(1):12365.

Konishi H, Isozaki S, Kashima S, Moriichi K, Ichikawa S, Yamamoto K, et al. Probiotic Aspergillus oryzae produces anti-tumor mediator and exerts anti-tumor effects in pancreatic cancer through the p38 MAPK signaling pathway. Sci Rep. 2021;11(1):11070.

Kostic AD, Chun E, Robertson L, Glickman JN, Gallini CA, Michaud M, et al. Fusobacterium nucleatum potentiates intestinal tumorigenesis and modulates the tumor-immune microenvironment. Cell Host Microbe. 2013;14(2):207–15.

Kumar M, Kumar A, Nagpal R, Mohania D, Behare P, Verma V, et al. Cancer-preventing attributes of probiotics: an update. Int J Food Sci Nutr. 2010;61(5):473–96.

Kumar RS, Kanmani P, Yuvaraj N, Paari KA, Pattukumar V, Thirunavukkarasu C, et al. Lactobacillus plantarum AS1 isolated from south Indian fermented food Kallappam suppress

1,2-dimethyl hydrazine (DMH)-induced colorectal cancer in male Wistar rats. Appl Biochem Biotechnol. 2012;166(3):620–31.

Kuno T, Takahashi S, Tomita H, Hisamatsu K, Hara A, Hirata A, et al. Preventive effects of fermented brown rice and rice bran against N-nitrosobis (2-oxopropyl) amine-induced pancreatic tumorigenesis in male hamsters. Oncol Lett. 2015;10(6):3377–84.

Kunz PL, Gubens M, Fisher GA, Ford JM, Lichtensztajn DY, Clarke CA. Long-term survivors of gastric cancer: a California population-based study. J Clin Oncol. 2012;30(28):3507–15.

Lauren P. The two histological main types of gastric carcinoma: diffuse and so-called intestinal-type carcinoma. An attempt at a histo-clinical classification. Acta Pathol Microbiol Scand. 1965;64:31–49.

Lebeer S, Vanderleyden J, De Keersmaecker SC. Genes and molecules of lactobacilli supporting probiotic action. Microbiol Mol Biol Rev. 2008;72(4):728–64, Table of Contents.

Lebeer S, Vanderleyden J, De Keersmaecker SC. Host interactions of probiotic bacterial surface molecules: comparison with commensals and pathogens. Nat Rev Microbiol. 2010;8(3):171–84.

Lee DK, Jang S, Kim MJ, Kim JH, Chung MJ, Kim KJ, et al. Anti-proliferative effects of Bifidobacterium adolescentis SPM0212 extract on human colon cancer cell lines. BMC Cancer. 2008;8:310.

Lee DK, Kang JY, Shin HS, Park IH, Ha NJ. Antiviral activity of Bifidobacterium adolescentis SPM0212 against hepatitis B virus. Arch Pharm Res. 2013;36(12):1525–32.

Lee N-K, Son S-H, Jeon EB, Jung GH, Lee J-Y, Paik H-D. The prophylactic effect of probiotic Bacillus polyfermenticus KU3 against cancer cells. J Funct Foods. 2015;14:513–8.

Li D, Morris JS, Liu J, Hassan MM, Day RS, Bondy ML, et al. Body mass index and risk, age of onset, and survival in patients with pancreatic cancer. JAMA. 2009;301(24):2553–62.

Li J, Sung CY, Lee N, Ni Y, Pihlajamäki J, Panagiotou G, et al. Probiotics modulated gut microbiota suppresses hepatocellular carcinoma growth in mice. Proc Natl Acad Sci U S A. 2016;113(9):E1306–15.

Li Q, Jin M, Liu Y, Jin L. Gut microbiota: its potential roles in pancreatic cancer. Front Cell Infect Microbiol. 2020;10:572492.

Li Q, Hu W, Liu WX, Zhao LY, Huang D, Liu XD, et al. Streptococcus thermophilus inhibits colorectal tumorigenesis through secreting β-galactosidase. Gastroenterology. 2021;160(4):1179–93.e14.

Lin RS, Lee FY, Lee SD, Tsai YT, Lin HC, Lu RH, et al. Endotoxemia in patients with chronic liver diseases: relationship to severity of liver diseases, presence of esophageal varices, and hyperdynamic circulation. J Hepatol. 1995;22(2):165–72.

Lin WJ, Su YW, Lu YC, Hao Z, Chio II, Chen NJ, et al. Crucial role for TNF receptor-associated factor 2 (TRAF2) in regulating NFκB2 signaling that contributes to autoimmunity. Proc Natl Acad Sci U S A. 2011;108(45):18354–9.

Lin PY, Li SC, Lin HP, Shih CK. Germinated brown rice combined with Lactobacillus acidophilus and Bifidobacterium animalis subsp. lactis inhibits colorectal carcinogenesis in rats. Food Sci Nutr. 2019;7(1):216–24.

Liu CT, Chu FJ, Chou CC, Yu RC. Antiproliferative and anticytotoxic effects of cell fractions and exopolysaccharides from Lactobacillus casei 01. Mutat Res. 2011;721(2):157–62.

Liu Y, Liu Q, Hesketh J, Huang D, Gan F, Hao S, et al. Protective effects of selenium-glutathione-enriched probiotics on CCl(4)-induced liver fibrosis. J Nutr Biochem. 2018;58:138–49.

Liu X, Shao L, Liu X, Ji F, Mei Y, Cheng Y, et al. Alterations of gastric mucosal microbiota across different stomach microhabitats in a cohort of 276 patients with gastric cancer. EBioMedicine. 2019;40:336–48.

Loo TM, Kamachi F, Watanabe Y, Yoshimoto S, Kanda H, Arai Y, et al. Gut microbiota promotes obesity-associated liver cancer through PGE(2)-mediated suppression of antitumor immunity. Cancer Discov. 2017;7(5):522–38.

Lu D, Yan J, Liu F, Ding P, Chen B, Lu Y, et al. Probiotics in preventing and treating chemotherapy-induced diarrhea: a meta-analysis. Asia Pac J Clin Nutr. 2019;28(4):701–10.

Lu K, Dong S, Wu X, Jin R, Chen H. Probiotics in cancer. Front Oncol. 2021;11:408.

Luan F, Li X, Cheng X, Huangfu L, Han J, Guo T, et al. TNFRSF11B activates Wnt/β-catenin signaling and promotes gastric cancer progression. Int J Biol Sci. 2020;16(11):1956–71.
Ma EL, Choi YJ, Choi J, Pothoulakis C, Rhee SH, Im E. The anticancer effect of probiotic Bacillus polyfermenticus on human colon cancer cells is mediated through ErbB2 and ErbB3 inhibition. Int J Cancer. 2010a;127(4):780–90.
Ma J, Sawai H, Matsuo Y, Ochi N, Yasuda A, Takahashi H, et al. IGF-1 mediates PTEN suppression and enhances cell invasion and proliferation via activation of the IGF-1/PI3K/Akt signaling pathway in pancreatic cancer cells. J Surg Res. 2010b;160(1):90–101.
Macfarlane S, Macfarlane GT. Regulation of short-chain fatty acid production. Proc Nutr Soc. 2003;62(1):67–72.
Maekawa T, Fukaya R, Takamatsu S, Itoyama S, Fukuoka T, Yamada M, et al. Possible involvement of Enterococcus infection in the pathogenesis of chronic pancreatitis and cancer. Biochem Biophys Res Commun. 2018;506(4):962–9.
Martín R, Chamignon C, Mhedbi-Hajri N, Chain F, Derrien M, Escribano-Vázquez U, et al. The potential probiotic Lactobacillus rhamnosus CNCM I-3690 strain protects the intestinal barrier by stimulating both mucus production and cytoprotective response. Sci Rep. 2019;9(1):5398.
Mejía-Caballero A, Salas-Villagrán VA, Jiménez-Serna A, Farrés A. Challenges in the production and use of probiotics as therapeuticals in cancer treatment or prevention. J Ind Microbiol Biotechnol. 2021;48(9–10):kuab052.
Meng C, Bai C, Brown TD, Hood LE, Tian Q. Human gut microbiota and gastrointestinal cancer. Genomics Proteomics Bioinformatics. 2018;16(1):33–49.
Mihailović M, Živković M, Jovanović JA, Tolinački M, Sinadinović M, Rajić J, et al. Oral administration of probiotic Lactobacillus paraplantarum BGCG11 attenuates diabetes-induced liver and kidney damage in rats. J Funct Foods. 2017;38:427–37.
Mima K, Nishihara R, Qian ZR, Cao Y, Sukawa Y, Nowak JA, et al. Fusobacterium nucleatum in colorectal carcinoma tissue and patient prognosis. Gut. 2016;65(12):1973–80.
Miro-Blanch J, Yanes O. Epigenetic regulation at the interplay between gut microbiota and host metabolism. Front Genet. 2019;10:638.
Molska M, Reguła J. Potential mechanisms of probiotics action in the prevention and treatment of colorectal cancer. Nutrients. 2019;11(10):2453.
Monteagudo-Mera A, Rastall RA, Gibson GR, Charalampopoulos D, Chatzifragkou A. Adhesion mechanisms mediated by probiotics and prebiotics and their potential impact on human health. Appl Microbiol Biotechnol. 2019;103(16):6463–72.
Mutlu EA, Gillevet PM, Rangwala H, Sikaroodi M, Naqvi A, Engen PA, et al. Colonic microbiome is altered in alcoholism. Am J Physiol Gastrointest Liver Physiol. 2012;302(9):G966–78.
Myllyluoma E, Veijola L, Ahlroos T, Tynkkynen S, Kankuri E, Vapaatalo H, et al. Probiotic supplementation improves tolerance to Helicobacter pylori eradication therapy—a placebo-controlled, double-blind randomized pilot study. Aliment Pharmacol Ther. 2005;21(10):1263–72.
Nabavi S, Rafraf M, Somi MH, Homayouni-Rad A, Asghari-Jafarabadi M. Effects of probiotic yogurt consumption on metabolic factors in individuals with nonalcoholic fatty liver disease. J Dairy Sci. 2014;97(12):7386–93.
Nair J, Ohshima H, Nair UJ, Bartsch H. Endogenous formation of nitrosamines and oxidative DNA-damaging agents in tobacco users. Crit Rev Toxicol. 1996;26(2):149–61.
Nanis GA, Mohamed LS, Hassan E, Maii MN. Lactobacillus acidophilus and Bifidobacteria spp having antibacterial and antiviral effects on chronic HCV infection. Afr J Microbiol Res. 2019;13(5):77–90.
O'Toole PW, Marchesi JR, Hill C. Next-generation probiotics: the spectrum from probiotics to live biotherapeutics. Nat Microbiol. 2017;2:17057.
Oh NS, Lee JY, Kim Y-T, Kim SH, Lee J-H. Cancer-protective effect of a synbiotic combination between Lactobacillus gasseri 505 and a Cudrania tricuspidata leaf extract on colitis-associated colorectal cancer. Gut Microbes. 2020;12(1):1785803.
Ohara T, Yoshino K, Kitajima M. Possibility of preventing colorectal carcinogenesis with probiotics. Hepatogastroenterology. 2010;57(104):1411–5.

Ojetti V, Bruno G, Ainora ME, Gigante G, Rizzo G, Roccarina D, et al. Impact of Lactobacillus reuteri supplementation on anti-Helicobacter pylori levofloxacin-based second-line therapy. Gastroenterol Res Pract. 2012;2012:740381.

Oo KM, Lwin AA, Kyaw YY, Tun WM, Fukada K, Goshima A, et al. Safety and long-term effect of the probiotic FK-23 in patients with hepatitis C virus infection. Biosci Microbiota Food Health. 2016;35(3):123–8.

Oppelt PJ, Hirbe AC, Van Tine BA. Gastrointestinal stromal tumors (GISTs): point mutations matter in management, a review. J Gastrointest Oncol. 2017;8(3):466–73.

Orlando A, Refolo MG, Messa C, Amati L, Lavermicocca P, Guerra V, et al. Antiproliferative and proapoptotic effects of viable or heat-killed Lactobacillus paracasei IMPC2.1 and Lactobacillus rhamnosus GG in HGC-27 gastric and DLD-1 colon cell lines. Nutr Cancer. 2012;64(7):1103–11.

Orlando A, Linsalata M, Russo F. Antiproliferative effects on colon adenocarcinoma cells induced by co-administration of vitamin K1 and Lactobacillus rhamnosus GG. Int J Oncol. 2016;48(6):2629–38.

Osterlund P, Ruotsalainen T, Korpela R, Saxelin M, Ollus A, Valta P, et al. Lactobacillus supplementation for diarrhoea related to chemotherapy of colorectal cancer: a randomised study. Br J Cancer. 2007;97(8):1028–34.

Pala V, Sieri S, Berrino F, Vineis P, Sacerdote C, Palli D, et al. Yogurt consumption and risk of colorectal cancer in the Italian European prospective investigation into cancer and nutrition cohort. Int J Cancer. 2011;129(11):2712–9.

Parisa A, Roya G, Mahdi R, Shabnam R, Maryam E, Malihe T. Anti-cancer effects of Bifidobacterium species in colon cancer cells and a mouse model of carcinogenesis. PLoS One. 2020;15(5):e0232930.

Perdigón G, de Moreno de LeBlanc A, Valdez J, Rachid M. Role of yoghurt in the prevention of colon cancer. Eur J Clin Nutr. 2002;56(Suppl 3):S65–8.

Ponziani FR, Bhoori S, Castelli C, Putignani L, Rivoltini L, Del Chierico F, et al. Hepatocellular carcinoma is associated with gut microbiota profile and inflammation in nonalcoholic fatty liver disease. Hepatology. 2019;69(1):107–20.

Rafter J, Bennett M, Caderni G, Clune Y, Hughes R, Karlsson PC, et al. Dietary synbiotics reduce cancer risk factors in polypectomized and colon cancer patients. Am J Clin Nutr. 2007;85(2):488–96.

Rahimi AM, Nabavizadeh F, Ashabi G, Halimi S, Rahimpour M, Vahedian J, et al. Probiotic Lactobacillus rhamnosus supplementation improved capecitabine protective effect against gastric cancer growth in male BALB/c mice. Nutr Cancer. 2021;73(10):2089–99.

Rahman F, Cotterchio M, Cleary SP, Gallinger S. Association between alcohol consumption and pancreatic cancer risk: a case-control study. PLoS One. 2015;10(4):e0124489.

Ravegnini G, Fosso B, Saverio VD, Sammarini G, Zanotti F, Rossi G, et al. Gastric adenocarcinomas and signet-ring cell carcinoma: unraveling gastric cancer complexity through microbiome analysis-deepening heterogeneity for a personalized therapy. Int J Mol Sci. 2020;21(24):9735.

Rawla P, Sunkara T, Barsouk A. Epidemiology of colorectal cancer: incidence, mortality, survival, and risk factors. Prz Gastroenterol. 2019a;14(2):89–103.

Rawla P, Sunkara T, Gaduputi V. Epidemiology of pancreatic cancer: global trends, etiology and risk factors. World J Oncol. 2019b;10(1):10–27.

Reis SAD, da Conceição LL, Peluzio M. Intestinal microbiota and colorectal cancer: changes in the intestinal microenvironment and their relation to the disease. J Med Microbiol. 2019;68(10):1391–407.

Risch HA. Etiology of pancreatic cancer, with a hypothesis concerning the role of N-nitroso compounds and excess gastric acidity. J Natl Cancer Inst. 2003;95(13):948–60.

Routy B, Le Chatelier E, Derosa L, Duong CPM, Alou MT, Daillère R, et al. Gut microbiome influences efficacy of PD-1-based immunotherapy against epithelial tumors. Science. 2018;359(6371):91–7.

Rozengurt E. Mechanistic target of rapamycin (mTOR): a point of convergence in the action of insulin/IGF-1 and G protein-coupled receptor agonists in pancreatic cancer cells. Front Physiol. 2014;5:357.

Rupasinghe HPV, Parmar I, Neir SV. Biotransformation of Cranberry proanthocyanidins to probiotic metabolites by *Lactobacillus rhamnosus* enhances their anticancer activity in HepG2 cells *in vitro*. Oxid Med Cell Longev. 2019;2019:4750795.

Sadeghi-Aliabadi H, Mohammadi F, Fazeli H, Mirlohi M. Effects of Lactobacillus plantarum A7 with probiotic potential on colon cancer and normal cells proliferation in comparison with a commercial strain. Iran J Basic Med Sci. 2014;17(10):815–9.

Salmaninejad A, Valilou SF, Shabgah AG, Aslani S, Alimardani M, Pasdar A, et al. PD-1/PD-L1 pathway: basic biology and role in cancer immunotherapy. J Cell Physiol. 2019;234(10):16824–37.

Sarhadi V, Mathew B, Kokkola A, Karla T, Tikkanen M, Rautelin H, et al. Gut microbiota of patients with different subtypes of gastric cancer and gastrointestinal stromal tumors. Gut Pathog. 2021;13(1):11.

Saxami G, Karapetsas A, Lamprianidou E, Kotsianidis I, Chlichlia A, Tassou C, et al. Two potential probiotic lactobacillus strains isolated from olive microbiota exhibit adhesion and anti-proliferative effects in cancer cell lines. J Funct Foods. 2016;24:461–71.

Schwabe RF, Greten TF. Gut microbiome in HCC—mechanisms, diagnosis and therapy. J Hepatol. 2020;72(2):230–8.

Shen L, Weber CR, Raleigh DR, Yu D, Turner JR. Tight junction pore and leak pathways: a dynamic duo. Annu Rev Physiol. 2011;73(1):283–309.

Sherman M. Hepatocellular carcinoma: epidemiology, surveillance, and diagnosis. Semin Liver Dis. 2010;30(1):3–16.

Sheu BS, Wu JJ, Lo CY, Wu HW, Chen JH, Lin YS, et al. Impact of supplement with Lactobacillus- and Bifidobacterium-containing yogurt on triple therapy for Helicobacter pylori eradication. Aliment Pharmacol Ther. 2002;16(9):1669–75.

Sheu B-S, Cheng H-C, Kao A-W, Wang S-T, Yang Y-J, Yang H-B, et al. Pretreatment with Lactobacillus- and Bifidobacterium-containing yogurt can improve the efficacy of quadruple therapy in eradicating residual Helicobacter pylori infection after failed triple therapy. Am J Clin Nutr. 2006;83(4):864–9.

Singhal B, Mukherjee A, Srivastav S. Role of probiotics in pancreatic cancer prevention: the prospects and challenges. Adv Biosci Biotechnol. 2016;7:468–500.

Sitaraman R. Helicobacter pylori DNA methyltransferases and the epigenetic field effect in cancerization. Front Microbiol. 2014;5:115.

Sivan A, Corrales L, Hubert N, Williams JB, Aquino-Michaels K, Earley ZM, et al. Commensal Bifidobacterium promotes antitumor immunity and facilitates anti-PD-L1 efficacy. Science. 2015;350(6264):1084–9.

Sivieri K, Spinardi-Barbisan ALT, Barbisan LF, Bedani R, Pauly ND, Carlos IZ, et al. Probiotic Enterococcus faecium CRL 183 inhibit chemically induced colon cancer in male Wistar rats. Eur Food Res Technol. 2008;228(2):231–7.

Sugimura N, Li Q, Chu ESH, Lau HCH, Fong W, Liu W, et al. *Lactobacillus gallinarum* modulates the gut microbiota and produces anti-cancer metabolites to protect against colorectal tumourigenesis. Gut. 2022;71:2011–21.

Sung H, Ferlay J, Siegel RL, Laversanne M, Soerjomataram I, Jemal A, et al. Global cancer statistics 2020: GLOBOCAN estimates of incidence and mortality worldwide for 36 cancers in 185 countries. CA Cancer J Clin. 2021;71(3):209–49.

Tanoue T, Morita S, Plichta DR, Skelly AN, Suda W, Sugiura Y, et al. A defined commensal consortium elicits CD8 T cells and anti-cancer immunity. Nature. 2019;565(7741):600–5.

Than NN, Newsome PN. A concise review of non-alcoholic fatty liver disease. Atherosclerosis. 2015;239(1):192–202.

The Cancer Genome Atlas Research Network. Comprehensive molecular characterization of gastric adenocarcinoma. Nature. 2014;513(7517):202–9.

Thirabunyanon M, Hongwittayakorn P. Potential probiotic lactic acid bacteria of human origin induce antiproliferation of colon cancer cells via synergic actions in adhesion to cancer cells and short-chain fatty acid bioproduction. Appl Biochem Biotechnol. 2013;169(2):511–25.
Thirabunyanon M, Boonprasom P, Niamsup P. Probiotic potential of lactic acid bacteria isolated from fermented dairy milks on antiproliferation of colon cancer cells. Biotechnol Lett. 2009;31(4):571–6.
Tiptiri-Kourpeti A, Spyridopoulou K, Santarmaki V, Aindelis G, Tompoulidou E, Lamprianidou EE, et al. Lactobacillus casei exerts anti-proliferative effects accompanied by apoptotic cell death and up-regulation of TRAIL in colon carcinoma cells. PLoS One. 2016;11(2):e0147960.
Tlaskalova-Hogenova H, Vannucci L, Klimesova K, Stepankova R, Krizan J, Kverka M. Microbiome and colorectal carcinoma: insights from germ-free and conventional animal models. Cancer J. 2014;20(3):217–24.
Toh JWT, Wilson RB. Pathways of gastric carcinogenesis, Helicobacter pylori virulence and interactions with antioxidant systems, vitamin C and phytochemicals. Int J Mol Sci. 2020;21(17):6451.
Touchefeu Y, Montassier E, Nieman K, Gastinne T, Potel G, Bruley des Varannes S, et al. Systematic review: the role of the gut microbiota in chemotherapy- or radiation-induced gastrointestinal mucositis—current evidence and potential clinical applications. Aliment Pharmacol Ther. 2014;40(5):409–21.
Tukenmez U, Aktas B, Aslim B, Yavuz S. The relationship between the structural characteristics of lactobacilli-EPS and its ability to induce apoptosis in colon cancer cells in vitro. Sci Rep. 2019;9(1):8268.
Tuomola EM, Ouwehand AC, Salminen SJ. The effect of probiotic bacteria on the adhesion of pathogens to human intestinal mucus. FEMS Immunol Med Microbiol. 1999;26(2):137–42.
Tursi A, Brandimarte G, Giorgetti GM, Modeo ME. Effect of Lactobacillus casei supplementation on the effectiveness and tolerability of a new second-line 10-day quadruple therapy after failure of a first attempt to cure Helicobacter pylori infection. Med Sci Monit. 2004;10(12):CR662–6.
Vauhkonen M, Vauhkonen H, Sajantila A, Sipponen P. Differences in genomic instability between intestinal- and diffuse-type gastric cancer. Gastric Cancer. 2005;8(4):238–44.
Vétizou M, Pitt JM, Daillère R, Lepage P, Waldschmitt N, Flament C, et al. Anticancer immunotherapy by CTLA-4 blockade relies on the gut microbiota. Science. 2015;350(6264):1079–84.
Vinasco K, Mitchell HM, Kaakoush NO, Castaño-Rodríguez N. Microbial carcinogenesis: lactic acid bacteria in gastric cancer. Biochim Biophys Acta Rev Cancer. 2019;1872(2):188309.
Wang X, Wei M, Sun Z. An association study of histological types of gastric carcinoma with Helicobacter pylori infection. Cell Biochem Biophys. 2014;70(2):1283–7.
Wang J, Wang W-J, Zhai L, Zhang D-F. Association of cholesterol with risk of pancreatic cancer: a meta-analysis. World J Gastroenterol. 2015;21(12):3711–9.
Wang CS, Li WB, Wang HY, Ma YM, Zhao XH, Yang H, et al. VSL#3 can prevent ulcerative colitis-associated carcinogenesis in mice. World J Gastroenterol. 2018;24(37):4254–62.
Wang Z, Gao X, Zeng R, Wu Q, Sun H, Wu W, et al. Changes of the gastric mucosal microbiome associated with histological stages of gastric carcinogenesis. Front Microbiol. 2020;11:997.
Wong SH, Yu J. Gut microbiota in colorectal cancer: mechanisms of action and clinical applications. Nat Rev Gastroenterol Hepatol. 2019;16(11):690–704.
Xie K. Interleukin-8 and human cancer biology. Cytokine Growth Factor Rev. 2001;12(4):375–91.
Xu M, Jung X, Hines OJ, Eibl G, Chen Y. Obesity and pancreatic cancer: overview of epidemiology and potential prevention by weight loss. Pancreas. 2018;47(2):158–62.
Xu Q, Xu P, Cen Y, Li W. Effects of preoperative oral administration of glucose solution combined with postoperative probiotics on inflammation and intestinal barrier function in patients after colorectal cancer surgery. Oncol Lett. 2019;18(1):694–8.
Xue L, He J, Gao N, Lu X, Li M, Wu X, et al. Probiotics may delay the progression of nonalcoholic fatty liver disease by restoring the gut microbiota structure and improving intestinal endotoxemia. Sci Rep. 2017;7(1):45176.

Yang Y, Weng W, Peng J, Hong L, Yang L, Toiyama Y, et al. Fusobacterium nucleatum increases proliferation of colorectal cancer cells and tumor development in mice by activating toll-like receptor 4 Signaling to nuclear factor-κB, and up-regulating expression of MicroRNA-21. Gastroenterology. 2017;152(4):851–66.e24.

Yang J, Zhou X, Liu X, Ling Z, Ji F. Role of the gastric microbiome in gastric cancer: from carcinogenesis to treatment. Front Microbiol. 2021;12(519):641322.

Yong X, Tang B, Li BS, Xie R, Hu CJ, Luo G, et al. Helicobacter pylori virulence factor CagA promotes tumorigenesis of gastric cancer via multiple signaling pathways. Cell Commun Signal. 2015;13:30.

Yu LX, Schwabe RF. The gut microbiome and liver cancer: mechanisms and clinical translation. Nat Rev Gastroenterol Hepatol. 2017;14(9):527–39.

Yue Y, Ye K, Lu J, Wang X, Zhang S, Liu L, et al. Probiotic strain Lactobacillus plantarum YYC-3 prevents colon cancer in mice by regulating the tumour microenvironment. Biomed Pharmacother. 2020;127:110159.

Zhang Z, Rigas B. NF-kappaB, inflammation and pancreatic carcinogenesis: NF-kappaB as a chemoprevention target (review). Int J Oncol. 2006;29(1):185–92.

Zhao R, Wang Y, Huang Y, Cui Y, Xia L, Rao Z, et al. Effects of fiber and probiotics on diarrhea associated with enteral nutrition in gastric cancer patients: a prospective randomized and controlled trial. Medicine (Baltimore). 2017;96(43):e8418.

Zheng D-W, Li R-Q, An J-X, Xie T-Q, Han Z-Y, Xu R, et al. Prebiotics-encapsulated probiotic spores regulate gut microbiota and suppress colon cancer. Adv Mater. 2020;32(45):2004529.

Zhu XY, Liu F. Probiotics as an adjuvant treatment in Helicobacter pylori eradication therapy. J Dig Dis. 2017;18(4):195–202.

Chapter 15
Gut Microbiota Impacts on the Efficacy of Anticancer Treatment of Colorectal Cancer

Jie Hong and Jing-Yuan Fang

Abstract Considering the stubbornly high morbidity and mortality and unsatisfactory clinical treatment efficacy of colorectal cancer (CRC), it is still urgent for exploring better therapy regimens. Various evidence have proved the important roles of gut microbiota in the development and treatment of CRC. Hence, the modulation of gut microbiota may be used as potential therapeutic approaches or adjuvants combined with other conventional treatments to prevent or treat CRC. Here, we summarize the diverse impacts of gut microbiota on different CRC therapeutic methods and discuss the potential clinical benefits of bacterial modulation with the goal of facilitating future research on the roles of the intestinal flora.

Keywords Colorectal cancer · Gut microbiota · Anticancer therapy · Probiotics Bacterial modulation

15.1 Introduction

CRC is the third most commonly diagnosed cancer in males and the second in females, with 1.9 million incidence cases and 0.9 million deaths in 2020 globally (Sung et al. 2021). Although increasing screening methods and treatment advances have lowered CRC incidence and mortality to some extent (Brenner et al. 2014), a rising trend is still observed worldwide. CRC is resulted from the accumulation of multifactorial abnormalities involving genetic, epigenetic, and environmental

J. Hong · J.-Y. Fang (✉)
State Key Laboratory for Oncogenes and Related Genes, Key Laboratory of Gastroenterology and Hepatology, Ministry of Health, Division of Gastroenterology and Hepatology, Shanghai Institute of Digestive Disease, Renji Hospital, School of Medicine, Shanghai Jiao Tong University, Shanghai, China
e-mail: jingyuanfang@sjtu.edu.cn

J. Yu (ed.), *Microbiome in Gastrointestinal Cancer*,
https://doi.org/10.1007/978-981-19-4492-5_15

aspects. Environmental factors, such as intake of food carcinogens, lack of exercise, and cigarette smoking, are known to play an important role in CRC occurrence and progression (Dekker et al. 2019; Keum and Giovannucci 2019). What is noteworthy is that the gut microbiota, often referred as the "forgotten organ," is a newly emerging yet important field to explore the environmental influences on CRC. Harboring about 100 trillion microorganisms, it is a complex combination of bacteria, fungi, protozoa, and viruses, of which bacteria are the predominant inhabitants (Pasolli et al. 2019). The development of high-throughput microbiome sequencing made it possible to profile gut microbiota comprehensively.

Accumulating evidence has suggested that enrichment of specific bacterial species in gut, including *Fusobacterium nucleatum* (*F. nucleatum*) (Mima et al. 2016; Brennan and Garrett 2019), *Peptostreptococcus anaerobius* (*P. anaerobius*) (Long et al. 2019), and enterotoxigenic *Bacteroides fragilis* (ETBF) (Cao et al. 2021), has been reported to contribute to colorectal carcinogenesis and progression through different pathways, including accelerating tumor proliferation, promoting inflammation, causing DNA damage, and so on. However, some bacteria, such as *Bifidobacterium animalis* (Liao et al. 2021) and *Streptococcus thermophilus* (Li et al. 2021), are found to be depleted in CRC patients. Suggesting that these bacteria play a protective role against CRC.

There are many methods for treatment of colon cancer, including surgery, chemotherapy, radiotherapy, and immunotherapy. However, most chemotherapeutic agents and radiation not only kill cancer cells, but also damage bone marrow and hair follicles, which called off-target effects. Moreover, chemoresistance diminishes the efficacy of chemotherapy and accounted for the high relapse rate partially (Sarmento-Ribeiro et al. 2019). Biopharmaceuticals, commonly used for targeted therapy, are more specific, less toxic, and side effects; however, the selectivity is often insufficient in practice (Perez-Ruiz et al. 2020).

Notably, the composition of the gut microbiota is affected by multiple host factors, including diet, lifestyle, and medications. Interaction between medications and microbiota can be bidirectional, including drug-induced changes in microbial composition and microbiota-mediated modulation of therapeutic effect (Javdan et al. 2020). Except from its important roles in carcinogenesis and tumor progression, there is numerous evidence showing that the gut microbiota mediates the efficacy and toxicity of therapy. For example, higher abundance of *F. nucleatum*, the well-known pro-tumorigenic gut bacteria, was associated with shorter survival. Meanwhile, it could also promote chemoresistance in CRC patients by activating autophagy, leading to treatment failure or disease recurrence consequently (Yu et al. 2017). With the increasing understanding of how gut microbiota affects carcinogenesis and therapeutic outcomes, gut microbiota modulation becomes a potential choice for CRC prevention and treatment.

Here we summarize diverse effects of gut microbiota on different therapeutic methods in CRC patients and discuss the potential values of bacterial modulation for CRC patients' treatment.

15.2 Effects of Gut Microbiota on Chemotherapy

Chemotherapy is a proficient therapeutic method and conducted by various chemotherapy agents such as COX-2 inhibitors and 5-fluorouracil (5-FU). Studies documented that gut microbiota could influence the anticancer effects of some chemotherapeutic agents, including 5-fluorouracil (5-FU), cyclophosphamide, gemcitabine, and oxaliplatin, mechanically through immunomodulation, metabolism, reduced ecological diversity, and so on (Biller and Schrag 2021). In antibiotic-treated or germ-free mice, tumor-infiltrating myeloid-derived cells responded poorly to therapy, resulting in deficient reactive oxygen production and cytotoxicity after chemotherapy (Iida et al. 2013). According to Yu et al., the higher abundance of *F. nucleatum* was related to higher recurrence rate after chemotherapy of CRC patients. Furthermore, *F. nucleatum* could confer weak responses to 5-FU, capecitabine, and oxaliplatin through the activation of autophagy (Yu et al. 2017). The studies by Zhang et al. showed that the expression of BIRC3 gene could upregulate TLR4/NF-κB pathway in CRC cells with the presence of *F. nucleatum* (Zhang et al. 2019), suggesting that *F. nucleatum* and BIRC3 could be the potential therapeutic targets for increasing the efficacy of chemotherapy.

To promote the outcomes in CRC patients, modulation of gut microbiota compositions has drawn increasing attention due to their potential influences on chemotherapy. Several studies showed that patients who administrated 5-FU with probiotics such as *Bifidobacterium bifidum* had better clinical response to chemotherapy. Further exploration through experiments in vitro found that cancer cell growth was greatly restrained under the treatment with the combination of 5-FU and metabolites extracted from probiotic *L. paracasei* compared with chemotherapeutic drug alone (Chang and Pan 2018; Genaro et al. 2019). Therefore, we can draw the conclusion positively that the combination of probiotics or prebiotics and chemotherapy is a useful therapeutic regimen for increasing the efficacy of chemotherapy.

However, chemotherapy would increase the risk of infections because of its toxicities, and then the drug efficacy inhibition followed. By directly altering the colonic environment, modulating the gut microbiota is a promising way to mitigate the adverse effects of chemotherapy. Myelosuppression is one of the important dose-limiting toxicities for many chemotherapeutic agents. One study found that *Lactobacillus casei* and *Lactobacillus rhamnosus* could stimulate the recovery of myeloid cells and neutrophils after cyclophosphamide treatment, facilitate phagocytosis in infection sites, and protect mice from opportunistic infection with *Candida albicans* (Salva et al. 2014). Meanwhile, various studies have also shown that some probiotics strains, or their metabolites, could alleviate chemotherapy-induced mucositis through suppressing inflammation, repairing gut barrier integrity and enhancing immunosurveillance (Klaenhammer et al. 2012; Alvarez et al. 2016). These studies have opened a new direction for the clinical implications of probiotics. What's more, by restoring gut microbiota homeostasis and promoting the integrity of intestinal barrier, FMT was shown to effectively protect mice from FOLFOX-induced diarrhea and intestinal mucositis (Chang et al. 2020).

15.3 Effects of Gut Microbiota on Immunotherapy

Immunotherapy is an effective treatment and has become a major pillar in cancer therapy. Targeting coinhibitory or costimulatory receptor–ligand systems, such as programmed death 1 (PD-1)–programmed death ligand 1 (PDL1) and cytotoxic T-lymphocyte-associated protein 4 (CTLA-4), the immune checkpoint inhibitors are effective methods to block inhibitory signals of immune cell activation and renew the host immune system in defending against cancer cells (Melero et al. 2021).

The gut microbiota is required for the effective immune response in immunotherapy. Specific bacteria, including *Akkermansia muciniphila* (Ansaldo et al. 2019), *Bifidobacterium spp.* (Sivan et al. 2015), and *Faecalibacterium spp.* (Gopalakrishnan et al. 2018) were positively correlated with immunotherapeutic response, a relative lack of *Akkermansia muciniphila* is associated with a weaker response to treatment in turn. Moreover, it has been found that commensal *Bifidobacterium* was able to increase apoptosis and promote immunotherapy by activating dendritic cells and CD8+ T cells (Sivan et al. 2015). No wonder that elimination of microbiota by antibiotics impairs the efficacy of immunotherapy. For instance, it was demonstrated that an antibiotic cocktail containing ampicillin, colistin, and streptomycin inhibited the CTLA-4 blockade and regained tumor progression in fibrosarcoma, melanoma, and CRC mouse models (Sivan et al. 2015; Gopalakrishnan et al. 2018; Routy et al. 2018). A recent study showed that *Bifidobacterium* could alleviate autoimmune toxicities in mice treated with anti-CTLA-4 therapy, while depletion by vancomycin results in more severe immunotherapy-associated colitis (Wang et al. 2018a). These findings made it possible to identify the important bacteria as predictive biomarkers for immunotherapy response. In fact, a study had identified a consortium consisting of 11 bacterial strains which could augment the effect of immunotherapy in a mouse colon adenocarcinoma model (Tanoue et al. 2019).

Interestingly, probiotics have also been evaluated as adjuvants in anticancer treatments. Combined administration of *L. acidophilus* cell lysates with an anti-CTLA-4 monoclonal antibody significantly increased CD8+ T cells, especially the effector memory T cells, and decreased Tregs in CRC mouse model. Moreover, the synergistic combination not only attenuated the abnormal enrichment of *Proteobacteria* in tumor microenvironment, but also restored CRC-induced dysbiosis in mice (Zhuo et al. 2019). Thus, immunotherapy in combination with probiotics may play an important role in the exploration of new therapeutic strategies against CRC.

The adverse effects of immunotherapy, such as immune checkpoint inhibitor-associated colitis were also influenced by gut microbiota. For example, enrichment of the *Bacteroidetes* phylum reduced the susceptibility to immune checkpoint inhibitor-associated colitis (Dubin et al. 2016). Furthermore, a report had showed that fecal microbiota transplantation (FMT) could mitigate refractory immunotherapy-associated colitis, with the complete resolution arise up to 78 days after two doses of FMT (Wang et al. 2018b).

15.4 Effects of Gut Microbiota on Radiotherapy

Given the fact that colorectal cancer cells were moderate sensitive to radiation, radiotherapy is often used as one of the comprehensive methods, combined with surgery and chemotherapy. Local irradiation can not only induce tumor cell death, but also promote systemic immunity and inflammation. However, adverse effects, including genomic instability, bystander effects on nearby cells, and alterations of commensal bacteria made the clinical application limited.

Studies have shown that gut microbiota could influence the efficacy of irradiation therapy effectively. Apoptosis of cancer cells and local infiltration of immunocytes were restrained in germ-free mice with irradiation, compared with conventional mice, which implied that commensal microbiota may play a positive role in regulating response to radiotherapy (Crawford and Gordon 2005). Further exploration indicated the core role of angiopoietin-like 4 (*ANGPTL4*), a protein inhibitor of lipoprotein lipase, in resistance to radiotherapy toxicity. The expression of *ANGPTL4* was activated by *Streptococcus, Lactobacillus,* and *Bifidobacterium spp*. to protect both germ-free mice and conventional mice against toxic effects of irradiation (Crawford and Gordon 2005). Furthermore, in preclinical patient derived CRC organoid models, butyrate, the well-known beneficial microbial metabolites, was proven to improve the efficacy of radiotherapy, which indicated the potential clinical application of butyrate in combination with other cancer therapies (Park et al. 2020). Besides, a clinical study proved that preparations containing *B. bifidum*, *L. acidophilus*, *Lactobacillus casei* could alleviate radiation-related intestinal side effects (Touchefeu et al. 2014).

Therefore, we could conclude that gut microbiota regulates the response and repair of irradiation-associated side effects. To better understand the regulation mechanisms and make use of gut microbiota to increase the efficacy and alleviate the toxicity of radiotherapy, further researches are needed to be done.

15.5 Effects of Gut Microbiota on Surgery

As the first curative treatment for CRC, surgery may alter the anatomical structure and function of the colorectum, increase the number of commensal microbiota and opportunistic pathogens (Guyton and Alverdy 2017). Thus, modulating the microbiota composition may preserve the intestinal mucosal barrier, prevent some postoperative complications, and alleviate CRC recurrence efficiently in patients who underwent surgery.

A clinical trial showed that preoperative consumption of prebiotics containing xylo-oligosaccharides, resistant dextrin, fructo-oligosaccharides, and polydextrose could recover the levels of immunological indicators, such as IgG, transferrin, and IgM, in the serum in CRC patients. More than that, it could also increase the abundance of *Bifidobacterium* and *Enterococcus* while reducing the abundance of *Bacteroides* (Xie et al. 2019). Similarly, according to a randomized controlled trial, patients those who took perioperative administration of probiotics showed lower risk of bacteremia after surgery and better bowel functions (Liu et al. 2013). Rafter et al. also revealed that preoperative administration of oligofructose-enriched inulin (SYN1), *L. rhamnosus* GG (LGG) and *Bifidobacterium lactis* Bb12 (BB12) could modify gut microbiota with more *Bifidobacterium* and *Lactobacillus* and less *Clostridium perfringens*, inhibit cancer cell proliferation, and enhance epithelial barrier function (Rafter et al. 2007). Collectively, application of single- or multi-strain probiotics to CRC patients prior to surgery can not only suppress gut-related complications but also recover the integrity of epithelial barrier and enhance their immunity.

There are also preclinical studies of supplementation of microbial metabolites to improve CRC surgery prognosis. Reduction of SCFAs-producing bacteria and butyrate levels, which was caused by the bowel preparation before CRC resection, could result in damage of the intestinal barrier, and subsequent bacterial translocation and possible infectious complications (Dalile et al. 2019). Evidence from rat models supported that postoperative intestinal butyrate supplementation enhances anastomotic bursting strength. Moreover, SCFAs could block the growth of pathogens related to anastomotic leakage (Bosmans et al. 2017; Netta et al. 2010).

15.6 Direct Effects of Gut Microbiota on Colorectal Cancer

15.6.1 Diet and Lifestyle

Diet is crucial in CRC genesis and development. In consideration of economical conditions and compliance of patients, dietary intervention is one of the best choices for CRC treatment. Previous studies have shown that different dietary habits could change intestinal microbial compositions markedly (Li et al. 2022; Wastyk et al. 2021), which indicate the potential ability to applying dietary strategies to CRC therapy. Dietary intervention increases the abundance of probiotics, whose fermentation could convert indigestible food composition into beneficial metabolites. A large population-based case-control study showed that compared with western diets, a healthy lifestyle including the healthy diet consumption lower CRC risk, regardless of the patient's genetic profile (Carr et al. 2018). Moreover, a polyposis mouse model showed that a high-fiber diet can enrich SCFA-producing bacteria and increase the expression of butyrate receptor GPR109A, thereby suppress colon carcinogenesis (So et al. 2018). These observations suggest the potential of diet-based cancer prevention strategies. Furthermore, regular alcohol consumption has been shown to change the intestinal microbiota composition which might account for the increased risk of CRC. In chronic alcoholism, anaerobic bacteria decrease, while anaerobes of the genus *Streptococcus* increase (Tsuruya et al. 2016). Therefore, dietary therapy and healthy lifestyles may be the most reasonable and cost-effective methods for CRC patients.

15.6.2 Microbial Products

Probiotics are live microorganisms that provide benefit to the health of the host (Hill et al. 2014). Probiotics executed antitumorigenic effect through variable mechanisms, such as altering intestinal microbiome composition, activating the immune system, modulating intestinal pH, and so on.

There have been numerous studies demonstrating the benefits for the host from probiotics A prospective controlled trial enrolling 22 CRC patients found that compared with the control group, patients those who received a mixture of *Bifidobacterium longum, Lactobacillus acidophilus, and Enterococcus faecalis* showed lower abundance of *Peptostreptococcus* and *Comamonas* and higher abundance of *Proteobacteria* and *Enterococcus*. Notably, the number of *F. nucleatum*, the taxa most related to CRC, was also reduced by five-fold after the administration (Gao et al. 2015). The results from Hibberd et al. showed that CRC patients receiving high concentrations of *Bifidobacterium lactis* and *Lactobacillus acidophilus* had less *Fusobacterium* and *Peptostreptococcus*, and more butyrate-producing bacteria *Clostridiales spp*, *Faecalibacterium*, and *Eubacterium* in stool (Hibberd et al. 2017). Moreover, specific *Lactobacillus* strains including *Lactobacillus rhamnosus*, *Lactobacillus acidophilus,* and *Lactobacillus fermentum* presented the ability to suppress cellular proliferation and carcinogenesis (Chou et al. 2020).

Probiotics or its components could recognize Toll-like receptors (TLRs) on dendritic cells (DCs), T regulatory cells, and natural killer (NK) cells to activate the host immune system. *Lactobacillus* and *Bifidobacterium* strains stimulate maturation of dendritic cells (DCs) and enhance the cytolytic potential of NK cells by producing interferon-γ (IFN-γ) (Fink et al. 2007). Furthermore, *Bifidobacterium pseudolongum* (Mager et al. 2020), *Akkermansia muciniphila* (Ansaldo et al. 2019), *Enterococcus hirae* (Daillere et al. 2016), and *Bacteroides fragilis* (Round et al. 2011) were proven to play a positive role in restoring antitumor immunity through the activation of T cells.

In addition to enhancing the immune system, probiotics help host generate beneficial properties such as SCFAs to exert the anti-tumor efficiency. It is generally acknowledged that lactic acid bacteria (LABs) such as *Lactobacillus, Lactococcus, Leuconostoc,* and *Pediococcus* are safe and ideal choices for bacterial therapy (Chung et al. 2021). The secretion of short-chain fatty acids (SCFAs) and lactic acid by probiotics like *Lactobacillus* (Wang et al. 2019a) and *Bifidobacterium* (Wang et al. 2020) can not only reduce the abundance of pathogenic bacteria by balancing the intestinal pH, but also restrain the growth of CRC through inhibition of inflammation and angiogenesis and repairing the damaged intestinal barrier. Similarly, the SCFAs-producing probiotic called *Propionibacterium freudenreichii* induce CRC cells apoptosis with the help of its metabolites too (Casanova et al. 2018).

15.6.3 Fecal Microbiota Transplantation

Fecal microbial transplantation (FMT), refilling receivers' lower gastrointestinal tract with feces from healthy donors, has emerged as a "natural" and promising therapeutic approach for patients with relapsed *Clostridium difficile* infection (CDI) (Youngster et al. 2014), IBD (Paramsothy et al. 2017), and CRC (Khoruts 2021). FMT is an effective way to restore the imbalanced gut microbiota composition without causing bacteremia. As a result, inflammatory cytokines like IL-1, IL-6, and TNF-a are decreased, while anti-inflammatory cytokines such as IL-10 and TGF-β are increased. Moreover, the accumulation of Tregs, the recognized negative immune regulator, is also triggered (Wang et al. 2019b).

Considering the severe dysbiosis caused by CDI, FMT is a worthy choice and has been proven to have a 90% clinical recovery rate (Kassam et al. 2013). In a CRC mouse model, FMT was used to normalize the gut microbiota to the limit tumor growth. However, studies on FMT for IBD mitigation have not showed satisfying results regarding the treatment's efficacy and safety, and further exploration is required (Grinspan and Kelly 2015). Similarly, the effectiveness of FMT in the clinical therapy for CRC is also not clarified.

It is worth noting that the complete impact of FMT on the host is complicated and unpredictable, and whether the treatment would cause dissemination of unknown pathogens cannot be answered certainly. In addition, vast questions are still unclear, such as the exact definition of a "good donor," the appropriate routes of administration, and the long-term effects of this therapy (Danne et al. 2021). Therefore, more exploration is needed to be done in the future to investigate the value of FMT in gastrointestinal diseases.

15.7 Prospect

As what mentioned before, gut microbiota plays a crucial role in CRC therapy (Fig. 15.1). It has provided an unprecedented opportunity to move microbiota discoveries toward clinical applications. Gut microbiota manipulation through a healthy dietary habit, the avoidance of unnecessary broad-spectrum antibiotics, the use of probiotics and prebiotics, and FMT accompanied by common therapies have the potential to exhibit better effects than conventional methods.

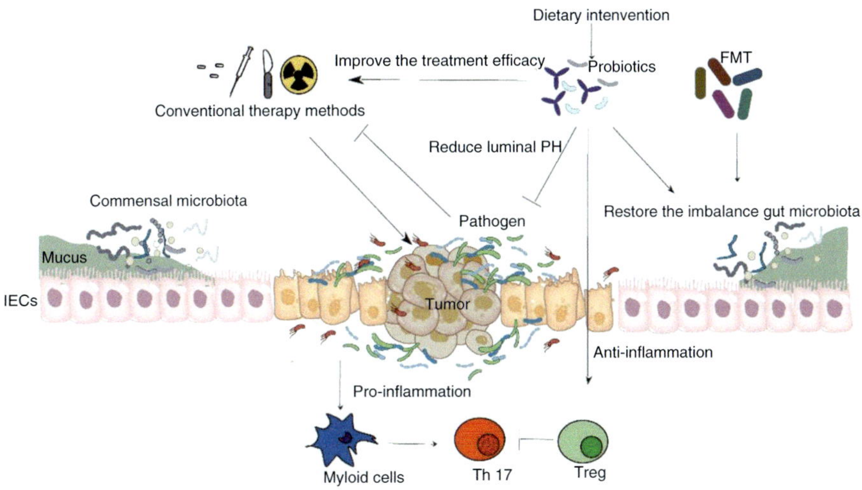

Fig. 15.1 Schematic representation of gut microbiome role in CRC therapy. The gut microbiota can affect the host response to different treatment methods by improving drug efficacy, promoting drug resistance, influencing the intestinal environmental homeostasis, and/or modulating host immune system directly. *FMT* Fecal microbiota transplantation, *Th17* T helper cell 17, *Treg* T regulatory cell, *IECs* Intestinal epithelial cell

Although accumulating preclinical evidence in microbiome research has gained satisfactory results to some extent, more complicated internal environment and regulatory mechanism make it more challenging to apply the academic findings to clinic. Therefore, before translating to bedside application, a clear definition and precise patient selection criteria are the priority among priorities. Once the most beneficial microbiota compositions in various clinical conditions have been identified, it may be a significant breakthrough in cancer treatment, especially for CRC. The ultimate goal is to develop a microbe therapy that both promotes anticancer therapy and reduces systemic toxicity. Thus, therapeutic intervention targeting the microbiota will be one of the next frontiers for precise and personalized therapies for CRC treatment.

Despite the many unknowns, we believe that gut microbiota modulation has the potential that deserves further investigation of its role in prevention and treatment of colon cancer. With more and more breakthroughs in CRC pathophysiology and medical techniques emerging, the increasing knowledge gain of gut microbiota will likely take us into a new realm of therapy for CRC in the near future.

References

Alvarez CS, Badia J, Bosch M, Gimenez R, Baldoma L. Outer membrane vesicles and soluble factors released by probiotic Escherichia coli Nissle 1917 and commensal ECOR63 enhance barrier function by regulating expression of tight junction proteins in intestinal epithelial cells. Front Microbiol. 2016;7:1981.

Ansaldo E, Slayden LC, Ching KL, Koch MA, Wolf NK, Plichta DR, et al. Akkermansia muciniphila induces intestinal adaptive immune responses during homeostasis. Science. 2019;364(6446):1179–84.

Biller LH, Schrag D. Diagnosis and treatment of metastatic colorectal cancer. JAMA. 2021;325(7):669–85.

Bosmans JW, Jongen AC, Boonen BT, van Rijn S, Scognamiglio F, Stucchi L, et al. Comparison of three different application routes of butyrate to improve colonic anastomotic strength in rats. Int J Color Dis. 2017;32(3):305–13.

Brennan CA, Garrett WS. Fusobacterium nucleatum—symbiont, opportunist and oncobacterium. Nat Rev Microbiol. 2019;17(3):156–66.

Brenner H, Stock C, Hoffmeister M. Effect of screening sigmoidoscopy and screening colonoscopy on colorectal cancer incidence and mortality: systematic review and meta-analysis of randomised controlled trials and observational studies. BMJ. 2014;348:g2467.

Cao Y, Wang Z, Yan Y, Ji L, He J, Xuan B, et al. Enterotoxigenic Bacteroides fragilis promotes intestinal inflammation and malignancy by inhibiting exosome-packaged miR-149-3pf. Gastroenterology. 2021;161(5):1552–1566.e12.

Carr PR, Weigl K, Jansen L, Walter V, Erben V, Chang-Claude J, et al. Healthy lifestyle factors associated with lower risk of colorectal cancer irrespective of genetic risk. Gastroenterology. 2018;155(6):1805–15.e5.

Casanova MR, Azevedo-Silva J, Rodrigues LR, Preto A. Colorectal cancer cells increase the production of short chain fatty acids by Propionibacterium freudenreichii impacting on cancer cells survival. Front Nutr. 2018;5:44.

Chang CY, Pan TM. Anticancer and antimigration effects of a combinatorial treatment of 5-fluorouracil and Lactobacillus paracasei subsp. paracasei NTU 101 fermented skim Milk extracts on colorectal cancer cells. J Agric Food Chem. 2018;66(22):5549–55.

Chang CW, Lee HC, Li LH, Chiang Chiau JS, Wang TE, Chuang WH, et al. Fecal microbiota transplantation prevents intestinal injury, upregulation of Toll-like receptors, and 5-fluorouracil/oxaliplatin-induced toxicity in colorectal cancer. Int J Mol Sci. 2020;21(2):386.

Chou YC, Ho PY, Chen WJ, Wu SH, Pan MH. Lactobacillus fermentum V3 ameliorates colitis-associated tumorigenesis by modulating the gut microbiome. Am J Cancer Res. 2020;10(4):1170–81.

Chung Y, Ryu Y, An BC, Yoon YS, Choi O, Kim TY, et al. A synthetic probiotic engineered for colorectal cancer therapy modulates gut microbiota. Microbiome. 2021;9(1):122.

Crawford PA, Gordon JI. Microbial regulation of intestinal radiosensitivity. Proc Natl Acad Sci U S A. 2005;102(37):13254–9.

Daillere R, Vetizou M, Waldschmitt N, Yamazaki T, Isnard C, Poirier-Colame V, et al. Enterococcus hirae and Barnesiella intestinihominis facilitate cyclophosphamide-induced therapeutic immunomodulatory effects. Immunity. 2016;45(4):931–43.

Dalile B, Van Oudenhove L, Vervliet B, Verbeke K. The role of short-chain fatty acids in microbiota-gut-brain communication. Nat Rev Gastroenterol Hepatol. 2019;16(8):461–78.

Danne C, Rolhion N, Sokol H. Recipient factors in faecal microbiota transplantation: one stool does not fit all. Nat Rev Gastroenterol Hepatol. 2021;18(7):503–13.

Dekker E, Tanis PJ, Vleugels JLA, Kasi PM, Wallace MB. Colorectal cancer. Lancet. 2019;394(10207):1467–80.

Dubin K, Callahan MK, Ren B, Khanin R, Viale A, Ling L, et al. Intestinal microbiome analyses identify melanoma patients at risk for checkpoint-blockade-induced colitis. Nat Commun. 2016;7:10391.

Fink LN, Zeuthen LH, Christensen HR, Morandi B, Frokiaer H, Ferlazzo G. Distinct gut-derived lactic acid bacteria elicit divergent dendritic cell-mediated NK cell responses. Int Immunol. 2007;19(12):1319–27.

Gao Z, Guo B, Gao R, Zhu Q, Wu W, Qin H. Probiotics modify human intestinal mucosa-associated microbiota in patients with colorectal cancer. Mol Med Rep. 2015;12(4):6119–27.

Genaro SC, de Souza L, Reis LS, Reis SK, Rabelo Socca EA, Favaro WJ. Probiotic supplementation attenuates the aggressiveness of chemically induced colorectal tumor in rats. Life Sci. 2019;237:116895.

Gopalakrishnan V, Spencer CN, Nezi L, Reuben A, Andrews MC, Karpinets TV, et al. Gut microbiome modulates response to anti-PD-1 immunotherapy in melanoma patients. Science. 2018;359(6371):97–103.

Grinspan AM, Kelly CR. Fecal microbiota transplantation for ulcerative colitis: not just yet. Gastroenterology. 2015;149(1):15–8.

Guyton K, Alverdy JC. The gut microbiota and gastrointestinal surgery. Nat Rev Gastroenterol Hepatol. 2017;14(1):43–54.

Hibberd AA, Lyra A, Ouwehand AC, Rolny P, Lindegren H, Cedgard L, et al. Intestinal microbiota is altered in patients with colon cancer and modified by probiotic intervention. BMJ Open Gastroenterol. 2017;4(1):e000145.

Hill C, Guarner F, Reid G, Gibson GR, Merenstein DJ, Pot B, et al. Expert consensus document. The International Scientific Association for Probiotics and Prebiotics consensus statement on the scope and appropriate use of the term probiotic. Nat Rev Gastroenterol Hepatol. 2014;11(8):506–14.

Iida N, Dzutsev A, Stewart CA, Smith L, Bouladoux N, Weingarten RA, et al. Commensal bacteria control cancer response to therapy by modulating the tumor microenvironment. Science. 2013;342(6161):967–70.

Javdan B, Lopez JG, Chankhamjon P, Lee YJ, Hull R, Wu Q, et al. Personalized mapping of drug metabolism by the human gut microbiome. Cell. 2020;181(7):1661–1679.e22.

Kassam Z, Lee CH, Yuan Y, Hunt RH. Fecal microbiota transplantation for clostridium difficile infection: systematic review and meta-analysis. Am J Gastroenterol. 2013;108(4):500–8.

Keum N, Giovannucci E. Global burden of colorectal cancer: emerging trends, risk factors and prevention strategies. Nat Rev Gastroenterol Hepatol. 2019;16(12):713–32.

Khoruts A. Can FMT. Cause or prevent CRC? Maybe, but there is more to consider. Gastroenterology. 2021;161(4):1103–5.

Klaenhammer TR, Kleerebezem M, Kopp MV, Rescigno M. The impact of probiotics and prebiotics on the immune system. Nat Rev Immunol. 2012;12(10):728–34.

Li Q, Hu W, Liu WX, Zhao LY, Huang D, Liu XD, et al. Streptococcus thermophilus inhibits colorectal tumorigenesis through secreting beta-galactosidase. Gastroenterology. 2021;160(4):1179–1193.e14.

Li J, Li Y, Ivey KL, Wang DD, Wilkinson JE, Franke A, et al. Interplay between diet and gut microbiome, and circulating concentrations of trimethylamine N-oxide: findings from a longitudinal cohort of US men. Gut. 2022;71(4):724–33.

Liao W, Khan I, Huang G, Chen S, Liu L, Leong WK, et al. Bifidobacterium animalis: the missing link for the cancer-preventive effect of Gynostemma pentaphyllum. Gut Microbes. 2021;13(1):1847629.

Liu ZH, Huang MJ, Zhang XW, Wang L, Huang NQ, Peng H, et al. The effects of perioperative probiotic treatment on serum zonulin concentration and subsequent postoperative infectious complications after colorectal cancer surgery: a double-center and double-blind randomized clinical trial. Am J Clin Nutr. 2013;97(1):117–26.

Long X, Wong CC, Tong L, Chu ESH, Ho Szeto C, Go MYY, et al. Peptostreptococcus anaerobius promotes colorectal carcinogenesis and modulates tumour immunity. Nat Microbiol. 2019;4(12):2319–30.

Mager LF, Burkhard R, Pett N, Cooke NCA, Brown K, Ramay H, et al. Microbiome-derived inosine modulates response to checkpoint inhibitor immunotherapy. Science. 2020;369(6510):1481–9.

Melero I, Castanon E, Alvarez M, Champiat S, Marabelle A. Intratumoural administration and tumour tissue targeting of cancer immunotherapies. Nat Rev Clin Oncol. 2021;18(9):558–76.

Mima K, Nishihara R, Qian ZR, Cao Y, Sukawa Y, Nowak JA, et al. Fusobacterium nucleatum in colorectal carcinoma tissue and patient prognosis. Gut. 2016;65(12):1973–80.

Netta S, Michalopoulos A, Apostolidis S, Paramythiotis D, Papavramidis T, Papadopoulos V, et al. Enhancement of colonic anastomotic strength in rats by short-chain fatty acids. Tech Coloproctol. 2010;14(Suppl 1):S53–5.

Paramsothy S, Kamm MA, Kaakoush NO, Walsh AJ, van den Bogaerde J, Samuel D, et al. Multidonor intensive faecal microbiota transplantation for active ulcerative colitis: a randomised placebo-controlled trial. Lancet. 2017;389(10075):1218–28.

Park M, Kwon J, Shin HJ, Moon SM, Kim SB, Shin US, et al. Butyrate enhances the efficacy of radiotherapy via FOXO3A in colorectal cancer patient derived organoids. Int J Oncol. 2020;57(6):1307–18.

Pasolli E, Asnicar F, Manara S, Zolfo M, Karcher N, Armanini F, et al. Extensive unexplored human microbiome diversity revealed by over 150,000 genomes from metagenomes spanning age, geography, and lifestyle. Cell. 2019;176(3):649–662.e20.

Perez-Ruiz E, Melero I, Kopecka J, Sarmento-Ribeiro AB, Garcia-Aranda M, De Las RJ. Cancer immunotherapy resistance based on immune checkpoints inhibitors: targets, biomarkers, and remedies. Drug Resist Updat. 2020;53:100718.

Rafter J, Bennett M, Caderni G, Clune Y, Hughes R, Karlsson PC, et al. Dietary synbiotics reduce cancer risk factors in polypectomized and colon cancer patients. Am J Clin Nutr. 2007;85(2):488–96.

Round JL, Lee SM, Li J, Tran G, Jabri B, Chatila TA, et al. The Toll-like receptor 2 pathway establishes colonization by a commensal of the human microbiota. Science. 2011;332(6032):974–7.

Routy B, Chatelier EL, Derosa L, Duong CPM, Alou MT, Daillère R, et al. Gut microbiome influences efficacy of PD-1-based immunotherapy against epithelial tumors. Science. 2018;359(6371):91–7.

Salva S, Marranzino G, Villena J, Aguero G, Alvarez S. Probiotic Lactobacillus strains protect against myelosuppression and immunosuppression in cyclophosphamide-treated mice. Int Immunopharmacol. 2014;22(1):209–21.

Sarmento-Ribeiro AB, Scorilas A, Goncalves AC, Efferth T, Trougakos IP. The emergence of drug resistance to targeted cancer therapies: clinical evidence. Drug Resist Updat. 2019;47:100646.

Sivan A, Corrales L, Hubert N, Williams JB, Aquino-Michaels K, Earley ZM, et al. Commensal Bifidobacterium promotes antitumor immunity and facilitates anti-PD-L1 efficacy. Science. 2015;350(6264):1084–9.

So D, Whelan K, Rossi M, Morrison M, Holtmann G, Kelly JT, et al. Dietary fiber intervention on gut microbiota composition in healthy adults: a systematic review and meta-analysis. Am J Clin Nutr. 2018;107(6):965–83.

Sung H, Ferlay J, Siegel RL, Laversanne M, Soerjomataram I, Jemal A, et al. Global cancer statistics 2020: GLOBOCAN estimates of incidence and mortality worldwide for 36 cancers in 185 countries. CA Cancer J Clin. 2021;71(3):209–49.

Tanoue T, Morita S, Plichta DR, Skelly AN, Suda W, Sugiura Y, et al. A defined commensal consortium elicits CD8 T cells and anti-cancer immunity. Nature. 2019;565(7741):600–5.

Touchefeu Y, Montassier E, Nieman K, Gastinne T, Potel G, Bruley des Varannes S, et al. Systematic review: the role of the gut microbiota in chemotherapy- or radiation-induced gastrointestinal mucositis—current evidence and potential clinical applications. Aliment Pharmacol Ther. 2014;40(5):409–21.

Tsuruya A, Kuwahara A, Saito Y, Yamaguchi H, Tsubo T, Suga S, et al. Ecophysiological consequences of alcoholism on human gut microbiota: implications for ethanol-related pathogenesis of colon cancer. Sci Rep. 2016;6:27923.

Wang F, Yin Q, Chen L, Davis MM. Bifidobacterium can mitigate intestinal immunopathology in the context of CTLA-4 blockade. Proc Natl Acad Sci U S A. 2018a;115(1):157–61.

Wang Y, Wiesnoski DH, Helmink BA, Gopalakrishnan V, Choi K, DuPont HL, et al. Fecal microbiota transplantation for refractory immune checkpoint inhibitor-associated colitis. Nat Med. 2018b;24(12):1804–8.

Wang Y, Li A, Zhang L, Waqas M, Mehmood K, Iqbal M, et al. Probiotic potential of Lactobacillus on the intestinal microflora against Escherichia coli induced mice model through high-throughput sequencing. Microb Pathog. 2019a;137:103760.

Wang Z, Hua W, Li C, Chang H, Liu R, Ni Y, et al. Protective role of fecal microbiota transplantation on colitis and colitis-associated colon cancer in mice is associated with Treg cells. Front Microbiol. 2019b;10:2498.

Wang Q, Wang K, Wu W, Lv L, Bian X, Yang L, et al. Administration of Bifidobacterium bifidum CGMCC 15068 modulates gut microbiota and metabolome in azoxymethane (AOM)/dextran sulphate sodium (DSS)-induced colitis-associated colon cancer (CAC) in mice. Appl Microbiol Biotechnol. 2020;104(13):5915–28.

Wastyk HC, Fragiadakis GK, Perelman D, Dahan D, Merrill BD, Yu FB, et al. Gut-microbiota-targeted diets modulate human immune status. Cell. 2021;184(16):4137–53.e14.

Xie X, He Y, Li H, Yu D, Na L, Sun T, et al. Effects of prebiotics on immunologic indicators and intestinal microbiota structure in perioperative colorectal cancer patients. Nutrition. 2019;61:132–42.

Youngster I, Russell GH, Pindar C, Ziv-Baran T, Sauk J, Hohmann EL. Oral, capsulized, frozen fecal microbiota transplantation for relapsing Clostridium difficile infection. JAMA. 2014;312(17):1772–8.

Yu T, Guo F, Yu Y, Sun T, Ma D, Han J, et al. Fusobacterium nucleatum promotes chemoresistance to colorectal cancer by modulating autophagy. Cell. 2017;170(3):548–63.e16.

Zhang S, Yang Y, Weng W, Guo B, Cai G, Ma Y, et al. Fusobacterium nucleatum promotes chemoresistance to 5-fluorouracil by upregulation of BIRC3 expression in colorectal cancer. J Exp Clin Cancer Res. 2019;38(1):14.

Zhuo Q, Yu B, Zhou J, Zhang J, Zhang R, Xie J, et al. Lysates of Lactobacillus acidophilus combined with CTLA-4-blocking antibodies enhance antitumor immunity in a mouse colon cancer model. Sci Rep. 2019;9(1):20128.

Chapter 16
Targeting Gut Microbiota in Colorectal Cancer

Sunny H. Wong

Abstract Colorectal cancer (CRC) is a prevalent cancer, accounting for about 10% of all new cases worldwide. The intestinal microbiota plays an increasingly important role in CRC. Recent studies have identified the role of several bacteria in the development of CRC. Metagenomic studies have revealed microbial changes in CRC patients, highlighting *Fusobacterium nucleatum*, *Peptostreptococcus anaerobius*, and specific strains of *Escherichia coli* and *Bacteroides fragilis*. These findings give new opportunities to utilize these microbes for clinical applications, such as detecting them as diagnostic or prognostic biomarkers. The importance of the microbiota in the development of CRC is increasingly evident, but identifying specific microbial features that influence CRC initiation and progression remains a central task for investigators. The next hurdle for the field is to demonstrate that the microbiota can be utilized to offer clinical benefits for CRC patients, by shrinking tumours, enhancing treatment, reducing treat side effects, and preventing cancer recurrence. The purpose of this chapter is to discuss the recent advances in the occurrence of microbial CRC and the translational potential of these findings.

Keywords Colorectal cancer · Gut microbiota · Probiotics · Faecal microbiota transplant · Oncology · Immunotherapy · Chemotherapy

16.1 Introduction

CRC is one of the most frequent malignancies, and it has a significant burden on global health. It is the third most diagnosed malignancy in the world, and it is also the second greatest cause of cancer death (Keum and Giovannucci 2019). In 2018, it resulted in around 1.8 million new cases and 900,000 fatalities per year (Bray

S. H. Wong (✉)
Centre for Microbiome Medicine, Lee Kong Chian School of Medicine,
Nanyang Technological University, Singapore, Singapore
e-mail: sunny.wong@ntu.edu.sg

J. Yu (ed.), *Microbiome in Gastrointestinal Cancer*,
https://doi.org/10.1007/978-981-19-4492-5_16

et al. 2018). CRC, like many other prevalent diseases, is complex in nature and is influenced by both hereditary and environmental factors. According to twin and family studies, the heritability of CRC is 35–40% (Graff et al. 2017; Lichtenstein et al. 2000). Genetic studies estimated that approximately 25% of CRC patients have a family history without an identifiable mutation (Jasperson et al. 2010), whereas approximately 5% are ascribed to hereditary cancer syndromes, such as hereditary nonpolyposis colorectal cancer (HNPCC, also known as Lynch syndrome) and familial adenomatous polyposis (FAP). These well-known cancer syndromes are caused by inherited germline mutations in susceptibility genes that are rare but have a high penetrance (for example, *MLH1* and *APC*, respectively). Common but low-penetrance genetic variants known to be related with CRC risk, which have been identified through genome-wide association studies, account for less than 1% of the heritability of CRC (Jiao et al. 2014). These findings imply that environmental variables are having a sizable impact on the development of CRC.

Physical inactivity, obesity, dietary factor, cigarette use, and excessive alcohol use are all recognized as risk factors for CRC (Keum and Giovannucci 2019). Furthermore, as an environmental factor, the importance of gut microbiota in the development of CRC is becoming increasingly recognized. Infectious agents are thought to be responsible for more than 15% of all malignancies, including the great majority of stomach cancers, hepatocellular carcinomas, and cervical cancers, according to estimates. While specific infectious agents (e.g. *Helicobacter pylori*, hepatitis B and C viruses, and human papillomavirus) have been studied for their oncogenic mechanisms, researchers have recently begun to investigate the collective microbial community present in the tumour environment for their effects on cancer. This community of microorganisms, referred to as the microbiota, has emerged as a significant environmental component in the development of certain cancers, including CRC. There is now a substantial amount of evidence to suggest that multiple bacteria play a collective mechanistic role in colorectal carcinogenesis. Understanding the mechanisms by which gut microbiota contribute to CRC development may lead to new insights into disease prevention and treatment. In this chapter, we will explore the mechanisms by which the microbiota associates with CRC and how this association can be modulated to prevent or treat the disease.

16.2 CRC Metagenomic Landscape

A total of around 40 trillion bacteria reside within the human body, which are greater than the total number of human cells (Ley et al. 2006; Sender et al. 2016). New evidence suggests that dysbiosis of the gut microbiota is a factor in the development of CRC. Animal studies provided the early evidence of the significance of the microbiome in colorectal cancer. In one experiment in which both germ-free and conventional mice were exposed to carcinogens, 93% of the conventional mice developed colon cancers, compared to only 21% of the germ-free mice (Reddy et al. 1974). Following this, it was discovered that the gut microbiota, which included certain species of the *Escherichia*, *Enterococcus*, *Bacteroides*, and *Clostridium* genera, might influence the colorectal carcinogenesis profiles generated by carcinogen (Onoue et al. 1997). It has also been shown that the transfer of stool from CRC patients to germ-free mice and azoxymethane (AOM) produced conventional animals can increase intestinal carcinogenesis (Wong et al. 2017a). Consistent results were observed in *Apc*$^{min/+}$ mice upon oral gavage of patients' stool (Li et al. 2019).

Using comparative metagenomic techniques in humans, researchers have consistently discovered that the CRC microbiome differs from that found in healthy controls. When the 16S ribosomal RNA sequencing technology was used to examine the microbiome of CRC, two separate teams of researchers discovered that Fusobacterium was significantly enriched in the microbiome of the disease (Kostic et al. 2012; Castellarin et al. 2012). After that, several metagenomic studies confirmed the findings (Zeller et al. 2014; Yu et al. 2017a; Feng et al. 2015a), demonstrating that the CRC microbiota exhibits an ecological shift in microbial structure, with decreased diversity and an altered microbial community, as well as enhanced pathobionts with potentially carcinogenic characteristics. Traditionally, CRC has been associated with *Bacteroides fragilis*, *Escherichia coli*, and *Streptococcus gallolyticus* strains; however, metagenomic research has revealed associations with *Fusobacterium nucleatum* (Castellarin et al. 2012), as well as species from the *Parvimonas*, *Peptostreptococcus*, *Porphyromonas*, and *Prevotella* genera (Zeller et al. 2014; Yu et al. 2017a; Ahn et al. 2013; Feng et al. 2015b; Chen et al. 2012; Allali et al. 2015; Flemer et al. 2017; Nakatsu et al. 2015). These species were shown to be more prevalent in patients with colorectal cancer. Despite the fact that population demography and geography have been shown to have an impact on microbiota (He et al. 2018; Zhernakova et al. 2016), several meta-analyses have discovered consistent signals with many of these bacteria across populations (Shah et al. 2018; Drewes et al. 2017; Dai et al. 2018), implying the presence of a carcinogenic core despite differences in genetics, diet, and other environmental variables.

In addition to bacteria, viruses, fungi, and archaea constitute important phylogenetic kingdoms in the gut microbiota (Collins et al. 2011). Targeted molecular or histological techniques have been used to detect cytomegalovirus (Harkins et al. 2002; Bender et al. 2009) and other viruses (Laghi et al. 1999; Grinstein et al. 2002; Cheng et al. 1995) in human CRC samples, although results from validation studies have been inconclusive (Knosel et al. 2004; Hart et al. 1982; Gornick et al. 2010). CRC patients have a different intestinal virome profile than healthy controls, with 22 viral taxa including cytomegalovirus serving as biomarkers to differentiate cases from healthy controls (Nakatsu et al. 2018). Other important differentiating taxa were *Orthobunyavirus*, *Inovirus* and *Tunalikevirus* (Risch and Merikangas 1996), the latter two known to infect Gram-negative bacteria such as *F nucleatum*, enterotoxigenic *B fragilis,* and genotoxic *E coli* which are implicated in CRC tumorigenesis. In a study with North American subjects which included healthy individuals and those with adenomas and cancers, bacteriophage signatures belonging to families Siphoviridae, Myoviridae, and other unclassified taxa were associated with individuals in a cancerous state (Hannigan et al. 2018). The investigators concluded that the cancer-associated virome was primarily composed of lysogenic bacteriophages, that played an indirect role in the progression of CRC by altering the bacterial populations which were present. It has also been discovered that changes in the mycobiome and archaeome are evident in the CRC microbiota, with an increase in the lipophilic *Malassezia* and the halophilic *Natrinema* (Coker et al. 2019, 2020; Gao et al. 2017). In these studies, correlation analysis revealed the possibility of trans-kingdom microbial interactions, including the loss of connectivity between numerous bacteriophages and oral bacteria in the gut (Nakatsu et al. 2018), and inter-kingdom bacterial fungal interactions in CRC (Coker et al. 2019; Liu et al. 2022).

16.3 Microbial Carcinogenesis in CRC

Colorectal carcinogenesis is a complex process to which hereditary and environmental factors both contribute through a variety of mechanisms. It is currently believed that microbial carcinogenesis of colorectal cancer is dependent on the interaction of keystone pathogens and the bacterial passengers (Hajishengallis et al. 2012; Tjalsma et al. 2012), both of which are critical in the formation of host–microbe interactions. Among these, inflammation, immunology, and genotoxicity are all intimately associated with the CRC microbiota (Tilg et al. 2018). Many cancers, including those of the colorectum (Brennan and Garrett 2016; Lasry et al. 2016), exhibit signs of chronic inflammation throughout their progression (Hanahan and Weinberg 2011). Several CRC-associated bacteria, such as *F nucleatum* (Kostic et al. 2013; Brennan et al. 2021), enterotoxigenic *B fragilis* (Wu et al. 2009; Kordahi et al. 2021), and genotoxic *E coli* (Arthur et al. 2012, 2014; Bonnet et al. 2014), have been shown to activate a signalling cascade and induce inflammation during CRC carcinogenesis in animal models. On the other hand, our immune system can recognize microbial molecules through pattern recognition receptors, such TLR2 and TLR4 for sensing *P anaerobius* (Tsoi et al. 2017) and *F nucleatum* (Yang et al. 2017; Wu et al. 2018). These bacteria may serve important mechanistic role in patients with inflammatory bowel diseases (IBD), who have a significantly higher risk of developing CRC (Beaugerie and Itzkowitz 2015) over the course of chronic inflammation.

Another important carcinogenic process is the generation of toxins by microorganisms with genotoxic effects. These toxins can damage DNA, creating double-strand breaks that accumulate over time and eventually lead to cancer. Several Enterobacteriaceae can produce cytolethal distending toxin (CDT), which, like colibactin, can cause double-strand DNA breaks (Nesic et al. 2004; Cuevas-Ramos et al. 2010; Shen et al. 2009; Buc et al. 2013). Furthermore, *bft* produced by enterotoxigenic *B fragilis* (Goodwin et al. 2011) and reactive oxygen species (ROS) produced by *E faecalis* have both been linked to colorectal neoplasia (Attene-Ramos et al. 2006; Huycke et al. 2002; Wang and Huycke 2007). Furthermore, CRC pathogenesis is also contributed by a number of other aberrations in gastrointestinal physiology, including abnormalities in lipid (Li et al. 2022; Kim et al. 2020), bile acid

(Ocvirk and O'Keefe 2021), and amino acid (Li et al. 2022; Kim et al. 2020; Coker et al. 2022) metabolism, as well as cellular senescence (Okumura et al. 2021) and biofilm formation (Tomkovich et al. 2019). Some bacteria are carcinogenic because they produce metabolites, such as secreted proteins or metabolites (termed secretome and metabolome), that interact between receptors in the host immune system and cancer cells (Ternes et al. 2020). These mechanisms can be better understood to get insight into how they can be modulated for therapeutic purposes.

16.4 Gut Microbiota as Biomarkers for CRC

The discovery of the gut microbiota is having an impact on the development of biomarkers. A biomarker is a biological marker that indicates the presence or severity of a disease. In light of the global health burden of CRC, there is an urgent need for a non-invasive CRC test that is accurate, inexpensive, and quick to perform, particularly for early neoplasia that can be treated with outstanding clinical outcomes. Because CRC is frequently asymptomatic in its early stages, non-invasive screening would be preferred over pro re nata colonoscopy for only symptomatic cases in order to detect the disease early. As high as 90% of patients with Stage I CRC will survive for at least 5 years, compared to just about 10% of those with Stage IV metastatic cancer (Etzioni et al. 2003). Current stool-based occult blood tests have limited sensitivity for the diagnosis of early CRC and advanced adenoma (Hundt et al. 2009). Despite the fact that the multi-target faecal DNA test may detect more malignancies than the faecal immunochemical test (FIT), its sensitivity to detect advanced adenomas is still less than optimal.

In this regard, some studies have made use of the abundance of bacterial species to differentiate between CRC and healthy individuals. This included two case-control studies that used more than 20 microbial biomarkers and yielded an area under the receiver operating characteristic (AUROC) curve of 0.84 (Zeller et al. 2014; Baxter et al. 2016). In a metagenomic study comparing CRC with healthy individuals in Hong Kong, a panel of 20 microbial genes were identified to be associated with disease status (Yu et al. 2017a). This collection of microbial markers can be reduced to two information-rich biomarkers that can be quantified by PCR, resulting in an AUC of 0.84 (Yu et al. 2017a). In another study using a Bayesian method, it was found that a logit model that combined data from six bacteria in the faeces could distinguish CRC from healthy persons with an AUC of 0.80, which further increased to 0.92 when age, race, and body mass index (BMI) were factored into the model (Zackular et al. 2014). A recent study has extended microbial biomarker discovery to early CRC and adenoma, using meta-analysis to identify unifying signals across different populations (Wu et al. 2021).

Among differentially abundant bacteria, *F nucleatum* appeared as a key marker that is critically informative to the diagnosis (Wong et al. 2017b). The presence of high levels of *F nucleatum* in the faeces can improve the sensitivity and specificity of FIT for the identification of CRC (Wong et al. 2017b; Liang et al. 2017). It has been demonstrated that the addition of faecal *F nucleatum* increases the AUC of FIT from 0.85 to 0.95, and that the combined test can save more than 75% of CRC samples that were missed by the solitary FIT (Wong et al. 2017b). Multiple markers were found to be beneficial in conjunction with one another in one study (Liang et al. 2017), and the addition of a *Lachnoclostridium* gene marker has been demonstrated to boost the sensitivity for advanced adenomas, which are otherwise difficult to detect (Liang et al. 2020). In this case, the advantage of multi-target testing across molecular entities is demonstrated, in which individual components may complement one another to improve test results. The best test may come from a panel that strikes a balance between the number of markers, the diagnostic performance, the logical feasibility, and the ease with which the test may be performed.

16.5 Modifying Gut Microbiota for Prophylaxis of CRC

There are some significant differences between the host genome and the microbial metagenome, particularly in terms of scalability and mobility. While the host's genetic factors cannot be changed, the gut microbiota can change very quickly in response to both external environmental influences and internal physiological situations. This opens us a valuable opportunity for manipulating the system for therapeutic objectives, and in the context of CRC, a possibility for cancer prevention and treatment (Fig. 16.1). In this light, tailoring probiotic cocktails for use as microbiome therapeutics is an area of research that should be pursued in further depth. Several probiotic bacteria have been identified and recently demonstrated to reduce tumorigenesis in animal models based on CRC metagenome data. These include *Streptococcus thermophilus*, which bacterium that could activate β-galactosidase-dependent metabolic switch (Li et al. 2021), and *Lactobacillus gallinarum* which could produce indole-3-lactic acid as a protective metabolite (Sugimura et al. 2021). Some other *Bifidobacterium* and *Lactobacillus* species have also been shown to have anti-cancer activities in CRC patients. In an interventional study which *Bifidobacterium lactis* and *Lactobacillus acidophilus* were given to patients with CRC, they were found to be able to enrich butyrate-producing bacteria and deplete pathobionts in the gut (Hibberd et al. 2017). According to the results of another study, which included 398 patients with a history of CRC, patients who received *Lactobacillus casei* had a lower rate of recurring tumours with moderate or higher-grade atypia (Ishikawa et al. 2005). Probiotic bacteria have the ability to mitigate CRC formation by lowering pro-inflammatory cytokines, slowing cell proliferation, and boosting apoptosis as well as the expression of tumour suppressor genes (Zeng et al. 2014). Given the importance of gut microbiota, there has been increased interest in developing next-generation probiotics (NGPs), understood as probiotics identified on the basis of comparative microbiota analyses (Kazmierczak-Siedlecka et al. 2022), as therapeutic agents that can have an impact on the development of CRC. These include bacteria such as *Akkermansia muciniphila* and *Faecalibacterium prausnitzii* that showed anti-inflammatory and short-chain fatty acid (SCFA)

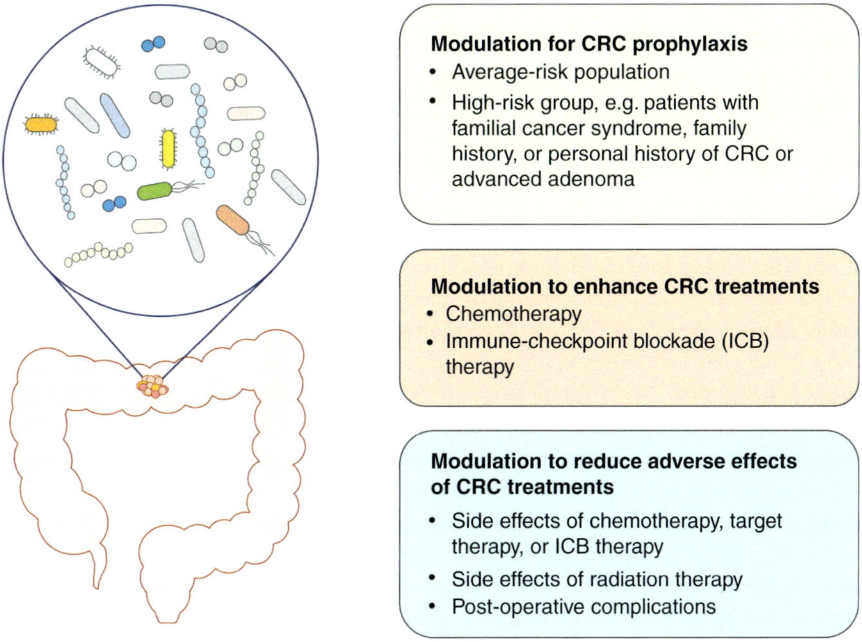

Fig. 16.1 A schematic diagram showing potential benefits of gut microbiota manipulation in management of CRC patients

producing abilities to maintain intestinal homeostasis (Kazmierczak-Siedlecka et al. 2020), giving potential to improve microbiome-related illnesses, such as CRC by delivering favourable gut microbiota changes (Dikeocha et al. 2021).

16.6 Modifying Gut Microbiota to Enhance CRC Treatments

Some studies have found evidence that the gut microbiota can influence the efficacy of some chemotherapy treatments, such as the chemotherapeutic drugs, cyclophosphamide (Viaud et al. 2013) and oxaliplatin (Iida et al. 2013). It has been demonstrated that the chemotherapy medication 5-fluorouracil causes its lethal effects in bacteria by inhibiting bacterial ribonucleotide metabolism (Garcia-Gonzalez et al. 2017). The role of gut microbiota to chemotherapy resistance has also been studied, as *F nucleatum* could activate autophagy to confer resistance to oxaliplatin and 5-fluorouracil (Yu et al. 2017b). Aside from that, the gut microbiota regulates the metabolism and influences the side effects of irinotecan (CPT-11), a prodrug of the topoisomerase inhibitor SN-38 that is commonly used to treat CRC. SN-38 is glucuronidated into an inactive conjugation by the host liver enzymes (SN-38G). In the human gut, β glucuronidase activity is present, especially in the Firmicutes phylum. When SN-38G enters the gut through biliary excretion, gut bacterial β-glucuronidase enzymes hydrolyse it back to SN-38, resulting in intestinal damage and severe diarrhoea (Wallace et al. 2010). SN-38 reactivation in the gut and its concomitant toxicity have been shown to be prevented in mice by administration of a selective inhibitor (Wallace et al. 2015), and a randomized trial found that probiotics derived from *Bifidobacterium* and *Lactobacillus* could reduce β-glucuronidase activity in order to reduce irinotecan-induced diarrhoea (Mego et al. 2015). In a randomized experiment, it was shown that the administration of *Lactobacillus rhamnosus* reduced abdominal discomfort as well as the frequency of severe diarrhoea in patients with CRC who were receiving 5-fluorouracil treatment (Osterlund et al. 2007). Larger studies are needed as some subsequent studies were unable to show significant clinical evidence (Wei et al. 2018); nevertheless, these data illustrate an approach to modify microbial activities in order to lessen side effects of chemotherapeutic medicines (Chang et al. 2018; Yeung et al. 2015; Kato et al. 2017).

While basic and clinical studies have demonstrated that the microbiota plays an important and targetable role in cancer immunotherapy, identifying the bacteria and their factors that are responsible for these effects or their mechanisms of action has proven to be a significant challenge for the microbiome field. There is great interest in modifying the microbiota to improve the efficacy of immune checkpoint blockade (ICB) treatment (Fig. 16.1). Immunotherapy with ICB is a highly effective treatment for many malignancies, although not all patients respond to the treatment. A study conducted on ICB therapy, particularly those targeting the programmed cell death protein (PD-1), found that the presence of unique and beneficial bacteria was associated with increased treatment efficacy (Sivan et al. 2015). For example, investigations have found a number of bacteria, including *A muciniphila* (Routy et al. 2018), *Bifidobacterium* (Sivan et al. 2015), *Faecalibacterium* (Chaput et al. 2017), and *Lachnospiraceae* (McCulloch et al. 2022), that have been linked to favourable immunotherapeutic response in patients. With the increasing use of immunotherapy in the treatment of metastatic CRC with high microsatellite instability (MSI-H) or DNA mismatch repair deficiency (dMMR) (Overman et al. 2017, 2018), manipulation of the gut microbiota may be a useful strategy to improve the immunotherapeutic response. Using animal models of colorectal cancer (CRC), researchers have discovered that specific consortia of multi-bacteria had a potent anti-tumour effect through activation of CD8+ T-cells (Montalban-Arques et al. 2021; Tanoue et al. 2019). A number of probiotic bacteria, such as *Lactobacillus paracasei* and *L rhamnosus*, have been identified in recent investigations as having the potential to improve the antitumor effect of anti-PD-1 in mice CRC models (Zhang et al. 2022; Si et al. 2022). Furthermore, intestinal *Bifidobacterium pseudolongum* was discovered to boost the immune therapeutic response against cytotoxic T lymphocyte-associated antigen 4 (CTLA-4) by the synthesis of the metabolite inosine (Mager et al. 2020). In addition to CRC, a probiotic *Clostridium butyricum* was shown to be useful in boosting immunotherapeutic response to metastatic renal cell carcinoma (Dizman et al. 2022), as well as faecal microbiota transplantation (FMT) in melanoma patients who are ICB resistant (Davar et al. 2021; Baruch et al. 2021). The gut microbiota may also play a role in modulating the side effects of ICB therapy, as specific bacteria such as *Bacteroides intestinalis* have been linked to the drug's toxicity (Dubin et al. 2016; Andrews et al. 2021). Patients with refractory immunotherapy-associated colitis have benefited from FMT, which has been shown to be effective.

16.7 Conclusion

Over the past decade, substantial research has revealed that the microbiota plays a role in the development of cancer, notably in CRC where tumours are strongly associated with the microbiota. It is believed that the microbiota plays a significant role in the development of CRC. This gives unparalleled prospects for novel applications of CRC diagnosis and management, while they are not without their own set of problems. A few obstacles to overcome include the validation of biomarkers in diverse populations to find the ideal biomarker combination, as well as the development of useful microbial products to be used in cancer treatment. Strategies like as mining clinical data, using omics, and developing clinically relevant preclinical models will aid in the transition from the identification of CRC-correlating microorganisms to the identification of variables that contribute to a pro-tumorigenic environment. Regardless, important microbiota research has advanced our understanding of cancer formation and opened the door to new avenues for the creation of innovative cancer detection and therapy applications.

References

Ahn J, Sinha R, Pei Z, Dominianni C, Wu J, Shi J, Goedert JJ, Hayes RB, Yang L. Human gut microbiome and risk for colorectal cancer. J Natl Cancer Inst. 2013;105:1907–11.

Allali I, Delgado S, Marron PI, Astudillo A, Yeh JJ, Ghazal H, Amzazi S, Keku T, Azcarate-Peril MA. Gut microbiome compositional and functional differences between tumor and non-tumor adjacent tissues from cohorts from the US and Spain. Gut Microbes. 2015;6:161–72.

Andrews MC, Duong CPM, Gopalakrishnan V, Iebba V, Chen WS, Derosa L, Khan MAW, Cogdill AP, White MG, Wong MC, Ferrere G, Fluckiger A, Roberti MP, Opolon P, Alou MT, Yonekura S, Roh W, Spencer CN, Curbelo IF, Vence L, Reuben A, Johnson S, Arora R, Morad G, Lastrapes M, Baruch EN, Little L, Gumbs C, Cooper ZA, Prieto PA, Wani K, Lazar AJ, Tetzlaff MT, Hudgens CW, Callahan MK, Adamow M, Postow MA, Ariyan CE, Gaudreau PO, Nezi L, Raoult D, Mihalcioiu C, Elkrief A, Pezo RC, Haydu LE, Simon JM, Tawbi HA, McQuade J, Hwu P, Hwu WJ, Amaria RN, Burton EM, Woodman SE, Watowich S, Diab A, Patel SP, Glitza IC, Wong MK, Zhao L, Zhang J, Ajami NJ, Petrosino J, Jenq RR, Davies MA, Gershenwald JE, Futreal PA, Sharma P, Allison JP, Routy B, Zitvogel L, Wargo JA. Gut microbiota signatures are associated with toxicity to combined CTLA-4 and PD-1 blockade. Nat Med. 2021;27:1432–41.

Arthur JC, Perez-Chanona E, Muhlbauer M, Tomkovich S, Uronis JM, Fan TJ, Campbell BJ, Abujamel T, Dogan B, Rogers AB, Rhodes JM, Stintzi A, Simpson KW, Hansen JJ, Keku TO, Fodor AA, Jobin C. Intestinal inflammation targets cancer-inducing activity of the microbiota. Science. 2012;338:120–3.

Arthur JC, Gharaibeh RZ, Muhlbauer M, Perez-Chanona E, Uronis JM, McCafferty J, Fodor AA, Jobin C. Microbial genomic analysis reveals the essential role of inflammation in bacteria-induced colorectal cancer. Nat Commun. 2014;5:4724.

Attene-Ramos MS, Wagner ED, Plewa MJ, Gaskins HR. Evidence that hydrogen sulfide is a genotoxic agent. Mol Cancer Res. 2006;4:9–14.

Baruch EN, Youngster I, Ben-Betzalel G, Ortenberg R, Lahat A, Katz L, Adler K, Dick-Necula D, Raskin S, Bloch N, Rotin D, Anafi L, Avivi C, Melnichenko J, Steinberg-Silman Y, Mamtani R, Harati H, Asher N, Shapira-Frommer R, Brosh-Nissimov T, Eshet Y, Ben-Simon S, Ziv O, Khan MAW, Amit M, Ajami NJ, Barshack I, Schachter J, Wargo JA, Koren O, Markel G, Boursi B. Fecal microbiota transplant promotes response in immunotherapy-refractory melanoma patients. Science. 2021;371:602–9.

Baxter NT, Koumpouras CC, Rogers MA, Ruffin MT 4th, Schloss PD. DNA from fecal immunochemical test can replace stool for detection of colonic lesions using a microbiota-based model. Microbiome. 2016;4:59.

Beaugerie L, Itzkowitz SH. Cancers complicating inflammatory bowel disease. N Engl J Med. 2015;373:195.

Bender C, Zipeto D, Bidoia C, Costantini S, Zamo A, Menestrina F, Bertazzoni U. Analysis of colorectal cancers for human cytomegalovirus presence. Infect Agent Cancer. 2009;4:6.

Bonnet M, Buc E, Sauvanet P, Darcha C, Dubois D, Pereira B, Dechelotte P, Bonnet R, Pezet D, Darfeuille-Michaud A. Colonization of the human gut by E. coli and colorectal cancer risk. Clin Cancer Res. 2014;20:859–67.

Bray F, Ferlay J, Soerjomataram I, Siegel RL, Torre LA, Jemal A. Global cancer statistics 2018: GLOBOCAN estimates of incidence and mortality worldwide for 36 cancers in 185 countries. CA Cancer J Clin. 2018;68:394–424.

Brennan CA, Garrett WS. Gut microbiota, inflammation, and colorectal cancer. Annu Rev Microbiol. 2016;70:395–411.

Brennan CA, Clay SL, Lavoie SL, Bae S, Lang JK, Fonseca-Pereira D, Rosinski KG, Ou N, Glickman JN, Garrett WS. Fusobacterium nucleatum drives a pro-inflammatory intestinal microenvironment through metabolite receptor-dependent modulation of IL-17 expression. Gut Microbes. 2021;13:1987780.

Buc E, Dubois D, Sauvanet P, Raisch J, Delmas J, Darfeuille-Michaud A, Pezet D, Bonnet R. High prevalence of mucosa-associated E. coli producing cyclomodulin and genotoxin in colon cancer. PLoS One. 2013;8:e56964.

Castellarin M, Warren RL, Freeman JD, Dreolini L, Krzywinski M, Strauss J, Barnes R, Watson P, Allen-Vercoe E, Moore RA, Holt RA. Fusobacterium nucleatum infection is prevalent in human colorectal carcinoma. Genome Res. 2012;22:299–306.

Chang CW, Liu CY, Lee HC, Huang YH, Li LH, Chiau JC, Wang TE, Chu CH, Shih SC, Tsai TH, Chen YJ. Lactobacillus casei variety rhamnosus probiotic preventively attenuates 5-fluorouracil/oxaliplatin-induced intestinal injury in a syngeneic colorectal cancer model. Front Microbiol. 2018;9:983.

Chaput N, Lepage P, Coutzac C, Soularue E, Le Roux K, Monot C, Boselli L, Routier E, Cassard L, Collins M, Vaysse T, Marthey L, Eggermont A, Asvatourian V, Lanoy E, Mateus C, Robert C, Carbonnel F. Baseline gut microbiota predicts clinical response and colitis in metastatic melanoma patients treated with ipilimumab. Ann Oncol. 2017;28:1368–79.

Chen W, Liu F, Ling Z, Tong X, Xiang C. Human intestinal lumen and mucosa-associated microbiota in patients with colorectal cancer. PLoS One. 2012;7:e39743.

Cheng JY, Sheu LF, Meng CL, Lee WH, Lin JC. Detection of human papillomavirus DNA in colorectal carcinomas by polymerase chain reaction. Gut. 1995;37:87–90.

Coker OO, Nakatsu G, Dai Z, Wu WKK, Ng SC, Wong SH, Chan FKK, Sung JJY, Yu J. Enteric fungal microbiota dysbiosis and ecological alterations in colorectal cancer. Gut. 2019;68(4):654–62.

Coker OO, Wu WKK, Wong SH, Sung JJY, Yu J. Altered gut archaea composition and interaction with bacteria are associated with colorectal cancer. Gastroenterology. 2020;159:1459–1470.e1455.

Coker OO, Liu C, Wu WKK, Wong SH, Jia W, Sung JJY, Yu J. Altered gut metabolites and microbiota interactions are implicated in colorectal carcinogenesis and can be non-invasive diagnostic biomarkers. Microbiome. 2022;10:35.

Collins D, Hogan AM, Winter DC. Microbial and viral pathogens in colorectal cancer. Lancet Oncol. 2011;12:504–12.

Cuevas-Ramos G, Petit CR, Marcq I, Boury M, Oswald E, Nougayrede JP. Escherichia coli induces DNA damage in vivo and triggers genomic instability in mammalian cells. Proc Natl Acad Sci U S A. 2010;107:11537–42.

Dai Z, Coker OO, Nakatsu G, Wu WKK, Zhao L, Chen Z, Chan FKL, Kristiansen K, Sung JJY, Wong SH, Yu J. Multi-cohort analysis of colorectal cancer metagenome identified altered bacteria across populations and universal bacterial markers. Microbiome. 2018;6:70.

Davar D, Dzutsev AK, McCulloch JA, Rodrigues RR, Chauvin JM, Morrison RM, Deblasio RN, Menna C, Ding Q, Pagliano O, Zidi B, Zhang S, Badger JH, Vetizou M, Cole AM, Fernandes MR, Prescott S, Costa RGF, Balaji AK, Morgun A, Vujkovic-Cvijin I, Wang H, Borhani AA, Schwartz MB, Dubner HM, Ernst SJ, Rose A, Najjar YG, Belkaid Y, Kirkwood JM, Trinchieri G, Zarour HM. Fecal microbiota transplant overcomes resistance to anti-PD-1 therapy in melanoma patients. Science. 2021;371:595–602.

Dikeocha IJ, Al-Kabsi AM, Eid EEM, Hussin S, Alshawsh MA. Probiotics supplementation in patients with colorectal cancer: a systematic review of randomized controlled trials. Nutr Rev. 2021;80:22–49.

Dizman N, Meza L, Bergerot P, Alcantara M, Dorff T, Lyou Y, Frankel P, Cui Y, Mira V, Llamas M, Hsu J, Zengin Z, Salgia N, Salgia S, Malhotra J, Chawla N, Chehrazi-Raffle A, Muddasani R, Gillece J, Reining L, Trent J, Takahashi M, Oka K, Higashi S, Kortylewski M, Highlander SK, Pal SK. Nivolumab plus ipilimumab with or without live bacterial supplementation in metastatic renal cell carcinoma: a randomized phase 1 trial. Nat Med. 2022;28:704–12.

Drewes JL, White JR, Dejea CM, Fathi P, Iyadorai T, Vadivelu J, Roslani AC, Wick EC, Mongodin EF, Loke MF, Thulasi K, Gan HM, Goh KL, Chong HY, Kumar S, Wanyiri JW, Sears CL. High-resolution bacterial 16S rRNA gene profile meta-analysis and biofilm status reveal common colorectal cancer consortia. NPJ Biofilms Microbiomes. 2017;3:34.

Dubin K, Callahan MK, Ren B, Khanin R, Viale A, Ling L, No D, Gobourne A, Littmann E, Huttenhower C, Pamer EG, Wolchok JD. Intestinal microbiome analyses identify melanoma patients at risk for checkpoint-blockade-induced colitis. Nat Commun. 2016;7:10391.

Etzioni R, Urban N, Ramsey S, McIntosh M, Schwartz S, Reid B, Radich J, Anderson G, Hartwell L. The case for early detection. Nat Rev Cancer. 2003;3:243–52.

Feng Q, Liang S, Jia H, Stadlmayr A, Tang L, Lan Z, Zhang D, Xia H, Xu X, Jie Z, Su L, Li X, Li X, Li J, Xiao L, Huber-Schonauer U, Niederseer D, Xu X, Al-Aama JY, Yang H, Wang J, Kristiansen K, Arumugam M, Tilg H, Datz C, Wang J. Gut microbiome development along the colorectal adenoma-carcinoma sequence. Nat Commun. 2015a;6:6528.

Feng Q, Liang S, Jia H, Stadlmayr A, Tang L, Lan Z, Zhang D, Xia H, Xu X, Jie Z, Su L, Li X, Li J, Xiao L, Huber-Schonauer U, Niederseer D, Al-Aama JY, Yang H, Wang J, Kristiansen K, Arumugam M, Tilg H, Datz C. Gut microbiome development along the colorectal adenoma-carcinoma sequence. Nat Commun. 2015b;6:6528.

Flemer B, Lynch DB, Brown JM, Jeffery IB, Ryan FJ, Claesson MJ, O'Riordain M, Shanahan F, O'Toole PW. Tumour-associated and non-tumour-associated microbiota in colorectal cancer. Gut. 2017;66:633–43.

Gao R, Kong C, Li H, Huang L, Qu X, Qin N, Qin H. Dysbiosis signature of mycobiota in colon polyp and colorectal cancer. Eur J Clin Microbiol Infect Dis. 2017;36:2457–68.

Garcia-Gonzalez AP, Ritter AD, Shrestha S, Andersen EC, Yilmaz LS, Walhout AJM. Bacterial metabolism affects the C. elegans response to cancer chemotherapeutics. Cell. 2017;169:431–441.e438.

Goodwin AC, Destefano Shields CE, Wu S, Huso DL, Wu X, Murray-Stewart TR, Hacker-Prietz A, Rabizadeh S, Woster PM, Sears CL, Casero RA Jr. Polyamine catabolism contributes to enterotoxigenic Bacteroides fragilis-induced colon tumorigenesis. Proc Natl Acad Sci U S A. 2011;108:15354–9.

Gornick MC, Castellsague X, Sanchez G, Giordano TJ, Vinco M, Greenson JK, Capella G, Raskin L, Rennert G, Gruber SB, Moreno V. Human papillomavirus is not associated with colorectal cancer in a large international study. Cancer Causes Control. 2010;21:737–43.

Graff RE, Moller S, Passarelli MN, Witte JS, Skytthe A, Christensen K, Tan Q, Adami HO, Czene K, Harris JR, Pukkala E, Kaprio J, Giovannucci EL, Mucci LA, Hjelmborg JB. Familial risk and heritability of colorectal cancer in the Nordic twin study of cancer. Clin Gastroenterol Hepatol. 2017;15:1256–64.

Grinstein S, Preciado MV, Gattuso P, Chabay PA, Warren WH, De Matteo E, Gould VE. Demonstration of Epstein-Barr virus in carcinomas of various sites. Cancer Res. 2002;62:4876–8.

Hajishengallis G, Darveau RP, Curtis MA. The keystone-pathogen hypothesis. Nat Rev Microbiol. 2012;10:717–25.

Hanahan D, Weinberg RA. Hallmarks of cancer: the next generation. Cell. 2011;144:646–74.

Hannigan GD, Duhaime MB, Ruffin MT 4th, Koumpouras CC, Schloss PD. Diagnostic potential and interactive dynamics of the colorectal cancer virome. mBio. 2018;9:e02248–18.

Harkins L, Volk AL, Samanta M, Mikolaenko I, Britt WJ, Bland KI, Cobbs CS. Specific localisation of human cytomegalovirus nucleic acids and proteins in human colorectal cancer. Lancet. 2002;360:1557–63.

Hart H, Neill WA, Norval M. Lack of association of cytomegalovirus with adenocarcinoma of the colon. Gut. 1982;23:21–30.

He Y, Wu W, Zheng HM, Li P, McDonald D, Sheng HF, Chen MX, Chen ZH, Ji GY, Zheng ZD, Mujagond P, Chen XJ, Rong ZH, Chen P, Lyu LY, Wang X, Wu CB, Yu N, Xu YJ, Yin J, Raes J, Knight R, Ma WJ, Zhou HW. Regional variation limits applications of healthy gut microbiome reference ranges and disease models. Nat Med. 2018;24:1532–5.

Hibberd AA, Lyra A, Ouwehand AC, Rolny P, Lindegren H, Cedgard L, Wettergren Y. Intestinal microbiota is altered in patients with colon cancer and modified by probiotic intervention. BMJ Open Gastroenterol. 2017;4:e000145.

Hundt S, Haug U, Brenner H. Comparative evaluation of immunochemical fecal occult blood tests for colorectal adenoma detection. Ann Intern Med. 2009;150:162–9.

Huycke MM, Abrams V, Moore DR. Enterococcus faecalis produces extracellular superoxide and hydrogen peroxide that damages colonic epithelial cell DNA. Carcinogenesis. 2002;23:529–36.

Iida N, Dzutsev A, Stewart CA, Smith L, Bouladoux N, Weingarten RA, Molina DA, Salcedo R, Back T, Cramer S, Dai RM, Kiu H, Cardone M, Naik S, Patri AK, Wang E, Marincola FM, Frank KM, Belkaid Y, Trinchieri G, Goldszmid RS. Commensal bacteria control cancer response to therapy by modulating the tumor microenvironment. Science. 2013;342:967–70.

Ishikawa H, Akedo I, Otani T, Suzuki T, Nakamura T, Takeyama I, Ishiguro S, Miyaoka E, Sobue T, Kakizoe T. Randomized trial of dietary fiber and Lactobacillus casei administration for prevention of colorectal tumors. Int J Cancer. 2005;116:762–7.

Jasperson KW, Tuohy TM, Neklason DW, Burt RW. Hereditary and familial colon cancer. Gastroenterology. 2010;138:2044–58.

Jiao S, Peters U, Berndt S, Brenner H, Butterbach K, Caan BJ, Carlson CS, Chan AT, Chang-Claude J, Chanock S, Curtis KR, Duggan D, Gong J, Harrison TA, Hayes RB, Henderson BE, Hoffmeister M, Kolonel LN, Le Marchand L, Potter JD, Rudolph A, Schoen RE, Seminara D, Slattery ML, White E, Hsu L. Estimating the heritability of colorectal cancer. Hum Mol Genet. 2014;23:3898–905.

Kato S, Hamouda N, Kano Y, Oikawa Y, Tanaka Y, Matsumoto K, Amagase K, Shimakawa M. Probiotic Bifidobacterium bifidum G9-1 attenuates 5-fluorouracil-induced intestinal mucositis in mice via suppression of dysbiosis-related secondary inflammatory responses. Clin Exp Pharmacol Physiol. 2017;44:1017–25.

Kazmierczak-Siedlecka K, Daca A, Fic M, van de Wetering T, Folwarski M, Makarewicz W. Therapeutic methods of gut microbiota modification in colorectal cancer management—

fecal microbiota transplantation, prebiotics, probiotics, and synbiotics. Gut Microbes. 2020;11:1518–30.
Kazmierczak-Siedlecka K, Skonieczna-Zydecka K, Hupp T, Duchnowska R, Marek-Trzonkowska N, Polom K. Next-generation probiotics—do they open new therapeutic strategies for cancer patients? Gut Microbes. 2022;14:2035659.
Keum N, Giovannucci E. Global burden of colorectal cancer: emerging trends, risk factors and prevention strategies. Nat Rev Gastroenterol Hepatol. 2019;16:713–32.
Kim M, Vogtmann E, Ahlquist DA, Devens ME, Kisiel JB, Taylor WR, White BA, Hale VL, Sung J, Chia N, Sinha R, Chen J. Fecal metabolomic signatures in colorectal adenoma patients are associated with gut microbiota and early events of colorectal cancer pathogenesis. mBio. 2020;11:e03186–19.
Knosel T, Schewe C, Dietel M, Petersen I. Cytomegalovirus is not associated with progression and metastasis of colorectal cancer. Cancer Lett. 2004;211:243–7.
Kordahi MC, Stanaway IB, Avril M, Chac D, Blanc MP, Ross B, Diener C, Jain S, McCleary P, Parker A, Friedman V, Huang J, Burke W, Gibbons SM, Willis AD, Darveau RP, Grady WM, Ko CW, DePaolo RW. Genomic and functional characterization of a mucosal symbiont involved in early-stage colorectal cancer. Cell Host Microbe. 2021;29:1589–1598.e1586.
Kostic AD, Gevers D, Pedamallu CS, Michaud M, Duke F, Earl AM, Ojesina AI, Jung J, Bass AJ, Tabernero J, Baselga J, Liu C, Shivdasani RA, Ogino S, Birren BW, Huttenhower C, Garrett WS, Meyerson M. Genomic analysis identifies association of fusobacterium with colorectal carcinoma. Genome Res. 2012;22:292–8.
Kostic AD, Chun E, Robertson L, Glickman JN, Gallini CA, Michaud M, Clancy TE, Chung DC, Lochhead P, Hold GL, El-Omar EM, Brenner D, Fuchs CS, Meyerson M, Garrett WS. Fusobacterium nucleatum potentiates intestinal tumorigenesis and modulates the tumor-immune microenvironment. Cell Host Microbe. 2013;14:207–15.
Laghi L, Randolph AE, Chauhan DP, Marra G, Major EO, Neel JV, Boland CR. JC virus DNA is present in the mucosa of the human colon and in colorectal cancers. Proc Natl Acad Sci U S A. 1999;96:7484–9.
Lasry A, Zinger A, Ben-Neriah Y. Inflammatory networks underlying colorectal cancer. Nat Immunol. 2016;17:230–40.
Ley RE, Peterson DA, Gordon JI. Ecological and evolutionary forces shaping microbial diversity in the human intestine. Cell. 2006;124:837–48.
Li L, Li X, Zhong W, Yang M, Xu M, Sun Y, Ma J, Liu T, Song X, Dong W, Liu X, Chen Y, Liu Y, Abla Z, Liu W, Wang B, Jiang K, Cao H. Gut microbiota from colorectal cancer patients enhances the progression of intestinal adenoma in Apc(min/+) mice. EBioMedicine. 2019;48:301–15.
Li Q, Hu W, Liu WX, Zhao LY, Huang D, Liu XD, Chan H, Zhang Y, Zeng JD, Coker OO, Kang W, Ng SSM, Zhang L, Wong SH, Gin T, Chan MTV, Wu JL, Yu J, Wu WKK. Streptococcus thermophilus inhibits colorectal tumorigenesis through secreting beta-galactosidase. Gastroenterology. 2021;160:1179–1193.e1114.
Li C, Wang Y, Liu D, Wong CC, Coker OO, Zhang X, Liu C, Zhou Y, Liu Y, Kang W, To KF, Sung JJ, Yu J. Squalene epoxidase drives cancer cell proliferation and promotes gut dysbiosis to accelerate colorectal carcinogenesis. Gut. 2022;71(11):2253–65.
Liang Q, Chiu J, Chen Y, Huang Y, Higashimori A, Fang J, Brim H, Ashktorab H, Ng SC, Ng SSM, Zheng S, Chan FKL, Sung JJY, Yu J. Fecal bacteria act as novel biomarkers for noninvasive diagnosis of colorectal cancer. Clin Cancer Res. 2017;23:2061–70.
Liang JQ, Li T, Nakatsu G, Chen YX, Yau TO, Chu E, Wong S, Szeto CH, Ng SC, Chan FKL, Fang JY, Sung JJY, Yu J. A novel faecal Lachnoclostridium marker for the non-invasive diagnosis of colorectal adenoma and cancer. Gut. 2020;69:1248–57.
Lichtenstein P, Holm NV, Verkasalo PK, Iliadou A, Kaprio J, Koskenvuo M, Pukkala E, Skytthe A, Hemminki K. Environmental and heritable factors in the causation of cancer—analyses of cohorts of twins from Sweden, Denmark, and Finland. N Engl J Med. 2000;343:78–85.

Liu NN, Jiao N, Tan JC, Wang Z, Wu D, Wang AJ, Chen J, Tao L, Zhou C, Fang W, Cheong IH, Pan W, Liao W, Kozlakidis Z, Heeschen C, Moore GG, Zhu L, Chen X, Zhang G, Zhu R, Wang H. Multi-kingdom microbiota analyses identify bacterial-fungal interactions and biomarkers of colorectal cancer across cohorts. Nat Microbiol. 2022;7:238–50.

Mager LF, Burkhard R, Pett N, Cooke NCA, Brown K, Ramay H, Paik S, Stagg J, Groves RA, Gallo M, Lewis IA, Geuking MB, McCoy KD. Microbiome-derived inosine modulates response to checkpoint inhibitor immunotherapy. Science. 2020;369:1481–9.

McCulloch JA, Davar D, Rodrigues RR, Badger JH, Fang JR, Cole AM, Balaji AK, Vetizou M, Prescott SM, Fernandes MR, Costa RGF, Yuan W, Salcedo R, Bahadiroglu E, Roy S, DeBlasio RN, Morrison RM, Chauvin JM, Ding Q, Zidi B, Lowin A, Chakka S, Gao W, Pagliano O, Ernst SJ, Rose A, Newman NK, Morgun A, Zarour HM, Trinchieri G, Dzutsev AK. Intestinal microbiota signatures of clinical response and immune-related adverse events in melanoma patients treated with anti-PD-1. Nat Med. 2022;28:545–56.

Mego M, Chovanec J, Vochyanova-Andrezalova I, Konkolovsky P, Mikulova M, Reckova M, Miskovska V, Bystricky B, Beniak J, Medvecova L, Lagin A, Svetlovska D, Spanik S, Zajac V, Mardiak J, Drgona L. Prevention of irinotecan induced diarrhea by probiotics: a randomized double blind, placebo controlled pilot study. Complement Ther Med. 2015;23:356–62.

Montalban-Arques A, Katkeviciute E, Busenhart P, Bircher A, Wirbel J, Zeller G, Morsy Y, Borsig L, Glaus Garzon JF, Muller A, Arnold IC, Artola-Boran M, Krauthammer M, Sintsova A, Zamboni N, Leventhal GE, Berchtold L, de Wouters T, Rogler G, Baebler K, Schwarzfischer M, Hering L, Olivares-Rivas I, Atrott K, Gottier C, Lang S, Boyman O, Fritsch R, Manz MG, Spalinger MR, Scharl M. Commensal Clostridiales strains mediate effective anti-cancer immune response against solid tumors. Cell Host Microbe. 2021;29:1573–1588.e1577.

Nakatsu G, Li X, Zhou H, Sheng J, Wong SH, Wu WK, Ng SC, Tsoi H, Dong Y, Zhang N, He Y, Kang Q, Cao L, Wang K, Zhang J, Liang Q, Yu J, Sung JJ. Gut mucosal microbiome across stages of colorectal carcinogenesis. Nat Commun. 2015;6:8727.

Nakatsu G, Zhou H, Wu WKK, Wong SH, Coker OO, Dai Z, Li X, Szeto CH, Sugimura N, Yuen-Tung Lam T, Chi-Shing Yu A, Wang X, Chen Z, Chi-Sang Wong M, Ng SC, Chan MTV, Chan PKS, Leung Chan FK, Jao-Yiu Sung J, Yu J. Alterations in enteric virome are associated with colorectal cancer and survival outcomes. Gastroenterology. 2018;155(2):529–541.e5.

Nesic D, Hsu Y, Stebbins CE. Assembly and function of a bacterial genotoxin. Nature. 2004;429:429–33.

Ocvirk S, O'Keefe SJD. Dietary fat, bile acid metabolism and colorectal cancer. Semin Cancer Biol. 2021;73:347–55.

Okumura S, Konishi Y, Narukawa M, Sugiura Y, Yoshimoto S, Arai Y, Sato S, Yoshida Y, Tsuji S, Uemura K, Wakita M, Matsudaira T, Matsumoto T, Kawamoto S, Takahashi A, Itatani Y, Miki H, Takamatsu M, Obama K, Takeuchi K, Suematsu M, Ohtani N, Fukunaga Y, Ueno M, Sakai Y, Nagayama S, Hara E. Gut bacteria identified in colorectal cancer patients promote tumourigenesis via butyrate secretion. Nat Commun. 2021;12:5674.

Onoue M, Kado S, Sakaitani Y, Uchida K, Morotomi M. Specific species of intestinal bacteria influence the induction of aberrant crypt foci by 1,2-dimethylhydrazine in rats. Cancer Lett. 1997;113:179–86.

Osterlund P, Ruotsalainen T, Korpela R, Saxelin M, Ollus A, Valta P, Kouri M, Elomaa I, Joensuu H. Lactobacillus supplementation for diarrhoea related to chemotherapy of colorectal cancer: a randomised study. Br J Cancer. 2007;97:1028–34.

Overman MJ, McDermott R, Leach JL, Lonardi S, Lenz HJ, Morse MA, Desai J, Hill A, Axelson M, Moss RA, Goldberg MV, Cao ZA, Ledeine JM, Maglinte GA, Kopetz S, Andre T. Nivolumab in patients with metastatic DNA mismatch repair-deficient or microsatellite instability-high colorectal cancer (CheckMate 142): an open-label, multicentre, phase 2 study. Lancet Oncol. 2017;18:1182–91.

Overman MJ, Lonardi S, Wong KYM, Lenz HJ, Gelsomino F, Aglietta M, Morse MA, Van Cutsem E, McDermott R, Hill A, Sawyer MB, Hendlisz A, Neyns B, Svrcek M, Moss RA, Ledeine JM, Cao ZA, Kamble S, Kopetz S, Andre T. Durable clinical benefit with nivolumab plus ipilimumab in DNA mismatch repair-deficient/microsatellite instability-high metastatic colorectal cancer. J Clin Oncol. 2018;36:773–9.

Reddy BS, Weisburger JH, Narisawa T, Wynder EL. Colon carcinogenesis in germ-free rats with 1,2-dimethylhydrazine and N-methyl-n'-nitro-N-nitrosoguanidine. Cancer Res. 1974;34:2368–72.

Risch N, Merikangas K. The future of genetic studies of complex human diseases. Science. 1996;273:1516–7.

Routy B, Le Chatelier E, Derosa L, Duong CPM, Alou MT, Daillere R, Fluckiger A, Messaoudene M, Rauber C, Roberti MP, Fidelle M, Flament C, Poirier-Colame V, Opolon P, Klein C, Iribarren K, Mondragon L, Jacquelot N, Qu B, Ferrere G, Clemenson C, Mezquita L, Masip JR, Naltet C, Brosseau S, Kaderbhai C, Richard C, Rizvi H, Levenez F, Galleron N, Quinquis B, Pons N, Ryffel B, Minard-Colin V, Gonin P, Soria JC, Deutsch E, Loriot Y, Ghiringhelli F, Zalcman G, Goldwasser F, Escudier B, Hellmann MD, Eggermont A, Raoult D, Albiges L, Kroemer G, Zitvogel L. Gut microbiome influences efficacy of PD-1-based immunotherapy against epithelial tumors. Science. 2018;359:91–7.

Sender R, Fuchs S, Milo R. Are we really vastly outnumbered? Revisiting the ratio of bacterial to host cells in humans. Cell. 2016;164:337–40.

Shah MS, DeSantis TZ, Weinmaier T, McMurdie PJ, Cope JL, Altrichter A, Yamal JM, Hollister EB. Leveraging sequence-based faecal microbial community survey data to identify a composite biomarker for colorectal cancer. Gut. 2018;67:882–91.

Shen Z, Feng Y, Rogers AB, Rickman B, Whary MT, Xu S, Clapp KM, Boutin SR, Fox JG. Cytolethal distending toxin promotes Helicobacter cinaedi-associated typhlocolitis in interleukin-10-deficient mice. Infect Immun. 2009;77:2508–16.

Si W, Liang H, Bugno J, Xu Q, Ding X, Yang K, Fu Y, Weichselbaum RR, Zhao X, Wang L. Lactobacillus rhamnosus GG induces cGAS/STING- dependent type I interferon and improves response to immune checkpoint blockade. Gut. 2022;71:521–33.

Sivan A, Corrales L, Hubert N, Williams JB, Aquino-Michaels K, Earley ZM, Benyamin FW, Lei YM, Jabri B, Alegre ML, Chang EB, Gajewski TF. Commensal Bifidobacterium promotes antitumor immunity and facilitates anti-PD-L1 efficacy. Science. 2015;350:1084–9.

Sugimura N, Li Q, Chu ESH, Lau HCH, Fong W, Liu W, Liang C, Nakatsu G, Su ACY, Coker OO, Wu WKK, Chan FKL, Yu J. Lactobacillus gallinarum modulates the gut microbiota and produces anti-cancer metabolites to protect against colorectal tumourigenesis. Gut. 2021;71(10):2011–21.

Tanoue T, Morita S, Plichta DR, Skelly AN, Suda W, Sugiura Y, Narushima S, Vlamakis H, Motoo I, Sugita K, Shiota A, Takeshita K, Yasuma-Mitobe K, Riethmacher D, Kaisho T, Norman JM, Mucida D, Suematsu M, Yaguchi T, Bucci V, Inoue T, Kawakami Y, Olle B, Roberts B, Hattori M, Xavier RJ, Atarashi K, Honda K. A defined commensal consortium elicits CD8 T cells and anti-cancer immunity. Nature. 2019;565:600–5.

Ternes D, Karta J, Tsenkova M, Wilmes P, Haan S, Letellier E. Microbiome in colorectal cancer: how to get from meta-omics to mechanism? Trends Microbiol. 2020;28:401–23.

Tilg H, Adolph TE, Gerner RR, Moschen AR. The intestinal microbiota in colorectal cancer. Cancer Cell. 2018;33:954–64.

Tjalsma H, Boleij A, Marchesi JR, Dutilh BE. A bacterial driver-passenger model for colorectal cancer: beyond the usual suspects. Nat Rev Microbiol. 2012;10:575–82.

Tomkovich S, Dejea CM, Winglee K, Drewes JL, Chung L, Housseau F, Pope JL, Gauthier J, Sun X, Muhlbauer M, Liu X, Fathi P, Anders RA, Besharati S, Perez-Chanona E, Yang Y, Ding H, Wu X, Wu S, White JR, Gharaibeh RZ, Fodor AA, Wang H, Pardoll DM, Jobin C, Sears CL. Human colon mucosal biofilms from healthy or colon cancer hosts are carcinogenic. J Clin Invest. 2019;129:1699–712.

Tsoi H, Chu ES, Zhang X, Sheng J, Nakatsu D, Ng SC, Chan AW, Chan FK, Sung JJ, Yu J. Peptostreptococcus anaerobius induces intracellular cholesterol biosynthesis in colon cells to induce proliferation and causes dysplasia in mice. Gastroenterology. 2017;152(6):1419–1433.e5.

Viaud S, Saccheri F, Mignot G, Yamazaki T, Daillere R, Hannani D, Enot DP, Pfirschke C, Engblom C, Pittet MJ, Schlitzer A, Ginhoux F, Apetoh L, Chachaty E, Woerther PL, Eberl G, Berard M, Ecobichon C, Clermont D, Bizet C, Gaboriau-Routhiau V, Cerf-Bensussan N, Opolon P, Yessaad N, Vivier E, Ryffel B, Elson CO, Dore J, Kroemer G, Lepage P, Boneca IG, Ghiringhelli F, Zitvogel L. The intestinal microbiota modulates the anticancer immune effects of cyclophosphamide. Science. 2013;342:971–6.

Wallace BD, Wang H, Lane KT, Scott JE, Orans J, Koo JS, Venkatesh M, Jobin C, Yeh LA, Mani S, Redinbo MR. Alleviating cancer drug toxicity by inhibiting a bacterial enzyme. Science. 2010;330:831–5.

Wallace BD, Roberts AB, Pollet RM, Ingle JD, Biernat KA, Pellock SJ, Venkatesh MK, Guthrie L, O'Neal SK, Robinson SJ, Dollinger M, Figueroa E, McShane SR, Cohen RD, Jin J, Frye SV, Zamboni WC, Pepe-Ranney C, Mani S, Kelly L, Redinbo MR. Structure and inhibition of microbiome beta-glucuronidases essential to the alleviation of cancer drug toxicity. Chem Biol. 2015;22:1238–49.

Wang X, Huycke MM. Extracellular superoxide production by Enterococcus faecalis promotes chromosomal instability in mammalian cells. Gastroenterology. 2007;132:551–61.

Wei D, Heus P, van de Wetering FT, van Tienhoven G, Verleye L, Scholten RJ. Probiotics for the prevention or treatment of chemotherapy- or radiotherapy-related diarrhoea in people with cancer. Cochrane Database Syst Rev. 2018;8:CD008831.

Wong SH, Zhao L, Zhang X, Nakatsu G, Han J, Xu W, Xiao X, Kwong TNY, Tsoi H, Wu WKK, Zeng B, Chan FKL, Sung JJY, Wei H, Yu J. Gavage of fecal samples from patients with colorectal cancer promotes intestinal carcinogenesis in germ-free and conventional mice. Gastroenterology. 2017a;153:1621–1633.e1626.

Wong SH, Kwong TNY, Chow TC, Luk AKC, Dai RZW, Nakatsu G, Lam TYT, Zhang L, Wu JCY, Chan FKL, Ng SSM, Wong MCS, Ng SC, Wu WKK, Yu J, Sung JJY. Quantitation of faecal fusobacterium improves faecal immunochemical test in detecting advanced colorectal neoplasia. Gut. 2017b;66:1441–8.

Wu S, Rhee KJ, Albesiano E, Rabizadeh S, Wu X, Yen HR, Huso DL, Brancati FL, Wick E, McAllister F, Housseau F, Pardoll DM, Sears CL. A human colonic commensal promotes colon tumorigenesis via activation of T helper type 17 T cell responses. Nat Med. 2009;15:1016–22.

Wu Y, Wu J, Chen T, Li Q, Peng W, Li H, Tang X, Fu X. Fusobacterium nucleatum potentiates intestinal tumorigenesis in mice via a toll-like receptor 4/p21-activated kinase 1 cascade. Dig Dis Sci. 2018;63:1210–8.

Wu Y, Jiao N, Zhu R, Zhang Y, Wu D, Wang AJ, Fang S, Tao L, Li Y, Cheng S, He X, Lan P, Tian C, Liu NN, Zhu L. Identification of microbial markers across populations in early detection of colorectal cancer. Nat Commun. 2021;12:3063.

Yang Y, Weng W, Peng J, Hong L, Yang L, Toiyama Y, Gao R, Liu M, Yin M, Pan C, Li H, Guo B, Zhu Q, Wei Q, Moyer MP, Wang P, Cai S, Goel A, Qin H, Ma Y. Fusobacterium nucleatum increases proliferation of colorectal cancer cells and tumor development in mice by activating toll-like receptor 4 signaling to nuclear factor-kappaB, and up-regulating expression of microRNA-21. Gastroenterology. 2017;152:851–866.e824.

Yeung CY, Chan WT, Jiang CB, Cheng ML, Liu CY, Chang SW, Chiang Chiau JS, Lee HC. Amelioration of chemotherapy-induced intestinal mucositis by orally administered probiotics in a mouse model. PLoS One. 2015;10:e0138746.

Yu J, Feng Q, Wong SH, Zhang D, Liang QY, Qin Y, Tang L, Zhao H, Stenvang J, Li Y, Wang X, Xu X, Chen N, Wu WK, Al-Aama J, Nielsen HJ, Kiilerich P, Jensen BA, Yau TO, Lan Z, Jia H, Li J, Xiao L, Lam TY, Ng SC, Cheng AS, Wong VW, Chan FK, Xu X, Yang H, Madsen L, Datz C, Tilg H, Wang J, Brunner N, Kristiansen K, Arumugam M, Sung JJ, Wang J. Metagenomic analysis of faecal microbiome as a tool towards targeted non-invasive biomarkers for colorectal cancer. Gut. 2017a;66:70–8.

Yu T, Guo F, Yu Y, Sun T, Ma D, Han J, Qian Y, Kryczek I, Sun D, Nagarsheth N, Chen Y, Chen H, Hong J, Zou W, Fang JY. Fusobacterium nucleatum promotes chemoresistance to colorectal cancer by modulating autophagy. Cell. 2017b;170:548–563.e516.

Zackular JP, Rogers MA, Ruffin MT 4th, Schloss PD. The human gut microbiome as a screening tool for colorectal cancer. Cancer Prev Res (Phila). 2014;7:1112–21.

Zeller G, Tap J, Voigt AY, Sunagawa S, Kultima JR, Costea PI, Amiot A, Bohm J, Brunetti F, Habermann N, Hercog R, Koch M, Luciani A, Mende DR, Schneider MA, Schrotz-King P, Tournigand C, Tran Van Nhieu J, Yamada T, Zimmermann J, Benes V, Kloor M, Ulrich CM, von Knebel Doeberitz M, Sobhani I, Bork P. Potential of fecal microbiota for early-stage detection of colorectal cancer. Mol Syst Biol. 2014;10:766.

Zeng H, Lazarova DL, Bordonaro M. Mechanisms linking dietary fiber, gut microbiota and colon cancer prevention. World J Gastrointest Oncol. 2014;6:41–51.

Zhang SL, Han B, Mao YQ, Zhang ZY, Li ZM, Kong CY, Wu Y, Chen GQ, Wang LS. Lacticaseibacillus paracasei sh2020 induced antitumor immunity and synergized with anti-programmed cell death 1 to reduce tumor burden in mice. Gut Microbes. 2022;14:2046246.

Zhernakova A, Kurilshikov A, Bonder MJ, Tigchelaar EF, Schirmer M, Vatanen T, Mujagic Z, Vila AV, Falony G, Vieira-Silva S, Wang J, Imhann F, Brandsma E, Jankipersadsing SA, Joossens M, Cenit MC, Deelen P, Swertz MA, LifeLines Cohort Study, Weersma RK, Feskens EJ, Netea MG, Gevers D, Jonkers D, Franke L, Aulchenko YS, Huttenhower C, Raes J, Hofker MH, Xavier RJ, Wijmenga C, Fu J. Population-based metagenomics analysis reveals markers for gut microbiome composition and diversity. Science. 2016;352:565–9.

Chapter 17
Microbiota in Cancer Immunotherapy: The Next Milestone of Immuno-oncology?

Nick Lung-Ngai Ting and Jun Yu

Abstract Immune checkpoint inhibitors (ICIs) have revolutionized the field of oncology since the last decade. However, heterogeneous treatment responses among patients and immune-related adverse effects (irAEs) are critical challenges and limitations in current clinical practice. Emerging studies have now indicated that microbiota may influence the clinical responses and toxicity of cancer therapy across multiple cancer types. Early evidence has demonstrated promising results by manipulating the gut microbial composition via faecal microbiota transplantation (FMT) to improve immunotherapeutic efficacy. This chapter will start from the basics by exploring the mechanisms of pharmacomicrobiomics interactions in the context of ICIs, which can be summarised by the "TIME" mechanistic framework—T cell modulation, innate immunity, metabolites & molecular mimicry, and epithelial injury. The chapter will further discuss the translational potential of these laboratory findings in clinical settings for truly benefiting cancer patients. Gut microbial features can potentially be predictive biomarkers for therapeutic responses, guiding treatment selection for patients. Importantly, unlike host genetics, the gut microbial composition can be easily modified by prebiotics, probiotics, antibiotics, dietary modulations, and FMT, which serves as a potential strategy to augment cancer therapeutic responses and toxicity. Pharmacomicrobiomics may play an essential role in future cancer therapeutic interventions opening a new avenue for precision medicine in oncology.

Keywords Gut microbiota · Immunotherapy · Pharmacomicrobiomics · Microbiota modulation

N. L.-N. Ting · J. Yu (✉)
Institute of Digestive Disease and The Department of Medicine and Therapeutics, State Key Laboratory of Digestive Disease, Li Ka Shing Institute of Health Sciences, CUHK Shenzhen Research Institute, The Chinese University of Hong Kong, Hong Kong, China
e-mail: junyu@cuhk.edu.hk

J. Yu (ed.), *Microbiome in Gastrointestinal Cancer*,
https://doi.org/10.1007/978-981-19-4492-5_17

17.1 Introduction

Since the last decade, the emergence of immune checkpoint inhibitors (ICIs) has led to a paradigm shift in the field of oncology and reshaped treatment guidelines for multiple cancer types. The concept of immunotherapy stems from our understanding of cancer immunology. Usually, cancer cells are recognised and eradicated by host immunity, a process known as immunosurveillance. However, cancer cells can gradually develop mechanisms to evade the anti-cancer immunity. One of the mechanisms is turning on the immune checkpoint molecules which include cytotoxic T lymphocyte associated protein 4 (CTLA-4) and programmed cell death 1 (PD-1). Immune checkpoint molecules are negative regulators of T cell activation (Waldman et al. 2020). Tumour cells can upregulate programmed cell death ligand-1 (PD-L1) to interact with PD-1 on T cells causing T cell exhaustion. Similarly, the CTLA-4 on regulatory T (Treg) cells and CD8+ T cells can compete with CD28 for co-stimulatory signals restraining T cell activation (Waldman et al. 2020; Qureshi et al. 2011; Wherry and Kurachi 2015). Drugs targeting these immune checkpoint molecules have been successfully developed to treat aggressive cancers such as metastatic melanoma earning Tasuku Honjo and James Patrick Allison the 2018 Nobel Prize in Physiology or Medicine (Hodi et al. 2010; Schadendorf et al. 2015; Bellmunt et al. 2017; Cohen et al. 2019; Garon et al. 2015). Ipilimumab, the first monoclonal antibody (mAb) inhibiting CTLA4, was authorized in 2011 by FDA for melanoma treatment which was followed by the approval of anti-PD1 mAb and anti-PDL1 mAb. Clinical trials have also demonstrated their superior effects on prolonging patients' survival compared to traditional chemotherapeutics on several cancer types (Cohen et al. 2019; Herbst et al. 2016; Reck et al. 2016).

Nevertheless, heterogeneous responses of ICIs among patients as well as the immune-related adverse effects (irAEs) such as colitis and pneumonitis are still major challenges in immuno-oncology (Gide et al. 2018; Martins et al. 2019; Wang et al. 2018a; Michot et al. 2016). Researchers are looking for ideal biomarkers to predict immunotherapeutic responses and strategies to optimise therapeutic outcomes. Recently, scientists and clinicians have discovered that our microbiota could explain some of the variability in therapeutic efficacy and toxicity among cancer patients and could be a potential candidate for both predictive biomarkers and intervention targets (Ting et al. 2022).

The human body harbours 40 trillion resident microorganisms, including bacteria, fungi, archaea, and viruses comprising the human microbiota (Sender et al. 2016). The gut microbiota has been shown to profoundly affect human physiology especially in shaping the immune system homeostasis (Rooks and Garrett 2016; Fung et al. 2017), which is therefore being studied as one of the factors contributing to immunotherapeutic effects. The relationship between the microbiota, immune system and cancer development has been extensively studied. The concept "immune-oncology-microbiome" axis has been introduced to illustrate the microbial immunomodulatory effects in promoting inflammation and weakening immunosurveillance, indirectly facilitating tumorigenesis (Sepich-Poore et al. 2021).

Although pharmacogenomics has been an active field of research studying the effects of genetic variants in pharmacological responses among individuals, it fails to explain the interindividual disparity fully. Pharmacomicrobiomics has, therefore, been recently proposed to answer the unresolved questions from pharmacogenomics by studying the interplay between our commensal microbes and drug responses. Emerging studies have demonstrated how gut microbiota can dictate the anti-cancer responses of different therapies including chemotherapy (Alexander et al. 2017), radiotherapy (Shiao et al. 2021), targeted therapy (Ianiro et al. 2020; Wong et al. 2021), and immunotherapy (Lau et al. 2021). This chapter will focus on the microbial effects on ICIs as well as the translational potential of these laboratory findings at the bedside (Table 17.1).

Table 17.1 Summary on the mechanisms and translational potential of important microbes in modulating the efficacy and toxicity of ICIs

Immunotherapy	Involved microbes	Mechanisms	Translational potential
PD-1/PD-L1 blockade	*Bifidobacterium*	• *B. breve* and *B. longum* promote CD8+ T cell priming and infiltration in TME, enhancing the therapeutic efficacy of PD-1/PD-L1 blockade (Sivan et al. 2015) • Molecular mimicry between *B. breve* SVY antigen and mouse melanoma SIY neoantigen leads to cross-reactive anti-cancer T cell response (Bessell et al. 2020) • *Bifidobacterium* activates NK cells via hippurate secretion and inhibition of PD-L1 expression (Rizvi et al. 2021)	• *B. longum* is enriched in metastatic melanoma patients who respond to PD-1/PD-L1 blockade (Matson et al. 2018) • NSCLC patients receiving both PD-1/PD-L1 blockade and CBM588 (a live bacterial product containing *Clostridium butyricum* which is bifidogenic) had longer progression-free survival and overall survival (Tomita et al. 2020)
	Enterococcus	• Bacteriophage infecting *E. hirae* expresses TMP which stimulates cross-reactive CD8+ T cell anti-cancer response against cancer antigen PSMB4 protein (Fluckiger et al. 2020)	• *E. faecium* is enriched in metastatic melanoma patients on PD-1/PD-L1 blockade (Matson et al. 2018)
	Ruminococcaceae	• Abundance of fibre-fermenting *Ruminococcaceae* is associated with increased intra-tumoral T lymphocytes infiltration and T cell activation in mice treated with PD-1/PD-L1 blockade (Spencer et al. 2021)	• *Ruminococcaceae* family is enriched in metastatic melanoma patients who respond to PD-1/PD-L1 blockade (Gopalakrishnan et al. 2018) • High-fibre diet can enrich fibre-fermenting *Ruminococcaceae* and is associated with better survival outcome among cancer patients on ICIs (Spencer et al. 2021)
CTLA-4 blockade	*Akkermansia muciniphila*	• *A. muciniphila* secretes inosine which binds to the adenosine 2A receptors on naïve T cells, enhancing Th1 cell differentiation for anti-cancer immune response (Mager et al. 2020)	N/A
	Bifidobacterium	• *B. pseudolongum* secretes inosine which binds to the adenosine 2A receptors on naïve T cells, enhancing Th1 cell differentiation for anti-cancer immune response (Mager et al. 2020) • *Bifidobacterium* reduces irAEs by enhancing the immunosuppressive effects of Treg cells (Wang et al. 2018b)	• A patient with ipilimumab-induced colitis was successfully treated by FMT. After the transplantation, there was enrichment of *Bifidobacterium* in the patient's gut, which have been associated with reduced intestinal inflammation (Wang et al. 2018c)
	Bacteroides	• *B. fragilis and B. thetaiotaomicron* activate DCs and improve IL-12-dependent Th1 cell immune response (Vétizou et al. 2015)	N/A

CTLA-4 cytotoxic T lymphocyte-associated antigen-4, *DCs* dendritic cells, *FMT* faecal microbiota transplantation, *ICI* immune checkpoint inhibitor, *IL* interleukin, *irAEs* immune-related adverse events, *NK* natural killer, *NSCLC* non-small cell lung cancer, *PD-1* programmed cell death protein-1, *PD-L1* programmed death-ligand 1, *PSMB4* proteasome subunit beta type-4, *SIY* SIYRYYGL; SVY, SVYRYYGL, *Th* T helper, *TME* tumour microenvironment, *TMP* tape measure protein, *Treg* regulatory T cells

17.2 Pharmacomicrobiomics Interactions Between Microbiota and ICIs

Commensal microbes can modulate the immune system in multiple ways, including direct interaction via microbial components or indirect interaction via microbial metabolites (Rooks and Garrett 2016). Furthermore, almost all subsets of immune cells have been implicated in cancer immunology (Hiam-Galvez et al. 2021). The mechanisms of how microbiota modulate immunotherapeutic responses are therefore extremely complex. With reference to a previous review article explaining how the microbiota influence chemotherapeutic effects (Alexander et al. 2017), our group has proposed a "TIME" mechanistic framework (T cell mediation, Innate immunity, Metabolites and molecular mimicry, and Epithelial injury) to better illustrate the microbes–immunotherapy interactions (Ting et al. 2022) (Fig. 17.1). More mechanistic insights are required for designing strategies to augment immunotherapeutic responses via modulation of microbiota.

17.2.1 T Cell Modulation

T cells are considered the major players in anti-cancer immunity. A high level of intra-tumoral T cell infiltration is associated with a favourable prognosis in a wide variety of tumour types (Dieu-Nosjean et al. 2008). If sufficient neoantigens are produced from the tumours, naïve CD8+ T cells will be primed and activated by antigen presenting cells (APCs) in the lymph nodes. The differentiated cytotoxic T lymphocytes (CTLs) will then be recruited to the tumour microenvironment (TME) to eliminate immunogenic cancer cells by exocytosis of perforin and granzymes (Gonzalez et al. 2018). Meanwhile, the differentiated CD4+ T helper 1 (Th1) cells will secrete proinflammatory cytokines including interleukin-2 (IL-2), tumour necrosis factor-α (TNF-α), and interferon-γ (IFN-γ) to not only promote cytotoxic T cell activation but also increase the tumoricidal effects of macrophage and natural killer (NK) cells as well as the presentation of neoantigens (Gonzalez et al. 2018; Palucka and Coussens 2016).

Recent studies have demonstrated how gut microbiota interact with ICIs to bolster anti-cancer T cell response showing the indispensability of our gut commensals in immunotherapy. A pioneering study in 2015 showed in animal models that *Bacteroides fragilis*, *Bacteroides thetaiotaomicron*, and *Burkholderia cepacia* could be induced by anti-CTLA4 mAbs to grow in the intestinal mucosa (Vétizou et al. 2015). The growth of these bacteria leads to the production of polysaccharides, further contributing to the activation of dendritic cells (DCs) in lamina propria and the improvement of IL-12-dependent Th1 cell immune response in cancer-draining lymph nodes (Vétizou et al. 2015). Interestingly, the response to CTLA-4 blockade is impaired in microbiota-depleted mice, which is however reversible by recolonisation of *B. fragilis* and *B. cepacia* (Vétizou et al. 2015). This has raised the possibility that probiotics may have the potential to be adjuvants to enhance the anti-cancer immunity induced by ICIs.

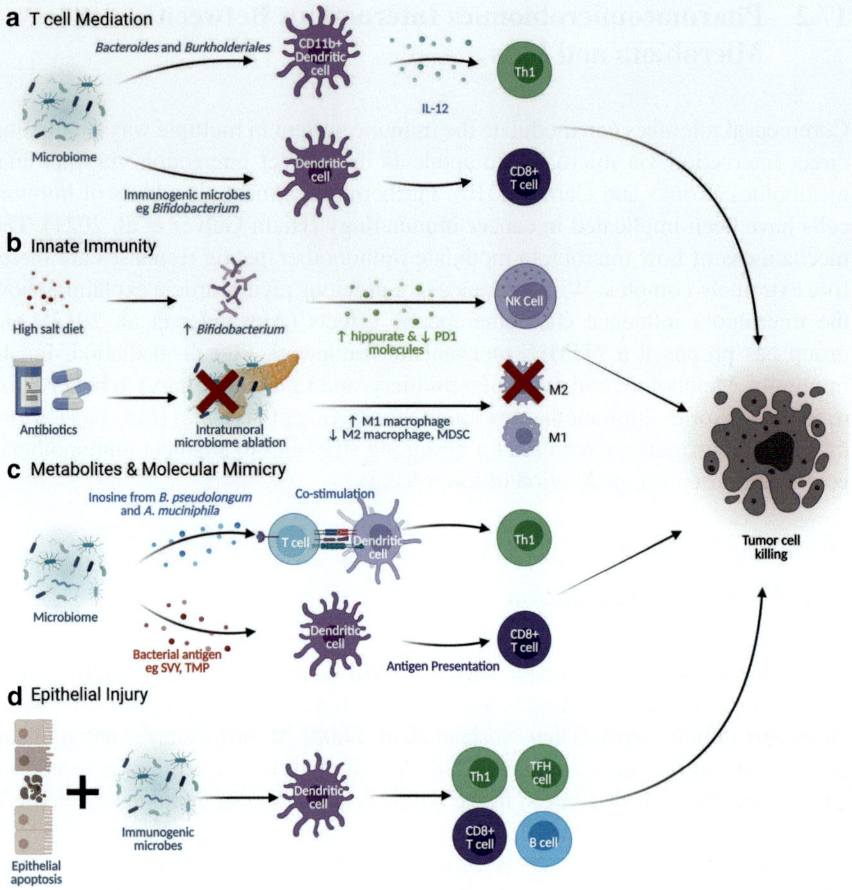

Fig. 17.1 'TIME' mechanistic framework. The figure is adapted with agreement from Ting NL-N, Lau HC-H, Yu J (2022) Cancer pharmacomicrobiomics: targeting microbiota to optimise cancer therapy outcomes. Gut 71:1412–1425. 'TIME' mechanistic framework: T cell mediation, Innate immunity, Metabolites, molecular mimicry, and Epithelial injury. (**a**) *Bacteroides*, *Burkholderiales,* and *Bifidobacterium* enhance anti-cancer T cell immunity to potentiate the efficacy of ICIs. (**b**) *Bifidobacterium* activates NK cells for anti-cancer immunity. Intra-tumoral bacterial ablation in PDAC increases proinflammatory M1 polarisation for cancer cell killing. Both actions improve the sensitivity of cancer cells to ICIs. (**c**) Inosine secreted by *Bifidobacterium pseudolongum* and *Akkermansia muciniphila* binds to adenosine 2A receptor to activate Th1 cell under DC co-stimulation. The SVY antigen from *Bifidobacterium breve* and TMP antigen from *Enterococcus hirae*-infecting bacteriophage are highly similar to tumour neoantigens. The molecular mimicry leads to cross-reactivity of CTL against cancer cells. (**d**) Epithelial injury and immunogenic bacteria stimulate DCs to bolster anti-cancer immunity. *CTL* cytotoxic T lymphocyte, *DC* dendritic cell, *ICI* immune checkpoint inhibitor, *NK* natural killer, *PDAC* pancreatic ductal adenocarcinoma, *SVY* SVYRYYGL, *Th* T helper, *TMP* tape measure protein

Apart from Th1 cells, gut commensals such as *Bifidobacterium longum* and *Bifidobacterium breve* also promote CD8+ T cell priming and infiltration in TME via activation of DCs, which enhance the therapeutic efficacy of PD-1/PD-L1 blockade (Sivan et al. 2015). *Lactobacillus rhamnosus* GG (LGG) is also able to augment the anti-cancer effects of PD-1 blockade, which is mediated by increased infiltration of DCs and T cells in TME (Si et al. 2022). Mechanistically, LGG increases INF-β production by DCs via the cGAS/STING/TBK1/IRF7-dependent signalling pathway. The secondary messenger cyclic GMP-AMP synthase (cGAS) is first involved in activating the stimulator of IFN genes (STING) which then recruits TANK binding kinase 1 (TBK1) for IFN regulatory factor 7 phosphorylation. This signalling pathway ultimately leads to the production of INF-β by DCs, enhancing the cross-priming of CD8+ T cells for anti-cancer immunity. Notably, a single microbe may not mediate the anti-cancer immune response on its own. LGG not only promotes intra-tumoral DCs and CD8+ T cells infiltration but also enriches tumour-suppressing microbes including *Lactobacillus murinus*, which is associated with the activation of DCs (Huang et al. 2016) and *Bacteroides uniformis*, which is associated with the enrichment of IFN-γ + CD8+ T cells (Tanoue et al. 2019).

T cell modulation is also implicated in therapeutic toxicity. *Bifidobacterium* has been shown to reduce irAEs induced by CTLA-4 blockade via Treg cell activation. *Bifidobacterium* enhances Treg cell immunosuppression via its surface β-glucan/galactan polysaccharides and IL-10 mediation to mitigate CTLA-4 blockade-induced colitis (Wang et al. 2018b; Sun et al. 2020; Verma et al. 2018). Since *Bifidobacterium* can also enhance the efficacy of PD-1/PD-L1 blockade, it is worth investigating whether it can simultaneously improve treatment efficacy and reduce irAEs in combined immune checkpoint blockade (CICB).

17.2.2 Innate Immunity

Although T cells are the key players in anti-cancer immunity, the role of innate immune response cannot be neglected. Activated macrophages can be either the proinflammatory M1 type or the anti-inflammatory M2 type. Although macrophages display a proinflammatory M1-like polarisation early on during carcinogenesis to eliminate immunogenic cancer cells, as cancer progresses, the TME recruits the protumorigenic tumour-associated macrophages (TAMs), which display M2-like polarisation. TAMs promote carcinogenesis via multiple mechanisms such as stimulating angiogenesis, lymphangiogenesis, cancer cell proliferation, and epithelial-mesenchymal transition (Gonzalez et al. 2018; Mantovani et al. 2017). NK cells are also innate immune cells but they display anti-cancer effects predominantly (Shimasaki et al. 2020).

Bifidobacterium has been shown to potentiate PD-1 blockade efficacy in melanoma mouse models by activating NK cells via hippurate secretion and inhibition of PD-L1 expression (Rizvi et al. 2021). Cancer cells are then eradicated by NK cells via perforin, granzymes, and IFN-γ mediation. However, the role of microbiota is not always desirable. Intra-tumoral bacterial ablation in pancreatic ductal adenocarcinoma (PDAC) mouse models has been shown to increase proinflammatory M1 macrophage polarisation and protect against tumour growth (Pushalkar et al. 2018). Therefore, the actions of different microbes must be carefully studied and the differences in cancer types should be considered if we hope to augment treatment responses via microbial modulation.

17.2.3 Metabolites and Molecular Mimicry

Immunomodulation can also be indirectly mediated by microbial-derived metabolites. *Bifidobacterium pseudolongum* and *Akkermansia muciniphila* secrete inosine in the gut. With intestinal barrier impairment induced by CTLA-4 blockade, inosine can enter systemic circulation and bind to the adenosine 2A receptors on naïve T cells (Mager et al. 2020). With the co-stimulation from DCs, inosine enhances Th1 cell differentiation and subsequent anti-cancer immune response (Mager et al. 2020). Moreover, glucose, an important energy source, is rapidly depleted by cancer cells in the TME, which limits the full functions of effector T cells. Inosine can be an alternative energy fuel to effector T cells, and inosine supplementation has been shown to improve the efficacy of PD-L1 blockade in melanoma mouse models (Wang et al. 2020). While inosine can promote anti-cancer immunity, the anti-inflammatory effects of short-chain fatty acids (SCFA) are associated with resistance to anti-CTLA-4 mAbs. Butyrate restrains the upregulation of CD80/86 co-stimulatory molecules on DCs induced by CTLA-4 blockade. High blood butyrate and propionate levels are also correlated with the enrichment of immunosuppressive Treg cells (Coutzac et al. 2020). Therefore, microbial-derived metabolites also show potential to affect both therapeutic efficacy and toxicity.

Molecular mimicry between commensals and cancer cells can also potentiate immune checkpoint blockade efficacy. As the SVY antigen of *B. breve* is homologous to mouse melanoma SIY neoantigen, SVY-specific T cells can cross-react with SIY-expressing melanoma leading to anti-cancer immune response and extended survival of mice (Bessell et al. 2020). Another recent study has identified that the bacteriophage infecting *Enterococcus hirae* expresses the tape measure protein (TMP) which contains a major histocompatibility complex (MHC) class I–restricted CD8+ T cell epitope. This microbial antigen shares structural homology with a cancer antigen proteasome subunit beta type-4 protein (PSMB4) which therefore induces a CD8+ memory T cell response to cross-react against cancer cells (Fluckiger et al. 2020). This cross-reactive immune response has also been shown to synergise with the immunotherapeutic effects of PD-1 blockade in mouse models (Fluckiger et al. 2020). Furthermore, recent studies also pointed out that several autoimmune conditions might be related to the cross-reactivity induced by microbial antigens (Gil-Cruz et al. 2019; Greiling et al. 2018; Konig et al. 2016). With the enormous amount of proteomes derived by human microbiota, it is highly possible that more microbial antigens mimicking cancer neoantigens will be discovered.

17.2.4 Epithelial Injury

The relationship between intestinal mucosal epithelium and microbial immunomodulation has recently been unveiled. RNF5 is a membrane anchored E3 ubiquitin ligase which controls the clearance of misfolded proteins. Rnf5$^{-/-}$ mice are shown to have activated endoplasmic reticulum stress response, decreased antimicrobial peptides secretion, and increased ileal crypts apoptosis (Li et al. 2019). These together lead to intestinal dysbiosis with the enrichment of *Bacteroides* and *Parabacteroides* promoting activation of DCs and infiltration of intra-tumoral effector T cells (Li et al. 2019). This observation is indeed similar to a recent study dissecting the mechanism of oxaliplatin-induced anti-cancer immunity. Immunogenic gut bacteria such as *Erysipelotrichaceae* and non-enterotoxigenic *B. fragilis*, together with the antigenicity provided by oxaliplatin-induced enterocyte apoptosis, stimulate migratory DCs to secrete IL-1β and IL-12 for follicular T (TFH) cell activation (Roberti et al. 2020). TFH cells then activate B cells for IgG2b response and enhanced CD8+ T cell anti-cancer activity (Roberti et al. 2020). Therefore, synergistic therapeutic effects can indeed be achieved by combining oxaliplatin and immune checkpoint blockade.

While certain microorganisms are shown to be essential for the anti-cancer immunity induced by ICIs, some other microbes play a protumorigenic role. Therefore, a thorough understanding of the microbial actions is crucial for the precise modulation of microbiota to optimise immunotherapeutic outcomes. It is now obvious that the emergence of pharmacomicrobiomics boasts impressive clinical potential and poses an opportunity to exploit the microbiota to treat cancer. Elucidating the mechanisms that mediate microbial immunomodulation will lead to personalised immunotherapy for patients, further unleashing the potential of immunotherapy in cancer treatment.

17.3 Clinical Potential—Predictive Biomarkers

Despite the unprecedented anti-cancer effects yielded by ICIs, clinical responses are restricted only to a subset of patients. Emerging evidence has now clearly indicated the roles of commensal microbes in influencing the therapeutic responses and irAEs of ICIs. Human metagenomic studies have revealed some potential microbes to be predictive biomarkers for treatment responses in both monotherapy and combined immune checkpoint blockade (CICB), which will be helpful in guiding patient selection for different types of immunotherapeutics.

17.3.1 Monotherapy

Three landmark studies published in 2018 identified response-associated species in melanoma and epithelial cancer patients receiving PD-1/PD-L1 blockade (Routy et al. 2018; Matson et al. 2018; Gopalakrishnan et al. 2018). While the enrichment of *Faecalibacterium*, *E. hirae*, *Collinsella aerofaciens*, *A. muciniphila*, *E. faecium*, and *B. longum* was observed in responders, *Bacteroidales*, *Roseburia intestinalis*, and *Ruminococcus obeum* were enriched in non-responders. The relative abundance of gut *Faecalibacterium* in patients is positively correlated with the level of tumour CD8+ T cell infiltration. In contrast, the relative abundance of *Bacteroidales* has an inverse relationship which might hint at their underlying mechanisms in affecting treatment responses (Gopalakrishnan et al. 2018). A more recent prospective multi-centric study with non-small lung carcinoma (NSCLC) patients was conducted to validate the value of *A. muciniphila* in predicting treatment response. A 'normal' abundance of *A. muciniphila* in stool (relative abundance <4.799%) is associated with longer OS, while either absence or overabundance of *A. muciniphila* (relative abundance >4.799%) is associated with shorter OS (Derosa et al. 2022). *A. muciniphila* even outperforms tumour PD-L1 expression, a clinically used biomarker, in predicting treatment response of NSCLC patients receiving ICIs suggesting the potential of microbiome studies in rewriting future oncology clinical guidelines (Derosa et al. 2022). Patients with higher faecal *A. muciniphila* abundance are observed to have higher intra-tumoral T cells which is also consistent with previous mechanistic studies in mouse models (Routy et al. 2018).

Distinct baseline gut microbial composition is also associated with therapeutic response and toxicity in CTLA-4 blockade. *Faecalibacterium*, *Gemmiger,* and *Clostridium* XIVa were enriched in responders of melanoma patients receiving ipilimumab, while *Bacteroides* were enriched in non-responders (Chaput et al. 2017). An important observation is that those bacteria enriched in responders are also correlated with a higher incidence of irAEs, particularly enterocolitis in the context of CTLA-4 blockade. At the same time, patients with the enrichment of *Bacteroides* are more likely to be colitis-free (Chaput et al. 2017; Dubin et al. 2016). The clinical implication behind this is how we can utilise the microbial markers to select the most appropriate patients for ICIs. If these microbial features are to be intervention targets, how can we maximise the immunotherapeutic effects while preventing the toxicity caused by an excessive immune response?

17.3.2 Combined Immune Checkpoint Blockade

The efficacy of ICIs can be further enhanced by targeting PD-1/PD-L1 and CTLA-4 at the same time. However, this inevitably leads to a higher incidence of irAEs due to an overactivated immune response causing off-target effects (Martins et al. 2019).

Researchers are therefore looking for baseline biomarkers that help identify patients who will be refractory to monotherapy and need the combined immune checkpoint blockade (CICB) while having minimal risk of developing severe irAEs. Andrews et al. have found that the response-specific species are different between monotherapy and CICB (Andrews et al. 2021). *Parabacteroides distasonis* is enriched in responders of CICB, which is, however, associated with poor response to either CTLA-4 blockade or PD-1 blockade monotherapy (Vétizou et al. 2015; Routy et al. 2018). Microbial features are also predictive of the incidence of therapeutic toxicity. *Intestinibacter bartlettii* and *Bacteroides intestinalis* are enriched in patients with high-grade irAEs, while *Dorea formicigenerans* is enriched in those with low-grade adverse events (Andrews et al. 2021). Mechanistic study in mice also demonstrated that *Bacteroides intestinalis* could cause an increased incidence of CICB-induced ileitis probably mediated by upregulation of ileal Il1b (Andrews et al. 2021). Unlike the results in the monotherapy study (Chaput et al. 2017), there is no overlapping microbial feature associated with both therapeutic efficacy and toxicity. Despite the small sample size of the study, it shows that microbiota also play a role in CICB, as in the case of monotherapy. However, further investigations are needed to study the different results yielded from monotherapy and CICB studies. A possible hypothesis is that microbes may switch their roles depending on the immunotherapy used as monotherapy, and CICB involves unique cellular mechanisms (Wei et al. 2019; Lam and Goldszmid 2021). The discrepancies may also be attributed to the small sample size, interpatient variability, and differences in study design.

Despite the promising results from these human studies, limitations and challenges remain. Inconsistent results among different human studies or between human and animal studies are major challenges to overcome. While human studies identified *Bacteroides* as being associated with poor response to CTLA-4 blockade (Chaput et al. 2017), preclinical animal studies demonstrated that *Bacteroides* genus (*B. fragilis* and *B. thetaiotaomicron*) could potentiate the anti-cancer immunity of CTLA-4 blockade (Vétizou et al. 2015). This might suggest that bacteria even in the same genus may play an opposite role in immunomodulation which still requires further investigations. Although different studies identified different response-specific microbes, a meta-analysis discovered that more overlaps are found in the microbial gene content instead of the microbial composition across studies (Routy et al. 2018; Matson et al. 2018; Gopalakrishnan et al. 2018; Gharaibeh and Jobin 2019). This indicates that there may be functional redundancy among the microbes. However, further efforts are still required to standardise the sample collection technique, sequencing methods, and bioinformatics analysis pipelines across studies, which may also be contributors to the existing discrepancies (Costea et al. 2017; Knight et al. 2018). Future studies are also needed to compare the microbial biomarkers to the existing predictive biomarkers such as tumour PD-L1 expression, tumour mutational burden, and intra-tumoral T cell infiltration. The predictive power of a combination of different biomarkers is also worth studying. Nevertheless, the current results are still encouraging and promising. Microbes such as

A. muciniphila (Routy et al. 2018), *B. thetaiotaomicron* (Frankel et al. 2017), and *B. intestinihominis* (Limeta et al. 2020) were consistently reported to be associated with improved immunotherapeutic response in both animal and human studies. More insights will be provided by future large-cohort studies with more in-depth functional analysis.

17.4 Clinical Potential: Microbiota Modulation

Beyond predictive biomarkers for guiding patient selection for ICIs, intervention strategies are also urgently needed to help overcome treatment resistance and reduce therapeutic toxicity. Microbiota serves as a potential target as it can easily be modulated via various methods, including dietary modulation, probiotics, antibiotics, and FMT, unlike our host genetics.

17.4.1 Dietary Modulation

A recent study has revealed that dietary fibre intake can ameliorate the clinical outcome of ICIs (Spencer et al. 2021). Melanoma patients with daily fibre intake >20 g/day have improved progressive-free survival (PFS) compared to those who do not meet the threshold. The study also revealed that for every increase of 5 g in daily fibre intake, there would be a 30% decrease in the risk of progression or death. A parallel mechanistic study in mice further supported this phenomenon by showing that mice fed with a high-fibre diet had delayed tumour growth compared with those provided with a low-fibre diet (Spencer et al. 2021). A high-fibre diet can enrich fibre-fermenting *Ruminococcaceae* in mice which is associated with increased intra-tumoral T lymphocytes infiltration and T cell activation in ICI-treated mice. Melanoma patients with high-fibre intake but no probiotics demonstrated enriched fibre-fermenting and butyrate-producing *Ruminococcaceae* family members and *Faecalibacterium* species (Spencer et al. 2021), which were reported to be associated with improved therapeutic response (Gopalakrishnan et al. 2018). Ketone diet is another way of dietary modulation which benefits the clinical outcome of ICIs (Ferrere et al. 2021). 3-hydroxybutyrate from ketone diet leads to increased CD8+ cells and restrained PD-L1 expression for T cell activation, contributing to enhanced immunotherapeutic responses (Ferrere et al. 2021). Other dietary modulations including caloric restriction and supplementation of micronutrients have also been shown to augment the anti-cancer immunity for cancer eradication in the context of ICIs (Wang et al. 2021; Pomatto-Watson et al. 2021).

17.4.2 Probiotics

From the aforementioned studies, several response-specific microbes have been identified. Researchers are investigating if it is possible to transplant a single microbe or a consortium of microbial species to enhance patients' response to ICIs. In preclinical models, probiotics have been shown to reduce Treg cell level, activate CD8+ T cell activation, and promote CD4+ T cell differentiation as well as NK cell intra-tumoral infiltration (Jacouton et al. 2017; Hu et al. 2015). As *Clostridium butyricum* is bifidogenic (Hagihara et al. 2020) and *Bifidobacterium* spp. could enhance the anti-cancer immunity induced by ICIs (Sivan et al. 2015; Matson et al. 2018), clinical studies have been done to investigate whether probiotics containing *Clostridium butyricum* could improve clinical response to ICIs. A retrospective study on NSCLC showed that patients receiving both ICIs and CBM588 (a live bacterial product containing *Clostridium butyricum*) had longer PFS and overall survival (Tomita et al. 2020). A recent prospective randomised phase 1 clinical trial further demonstrated that metastatic renal cell carcinoma patients receiving nivolumab-ipilimumab together with CBM588 had significantly longer PFS. Although statistical significance was not achieved, patients receiving CBM588 also had a higher response rate to ICIs (50% vs 20%) (Dizman et al. 2022). Despite the promising early evidence, caution should still be taken in using probiotics with ICIs. A recent study has demonstrated that the use of commercially available probiotics is associated with worse treatment outcomes in both animal models and human cohorts (Spencer et al. 2021). Potential risks of probiotics such as bacteraemia should also be considered especially in critically ill cancer patients (Yelin et al. 2019).

17.4.3 Antibiotics

Prophylactic antibiotics are commonly used to prevent life-threatening infections in cancer patients. However, as previously noted, broad-spectrum antibiotics can lead to dysbiosis, which is associated with worse outcomes of ICIs. Preclinical animal models (Vétizou et al. 2015; Sivan et al. 2015), retrospective (Derosa et al. 2018; Tinsley et al. 2020) and prospective (Pinato et al. 2019) clinical studies have observed the worse clinical outcomes of ICIs in patients receiving concurrent antibiotics. Notably, recent evidence has revealed that this is not always the case. Carefully selected antibiotics targeting pathogenic microbes may be possible to bolster the immunotherapeutic response of cancer patients. In mouse models of PDAC, intra-tumoral bacterial ablation using antibiotics could reprogramme the tumour microenvironment and protect against tumour growth. Intra-tumoral bacterial ablation has been shown to increase tumour protective M1 macrophage polarisation, infiltration of T helper cells and CTLs. PD-1 expression is also upregulated, suggesting potential synergistic effects of concurrent bacterial ablation and PD-1/PD-L1 blockade in cancer eradication. More advanced approaches, such as using bacteriophage to selectively modulate gut or tumour microbiota are also under investigation (Selle et al. 2020; Zheng et al. 2019). However, the development of these approaches is still in its infancy which is expected to expand and reshape the therapeutics landscape in immuno-oncology.

17.4.4 Faecal Microbiota Transplantation

FMT is probably the most drastic and effective approach to modulate gut microbial composition, which involves the transfer of the entire gut microbial community from a healthy donor to the recipient. The clinical application of FMT has already been demonstrated before, as it is an FDA-approved treatment for recurrent *Clostridium difficile* infection (Borody and Khoruts 2012). Two recent proof-of-concept clinical trials have shown that FMT is safe and effective in boosting immunotherapeutic response to PD-1 blockade in refractory metastatic melanoma patients (Baruch et al. 2021; Davar et al. 2021). Recipients with successful colonisation of gut microbes from donor microbiota showed enrichment of beneficial bacteria in gut such as *Ruminococcaceae* and *Bifidobacteriaceae*, which were previously shown to be associated with better immunotherapeutic outcomes. Recipients with improved response to ICIs after FMT also showed increased intra-tumoral infiltration of immune cells. The clinical application of FMT has also extended to mitigate the therapeutic toxicity of ICIs. Common ICI-induced irAEs such as enterocolitis are normally treated with immunosuppressive agents such as corticosteroids. Wang et al. reported the first case of using FMT to treat patients with ICI-induced enterocolitis who were refractory to conventional immunosuppressive therapy (Wang et al. 2018c). FMT has been shown to have promising effects in augmenting the efficacy and toxicity of ICIs. However, current studies are of pioneering nature, containing only cohorts with a small sample size. Future large-scale clinical trials are warranted to investigate further the effects of FMT on patients and its underlying mechanism of action.

17.5 Challenges and Future Prospects

Scientists and clinicians are searching for strategies to overcome the therapeutic resistance and toxicity of ICIs, which are the major stumbling blocks in immuno-oncology. Our understanding of the impacts of host microbiota on normal physiology and disease pathogenesis has evoked significantly over the past years. Given the current promising results, the gut and tumour microbial features are undeniably potential candidates for being both predictive biomarkers and intervention targets to optimise and personalise future cancer treatments. However, several important limitations have to be overcome before translating current findings into clinical application. These include the lack of consensus on the microbial features for being the predictive biomarkers, insufficient mechanistic understanding of the role of microbiota on cancer immunology, as well as the optimised methods for microbiota modulation.

First, large-cohort studies with deep functional investigations and standardised methodology are required to identify reliable microbial features for predicting treatment outcomes. Although a recent meta-analysis on previously published data identified a panel of response-specific species, no single species was fully consistent across all studies (Lee et al. 2022). This means that the identified panel of microbes is predictive of treatment response in some but not all cohorts. The role of microbiota in ICI response is complex. We should go beyond identifying the differentially abundant microbes and investigate deeper how microbes interact with different clinical predictors and biological factors. Factors affecting gut microbiota such as medication use, diet, and systemic inflammatory markers should be considered in future studies (Bhutiani and Wargo 2022). Multi-omics approaches, including metagenomics, meta-transcriptomics, and metabolomics, should also be used to study the multi-faceted actions of microbiota. Second, future microbiome studies should expand beyond bacteria. Existing studies on microbiota and ICIs mainly focus on the bacterial component. However, a recent study demonstrated the antagonistic effects between gut bacteria and fungi in the anti-cancer immune response triggered by radiotherapy (Shiao et al. 2021). Depletion of fungi was shown to improve radiotherapeutic effects while depletion of bacteria could lead to fungal overgrowth and poor treatment response (Shiao et al. 2021). Lastly, emerging technological advances such as capsule endoscopy for sampling the microbiome (Kalantar-Zadeh et al. 2018; Song and Shim 2016), artificial gut-on-a-chip models (Jalili-Firoozinezhad et al. 2019), and multi-omics profiling will enable researchers to study the microbiome along different regions of the gastrointestinal tract with in-depth functional investigation.

Despite the aforementioned challenges and limitations, our understanding of the microbiome has evoked tremendously over the last decade. We can foresee that apart from profiling of the tumour tissue for histopathology, genomic or proteomic alterations (such as HER2), and immune cell profiling (such as PD-L1 expression), microbiome profiling will be incorporated into personalised cancer care. With concerted efforts from scientists and clinicians, microbiota is expected to play an important role in immuno-oncology.

Funding This study was supported by National Key R&D Program of China (No. 2020YFA0509200/2020YFA0509203), RGC Theme-based Res Scheme Hong Kong (T21-705/20-N), RGC Collaborative Research Fund (C4039-19GF, C7065-18GF), RGC-GRF Hong Kong (14163817), Vice-Chancellor's Discretionary Fund Chinese University of Hong Kong.

References

Alexander JL, Wilson ID, Teare J, Marchesi JR, Nicholson JK, Kinross JM. Gut microbiota modulation of chemotherapy efficacy and toxicity. Nat Rev Gastroenterol Hepatol. 2017;14:356–65.

Andrews MC, Duong CPM, Gopalakrishnan V, et al. Gut microbiota signatures are associated with toxicity to combined CTLA-4 and PD-1 blockade. Nat Med. 2021;27:1432–41.

Baruch EN, Youngster I, Ben-Betzalel G, et al. Fecal microbiota transplant promotes response in immunotherapy-refractory melanoma patients. Science. 2021;371:602–9.

Bellmunt J, de Wit R, Vaughn DJ, et al. Pembrolizumab as second-line therapy for advanced urothelial carcinoma. N Engl J Med. 2017;376:1015–26.

Bessell CA, Isser A, Havel JJ, et al. Commensal bacteria stimulate antitumor responses via T cell cross-reactivity. JCI Insight. 2020;5(8):e135597. https://doi.org/10.1172/jci.insight.135597.

Bhutiani N, Wargo JA. Gut microbes as biomarkers of ICI response—sharpening the focus. Nat Rev Clin Oncol. 2022;19(8):495–6.

Borody TJ, Khoruts A. Fecal microbiota transplantation and emerging applications. Nat Rev Gastroenterol Hepatol. 2012;9:88–96.

Chaput N, Lepage P, Coutzac C, et al. Baseline gut microbiota predicts clinical response and colitis in metastatic melanoma patients treated with ipilimumab. Ann Oncol. 2017;28:1368–79.

Cohen EEW, Soulières D, Tourneau CL, et al. Pembrolizumab versus methotrexate, docetaxel, or cetuximab for recurrent or metastatic head-and-neck squamous cell carcinoma (KEYNOTE-040): a randomised, open-label, phase 3 study. Lancet. 2019;393:156–67.

Costea PI, Zeller G, Sunagawa S, et al. Towards standards for human fecal sample processing in metagenomic studies. Nat Biotechnol. 2017;35:1069–76.

Coutzac C, Jouniaux J-M, Paci A, et al. Systemic short chain fatty acids limit antitumor effect of CTLA-4 blockade in hosts with cancer. Nat Commun. 2020;11:2168.

Davar D, Dzutsev AK, McCulloch JA, et al. Fecal microbiota transplant overcomes resistance to anti–PD-1 therapy in melanoma patients. Science. 2021;371:595–602.

Derosa L, Hellmann MD, Spaziano M, et al. Negative association of antibiotics on clinical activity of immune checkpoint inhibitors in patients with advanced renal cell and non-small-cell lung cancer. Ann Oncol. 2018;29:1437–44.

Derosa L, Routy B, Thomas AM, et al. Intestinal Akkermansia muciniphila predicts clinical response to PD-1 blockade in patients with advanced non-small-cell lung cancer. Nat Med. 2022;28:315–24.

Dieu-Nosjean M-C, Antoine M, Danel C, et al. Long-term survival for patients with non–small-cell lung cancer with intratumoral lymphoid structures. JCO. 2008;26:4410–7.

Dizman N, Meza L, Bergerot P, et al. Nivolumab plus ipilimumab with or without live bacterial supplementation in metastatic renal cell carcinoma: a randomized phase 1 trial. Nat Med. 2022;28:704–12.

Dubin K, Callahan MK, Ren B, et al. Intestinal microbiome analyses identify melanoma patients at risk for checkpoint-blockade-induced colitis. Nat Commun. 2016;7:10391.

Ferrere G, Alou MT, Liu P, et al. Ketogenic diet and ketone bodies enhance the anticancer effects of PD-1 blockade. JCI Insight. 2021;6(2):e145207. https://doi.org/10.1172/jci.insight.145207.

Fluckiger A, Daillère R, Sassi M, et al. Cross-reactivity between tumor MHC class I–restricted antigens and an enterococcal bacteriophage. Science. 2020;369:936–42.

Frankel AE, Coughlin LA, Kim J, Froehlich TW, Xie Y, Frenkel EP, Koh AY. Metagenomic shotgun sequencing and unbiased metabolomic profiling identify specific human gut microbiota and metabolites associated with immune checkpoint therapy efficacy in melanoma patients. Neoplasia. 2017;19:848–55.

Fung TC, Olson CA, Hsiao EY. Interactions between the microbiota, immune and nervous systems in health and disease. Nat Neurosci. 2017;20:145–55.

Garon EB, Rizvi NA, Hui R, et al. Pembrolizumab for the treatment of non–small-cell lung cancer. N Engl J Med. 2015;372:2018–28.

Gharaibeh RZ, Jobin C. Microbiota and cancer immunotherapy: in search of microbial signals. Gut. 2019;68:385–8.
Gide TN, Wilmott JS, Scolyer RA, Long GV. Primary and acquired resistance to immune checkpoint inhibitors in metastatic melanoma. Clin Cancer Res. 2018;24:1260–70.
Gil-Cruz C, Perez-Shibayama C, Martin AD, et al. Microbiota-derived peptide mimics drive lethal inflammatory cardiomyopathy. Science. 2019;366:881–6.
Gonzalez H, Hagerling C, Werb Z. Roles of the immune system in cancer: from tumor initiation to metastatic progression. Genes Dev. 2018;32:1267–84.
Gopalakrishnan V, Spencer CN, Nezi L, et al. Gut microbiome modulates response to anti–PD-1 immunotherapy in melanoma patients. Science. 2018;359:97–103.
Greiling TM, Dehner C, Chen X, et al. Commensal orthologs of the human autoantigen Ro60 as triggers of autoimmunity in lupus. Sci Transl Med. 2018;10(434):eaan2306. https://doi.org/10.1126/scitranslmed.aan2306.
Hagihara M, Kuroki Y, Ariyoshi T, et al. Clostridium butyricum modulates the microbiome to protect intestinal barrier function in mice with antibiotic-induced dysbiosis. iScience. 2020;23:100772.
Herbst RS, Baas P, Kim D-W, et al. Pembrolizumab versus docetaxel for previously treated, PD-L1-positive, advanced non-small-cell lung cancer (KEYNOTE-010): a randomised controlled trial. Lancet. 2016;387:1540–50.
Hiam-Galvez KJ, Allen BM, Spitzer MH. Systemic immunity in cancer. Nat Rev Cancer. 2021;21:345–59.
Hodi FS, O'Day SJ, McDermott DF, et al. Improved survival with ipilimumab in patients with metastatic melanoma. N Engl J Med. 2010;363:711–23.
Hu J, Wang C, Ye L, Yang W, Huang H, Meng F, Shi S, Ding Z. Anti-tumour immune effect of oral administration of Lactobacillus plantarum to CT26 tumour-bearing mice. J Biosci. 2015;40:269–79.
Huang C-H, Shen C-C, Liang Y-C, Jan T-R. The probiotic activity of Lactobacillus murinus against food allergy. J Funct Foods. 2016;25:231–41.
Ianiro G, Rossi E, Thomas AM, et al. Faecal microbiota transplantation for the treatment of diarrhoea induced by tyrosine-kinase inhibitors in patients with metastatic renal cell carcinoma. Nat Commun. 2020;11:4333.
Jacouton E, Chain F, Sokol H, Langella P, Bermúdez-Humarán LG. Probiotic strain Lactobacillus casei BL23 prevents colitis-associated colorectal cancer. Front Immunol. 2017;8:1553.
Jalili-Firoozinezhad S, Gazzaniga FS, Calamari EL, et al. A complex human gut microbiome cultured in an anaerobic intestine-on-a-chip. Nat Biomed Eng. 2019;3:520–31.
Kalantar-Zadeh K, Berean KJ, Ha N, et al. A human pilot trial of ingestible electronic capsules capable of sensing different gases in the gut. Nat Electron. 2018;1:79–87.
Knight R, Vrbanac A, Taylor BC, et al. Best practices for analysing microbiomes. Nat Rev Microbiol. 2018;16:410–22.
Konig MF, Abusleme L, Reinholdt J, et al. Aggregatibacter actinomycetemcomitans–induced hypercitrullination links periodontal infection to autoimmunity in rheumatoid arthritis. Sci Transl Med. 2016;8:369ra176.
Lam KC, Goldszmid RS. Can gut microbes predict efficacy and toxicity of combined immune checkpoint blockade? Cancer Cell. 2021;39:1314–6.
Lau HCH, Sung JJ-Y, Yu J. Gut microbiota: impacts on gastrointestinal cancer immunotherapy. Gut Microbes. 2021;13:1–21.
Lee KA, Thomas AM, Bolte LA, et al. Cross-cohort gut microbiome associations with immune checkpoint inhibitor response in advanced melanoma. Nat Med. 2022;28:535–44.
Li Y, Tinoco R, Elmén L, et al. Gut microbiota dependent anti-tumor immunity restricts melanoma growth in Rnf5−/− mice. Nat Commun. 2019;10:1492.
Limeta A, Ji B, Levin M, Gatto F, Nielsen J. Meta-analysis of the gut microbiota in predicting response to cancer immunotherapy in metastatic melanoma. JCI Insight. 2020;5(23):e140940. https://doi.org/10.1172/jci.insight.140940.

Mager LF, Burkhard R, Pett N, et al. Microbiome-derived inosine modulates response to checkpoint inhibitor immunotherapy. Science. 2020;369:1481–9.

Mantovani A, Marchesi F, Malesci A, Laghi L, Allavena P. Tumour-associated macrophages as treatment targets in oncology. Nat Rev Clin Oncol. 2017;14:399–416.

Martins F, Sofiya L, Sykiotis GP, et al. Adverse effects of immune-checkpoint inhibitors: epidemiology, management and surveillance. Nat Rev Clin Oncol. 2019;16:563–80.

Matson V, Fessler J, Bao R, Chongsuwat T, Zha Y, Alegre M-L, Luke JJ, Gajewski TF. The commensal microbiome is associated with anti–PD-1 efficacy in metastatic melanoma patients. Science. 2018;359:104–8.

Michot JM, Bigenwald C, Champiat S, et al. Immune-related adverse events with immune checkpoint blockade: a comprehensive review. Eur J Cancer. 2016;54:139–48.

Palucka AK, Coussens LM. The basis of oncoimmunology. Cell. 2016;164:1233–47.

Pinato DJ, Howlett S, Ottaviani D, et al. Association of prior antibiotic treatment with survival and response to immune checkpoint inhibitor therapy in patients with cancer. JAMA Oncol. 2019;5:1774.

Pomatto-Watson LCD, Bodogai M, Bosompra O, et al. Daily caloric restriction limits tumor growth more effectively than caloric cycling regardless of dietary composition. Nat Commun. 2021;12:6201.

Pushalkar S, Hundeyin M, Daley D, et al. The pancreatic cancer microbiome promotes oncogenesis by induction of innate and adaptive immune suppression. Cancer Discov. 2018;8:403–16.

Qureshi OS, Zheng Y, Nakamura K, et al. Trans-endocytosis of CD80 and CD86: a molecular basis for the cell-extrinsic function of CTLA-4. Science. 2011;332:600–3.

Reck M, Rodríguez-Abreu D, Robinson AG, et al. Pembrolizumab versus chemotherapy for PD-L1–positive non–small-cell lung cancer. N Engl J Med. 2016;375:1823–33.

Rizvi ZA, Dalal R, Sadhu S, Kumar Y, Kumar S, Gupta SK, Tripathy MR, Rathore DK, Awasthi A. High-salt diet mediates interplay between NK cells and gut microbiota to induce potent tumor immunity. Sci Adv. 2021;7(37):eabg5016. https://doi.org/10.1126/sciadv.abg5016.

Roberti MP, Yonekura S, Duong CPM, et al. Chemotherapy-induced ileal crypt apoptosis and the ileal microbiome shape immunosurveillance and prognosis of proximal colon cancer. Nat Med. 2020;26:919–31.

Rooks MG, Garrett WS. Gut microbiota, metabolites and host immunity. Nat Rev Immunol. 2016;16:341–52.

Routy B, Chatelier EL, Derosa L, et al. Gut microbiome influences efficacy of PD-1–based immunotherapy against epithelial tumors. Science. 2018;359:91–7.

Schadendorf D, Hodi FS, Robert C, Weber JS, Margolin K, Hamid O, Patt D, Chen T-T, Berman DM, Wolchok JD. Pooled analysis of long-term survival data from phase II and phase III trials of ipilimumab in unresectable or metastatic melanoma. JCO. 2015;33:1889–94.

Selle K, Fletcher JR, Tuson H, et al. In vivo targeting of Clostridioides difficile using phage-delivered CRISPR-Cas3 antimicrobials. mBio. 2020;11:e00019–20.

Sender R, Fuchs S, Milo R. Revised estimates for the number of human and bacteria cells in the body. PLoS Biol. 2016;14:e1002533.

Sepich-Poore GD, Zitvogel L, Straussman R, Hasty J, Wargo JA, Knight R. The microbiome and human cancer. Science. 2021;371(6536):eabc4552. https://doi.org/10.1126/science.abc4552.

Shiao SL, Kershaw KM, Limon JJ, et al. Commensal bacteria and fungi differentially regulate tumor responses to radiation therapy. Cancer Cell. 2021;39:1202–1213.e6.

Shimasaki N, Jain A, Campana D. NK cells for cancer immunotherapy. Nat Rev Drug Discov. 2020;19:200–18.

Si W, Liang H, Bugno J, Xu Q, Ding X, Yang K, Fu Y, Weichselbaum RR, Zhao X, Wang L. Lactobacillus rhamnosus GG induces cGAS/STING- dependent type I interferon and improves response to immune checkpoint blockade. Gut. 2022;71(3):521–33. https://doi.org/10.1136/gutjnl-2020-323426.

Sivan A, Corrales L, Hubert N, et al. Commensal Bifidobacterium promotes antitumor immunity and facilitates anti–PD-L1 efficacy. Science. 2015;350:1084–9.

Song HJ, Shim K-N. Current status and future perspectives of capsule endoscopy. Intest Res. 2016;14:21–9.
Spencer CN, McQuade JL, Gopalakrishnan V, et al. Dietary fiber and probiotics influence the gut microbiome and melanoma immunotherapy response. Science. 2021;374:1632–40.
Sun S, Luo L, Liang W, et al. Bifidobacterium alters the gut microbiota and modulates the functional metabolism of T regulatory cells in the context of immune checkpoint blockade. PNAS. 2020;117:27509–15.
Tanoue T, Morita S, Plichta DR, et al. A defined commensal consortium elicits CD8 T cells and anti-cancer immunity. Nature. 2019;565:600–5.
Ting NL-N, Lau HC-H, Yu J. Cancer pharmacomicrobiomics: targeting microbiota to optimise cancer therapy outcomes. Gut. 2022;71:1412–25.
Tinsley N, Zhou C, Tan G, et al. Cumulative antibiotic use significantly decreases efficacy of checkpoint inhibitors in patients with advanced cancer. Oncologist. 2020;25:55–63.
Tomita Y, Ikeda T, Sakata S, et al. Association of probiotic Clostridium butyricum therapy with survival and response to immune checkpoint blockade in patients with lung cancer. Cancer Immunol Res. 2020;8:1236–42.
Verma R, Lee C, Jeun E-J, et al. Cell surface polysaccharides of Bifidobacterium bifidum induce the generation of Foxp3+ regulatory T cells. Sci Immunol. 2018;3(28):eaat6975. https://doi.org/10.1126/sciimmunol.aat6975.
Vétizou M, Pitt JM, Daillère R, et al. Anticancer immunotherapy by CTLA-4 blockade relies on the gut microbiota. Science. 2015;350:1079–84.
Waldman AD, Fritz JM, Lenardo MJ. A guide to cancer immunotherapy: from T cell basic science to clinical practice. Nat Rev Immunol. 2020;20:651–68.
Wang DY, Salem J-E, Cohen JV, et al. Fatal toxic effects associated with immune checkpoint inhibitors: a systematic review and meta-analysis. JAMA Oncol. 2018a;4:1721–8.
Wang F, Yin Q, Chen L, Davis MM. Bifidobacterium can mitigate intestinal immunopathology in the context of CTLA-4 blockade. Proc Natl Acad Sci U S A. 2018b;115:157–61.
Wang Y, Wiesnoski DH, Helmink BA, et al. Fecal microbiota transplantation for refractory immune checkpoint inhibitor-associated colitis. Nat Med. 2018c;24:1804–8.
Wang T, Gnanaprakasam JNR, Chen X, et al. Inosine is an alternative carbon source for CD8 + -T-cell function under glucose restriction. Nat Metab. 2020;2:635–47.
Wang Y, Wang F, Wang L, et al. NAD+ supplement potentiates tumor-killing function by rescuing defective TUB-mediated NAMPT transcription in tumor-infiltrated T cells. Cell Rep. 2021;36(6):109516. https://doi.org/10.1016/j.celrep.2021.109516.
Wei SC, Anang N-AAS, Sharma R, et al. Combination anti–CTLA-4 plus anti–PD-1 checkpoint blockade utilizes cellular mechanisms partially distinct from monotherapies. Proc Natl Acad Sci. 2019;116:22699–709.
Wherry EJ, Kurachi M. Molecular and cellular insights into T cell exhaustion. Nat Rev Immunol. 2015;15:486–99.
Wong CW, Yost SE, Lee JS, Gillece JD, Folkerts M, Reining L, Highlander SK, Eftekhari Z, Mortimer J, Yuan Y. Analysis of gut microbiome using explainable machine learning predicts risk of Diarrhea associated with tyrosine kinase inhibitor neratinib: a pilot study. Front Oncol. 2021;11:604584. https://doi.org/10.3389/fonc.2021.604584.
Yelin I, Flett KB, Merakou C, et al. Genomic and epidemiological evidence of bacterial transmission from probiotic capsule to blood in ICU patients. Nat Med. 2019;25:1728–32.
Zheng D-W, Dong X, Pan P, Chen K-W, Fan J-X, Cheng S-X, Zhang X-Z. Phage-guided modulation of the gut microbiota of mouse models of colorectal cancer augments their responses to chemotherapy. Nat Biomed Eng. 2019;3:717–28.

Chapter 18
Gut Microbiota in Coronavirus Disease 2019

Harry Cheuk-Hay Lau and Jun Yu

Abstract Coronavirus disease 2019 (COVID-19) pandemic has changed the globe ever since its first appearance in December 2019. It is an acute respiratory illness caused by severe acute respiratory syndrome coronavirus 2 (SARS-CoV-2), and over 540 million people have contracted COVID-19 as of mid-2022. For COVID-19 patients, gastrointestinal symptoms including anorexia and diarrhoea are frequently occurred, implicating the involvement of gut microbiota in the pathogenesis of COVID-19. Indeed, accumulating evidence has reported the association of altered microbiota with SARS-CoV-2 infection, disease severity, and post-acute COVID-19 syndrome. In this chapter, the roles of gut microbiota in COVID-19 as well as its mechanistic interplays with host after SARS-CoV-2 infection are explored. Given its importance to this disease, approaches to restore the altered microbiota may be utilised as potential treatments of COVID-19. Hence, different strategies to modulate the microbiota including dietary intervention, prebiotics, and probiotics against SARS-CoV-2 infection are also discussed.

Keywords COVID-19 · Gut microbiota · Microbiota modulation

18.1 Introduction

It is no doubt that Coronavirus disease 2019 (COVID-19), an acute respiratory illness caused by novel severe acute respiratory syndrome coronavirus 2 (SARS-CoV-2), has changed the globe since December 2019. As of early July 2022, over 540 million people have contracted COVID-19 with over 6.3 million deaths

H. C.-H. Lau · J. Yu (✉)
Institute of Digestive Disease, Department of Medicine and Therapeutics, State Key Laboratory of Digestive Disease, Li Ka Shing Institute of Health Sciences, CUHK Shenzhen Research Institute, Prince of Wales Hospital, The Chinese University of Hong Kong, Hong Kong, China
e-mail: junyu@cuhk.edu.hk

J. Yu (ed.), *Microbiome in Gastrointestinal Cancer*,
https://doi.org/10.1007/978-981-19-4492-5_18

globally (https://coronavirus.jhu.edu/map.html). Typical presentations of this infection include fever, cough, fatigue, pneumonia, and loss of taste or smell (Huang et al. 2020). Different variants of SARS-CoV-2 such as Alpha (B.1.1.7), Beta (B.1.351), Gamma (P.1), and Delta (B.1.617.2) have emerged since the pandemic. To date, Omicron (B.1.1529) is the most dominant variant of SARS-CoV-2 which is most likely attributed to its extremely high infectivity, thereby supporting its rapid transmission among populations (Shuai et al. 2022). Fortunately, lots of evidence has reported that patients infected with Omicron have lower severity and less symptoms in the lung airways, compared to Delta or other previous variants. The risk of severe outcomes including death following infection was also found to be significantly lower for Omicron than for Delta (Nyberg et al. 2022).

Although being relatively less common, gastrointestinal symptoms including anorexia, diarrhoea, vomiting, and abdominal discomfort were reported to occur in approximate 18% of COVID-19 patients (Cheung et al. 2020). Indeed, virus RNA was detected in faecal samples of up to 50% of COVID-19 patients, implicating the presence of gastrointestinal infection (Cheung et al. 2020). Gastrointestinal symptoms could also occur before the appearance of any respiratory conditions, thus indicating the viral involvement in the gastrointestinal tract during SARS-CoV-2 infection (Kotfis and Skonieczna-Zydecka 2020). Given that human gastrointestinal tract is full of commensal microbes, these findings therefore suggested that gut microbes may have close links with these symptoms and contribute to COVID-19 pathogenesis. In this chapter, the role of gut microbiota in SARS-CoV-2 infection is explored. Approaches to modulate the microbiota including dietary intervention, prebiotics, and probiotics as potential therapeutics against COVID-19 are also discussed.

18.2 SARS-CoV-2 Infection and Gut Microbiota

18.2.1 Gut Dysbiosis and COVID-19 Severity

Human gastrointestinal tract harbours trillions of microbes with bacteria being the most predominant taxonomic kingdom (about 93% of total microbial DNA), following by viruses and fungi (Shkoporov and Hill 2019). Together, these commensal microbes form an ecological community known as the gut microbiota. In healthy or non-disease condition, the composition of gut microbiota is maintained to achieve intestinal homeostasis with balanced abundance between beneficial commensals and opportunistic pathobionts. Whereas pathogenic alterations in the gut microbiota (commonly termed as dysbiosis) have been associated with various human diseases, especially inflammatory bowel disease and colorectal cancer.

In SARS-CoV-2 infection, microbial diversity was found to be decreased in faecal samples of patients and accompanied by the enrichment of opportunistic pathobionts including *Clostridium hathewayi* and *Ruminococcus* species (Ren et al. 2021;

Yeoh et al. 2021; Zuo et al. 2020). Through performing faecal metagenomic sequencing, two studies reported that several beneficial commensals such as *Faecalibacterium prausnitzii* and *Eubacterium rectale* were depleted in patients with COVID-19 (Yeoh et al. 2021; Zuo et al. 2020). *F. prausnitzii* which is a major producer of short-chain fatty acids (SCFAs; crucial for maintaining intestinal homeostasis) in the gut and has anti-inflammatory potential via inducing IL-10 production (Alameddine et al. 2019) was depleted in patients with COVID-19 and had inverse correlation with disease severity. In contrast, *C. hathewayi* and *Clostridium ramosum*, two species that are well acknowledged for their associations with bacteraemia and inflammation, were positively correlated to COVID-19 severity. Another study revealed that faecal samples with high SARS-CoV-2 infectivity were enriched with opportunistic pathogenic bacteria (e.g. *Collinsella* species, *Morganella morganii*) with reduced abundance of SCFA-producing bacteria (e.g. *Parabacteroides merdae, Lachnospiraceae bacterium*), compared to samples with low SARS-CoV-2 viral infectivity (Zuo et al. 2021). Moreover, faecal samples of deceased patients with COVID-19 were also identified to be enriched with pathobionts (e.g. *Enterococcus*) with significantly lower abundance of SCFAs and anti-inflammatory microbes (e.g. *Bifidobacterium, Ruminococcus*) than faeces retrieved from COVID-19 patients with mild or moderate severity (Albrich et al. 2022). Altogether, these findings indicate that gut dysbiosis with enrichment of pathogenic bacteria and depletion of beneficial commensals is closely related to the disease severity of COVID-19.

18.2.2 Persistent Dysbiosis after SARS-CoV-2 Clearance

Apart from acute infection caused by SARS-CoV-2, it is common for infected patients to have long-term complications. A study reported that persistent symptoms known as the post-acute COVID-19 syndrome (PACS) were observed in more than 80% of COVID-19 patients after viral clearance, and some individuals even developed multisystem inflammation (Carfi et al. 2020). Although the cause for persistent symptoms after viral clearance could be varied among individuals, numerous evidence has illustrated the potential contribution of gut dysbiosis to PACS. For instance, the gut microbiota between recovered COVID-19 patients and healthy adults was found to be markedly different, of which dysbiosis could persist over 30 days after disease resolution (Yeoh et al. 2021; Zuo et al. 2020). Infectious bacteria such as *Bifidobacterium dentium* and *Klebsiella pneumoniae* were enriched in recovered patients, whilst the anti-inflammatory *F. prausnitzii* was depleted (Ren et al. 2021; Yeoh et al. 2021; Zuo et al. 2020, 2021). Moreover, two independent studies longitudinally monitored the microbial alterations in patients with COVID-19, and their consistent results identified that the composition of gut microbiota was still not restored after 6 months of viral clearance (Chen et al. 2022; Liu et al. 2022). Particularly, the gut microbiota of patients with PACS was associated with the enrichment of opportunistic pathobionts *Ruminococcus gnavus* and *Bacteroides vulgatus*, while the depletion of beneficial *F. prausnitzii* was once again characterised in PACS patients (Liu et al. 2022). In general, prolonged dysbiosis in COVID-19 patients despite viral clearance may contribute to persistent illness of which secondary invasion of bacterial pathogens and reduction of beneficial commensals may become paramount for complete disease resolution.

18.2.3 Mechanistic Link Between SARS-CoV-2 Infection and Gut Microbiota

Pathogenesis starts with the interaction between SARS-CoV-2 and the viral entry receptor, angiotensin-converting enzyme (ACE)-2. ACE2 is a membrane-bound protein with high expression in intestinal enterocytes, and it is a crucial regulator of dietary amino acid homeostasis, microbial ecology, and innate immunity (Hashimoto et al. 2012). ACE2 also works with its countering opponent ACE to control the Renin–Angiotensin System (RAS; mediator of fluid and electrolyte balance). During infection, ACE2 is hijacked to become a receptor of SARS-CoV-2 which allows the viruses to undergo replication and initiate infection (Shang et al. 2020; Lamers et al. 2020; Zhou et al. 2020; Zang et al. 2020). This viral-mediated reduction of ACE2 causes the accumulation of its ligand angiotensin II and the imbalance of RAS, leading to increased intestinal permeability and impaired gut barrier, all of which are features of the so-called leaky gut syndrome (Penninger et al. 2021). As a consequence, bacteria and endotoxins (e.g. lipopolysaccharides) have easier access to the systemic circulation through the disrupted gut barrier, thereby contributing to exaggerated cytokine production and eventually triggering endotoxemia and inflammation. Meanwhile, SARS-CoV-2 infection also affects the composition of gut microbiota as aforementioned. The enrichment of bacterial pathogens and depletion of beneficial commensals in the dysbiotic microbiota could result in immunomodulation and local inflammation. For example, both *F. prausnitzii* and *E. rectale* were found to have negative association with the pro-inflammatory cytokines CXCL10 and TNF-α (Yeoh et al. 2021), implicating their anti-inflammatory potential against SARS-CoV-2 infection. Interestingly, several studies reported that SARS-CoV-2 infection could reduce local inflammation in the gut, while hospitalised COVID-19 patients with gastrointestinal symptoms were benefited from significant reduction in disease severity (Livanos et al. 2021). These findings therefore indicate the potential of gastrointestinal tract as well as the gut microbiota in attenuating symptoms of COVID-19.

Besides microbes themselves, SARS-CoV-2 infection can also affect the profile of gut metabolites, the intermediate or end products of microbes-mediated metabolism. For instance, patients with COVID-19 were found to have increased levels of guanosine and its derivatives 8-hydroxydeoxyguanosine which are involved in the upregulation of oxidative DNA damage and cytokine production (Zuo et al. 2021).

Glycolysis and its intermediate product L-serine were also increased in patients with COVID-19, of which pathogenic bacteria could catabolise L-serine to confer growth advantage against other bacterial competitors in the inflamed gut (Kitamoto et al. 2020). In addition, given the significant depletion of SCFA-producing bacteria particularly *F. prausnitzii* after viral infection, the synthesis of anti-inflammatory SCFAs is inevitably reduced, further contributing to persistent inflammation. Collectively, SARS-CoV-2 invades intestinal enterocytes via ACE2 and alters the gut microbiota and their metabolites, consequently leading to impaired barrier function, bacterial translocation into the circulation, and eventually aggravated systemic inflammation and multiple-organ involvement (Fig. 18.1).

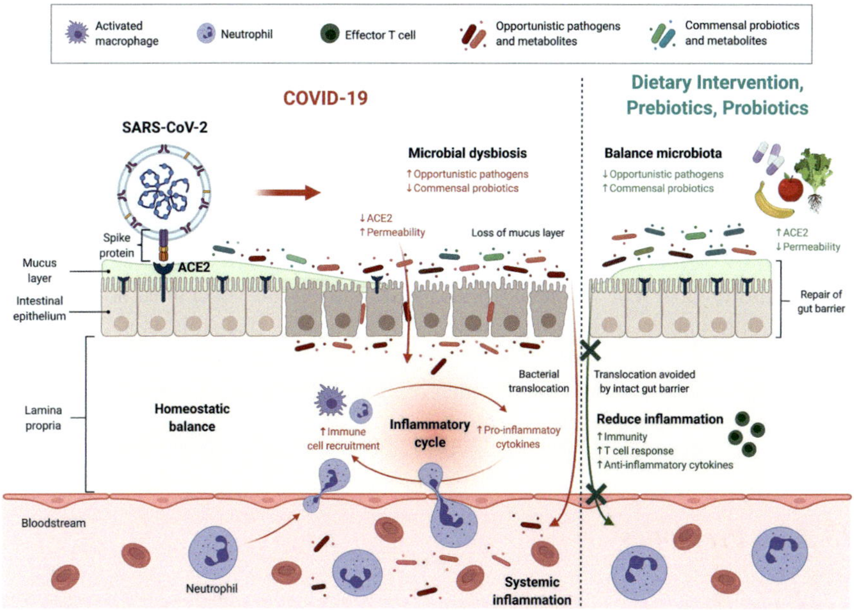

Fig. 18.1 The mechanism of SARS-CoV-2 infection in human gut. Infection begins with the binding of SARS-CoV-2 to ACE2 expressed in the membrane of intestinal epithelial cells. Enrichment of opportunistic pathogens (e.g. *Clostridium hathewayi*) and depletion of commensal probiotics (e.g. *Faecalibacterium prausnitzii*) occur after viral infection. Reduced ACE2 leads to increased permeability of gut barrier and impaired mucus layer. Pathogens and harmful metabolites (e.g. guanosine, L-serine) can therefore have easier access to the systemic circulation, contributing to inflammation with overproduction of pro-inflammatory cytokines (e.g. CXCL10, TNFα). Dietary intervention, prebiotics, and probiotics can restore the gut microbiota and replenish the loss of ACE2 upon SARS-CoV-2 infection. These facilitate the repair of gut barrier thus reducing bacterial translocation and alleviating inflammation. The growth of probiotics and synthesis of beneficial metabolites (e.g. SCFAs) can also be stimulated, thereby hastening recovery. (Figure was adopted in agreement with Lau et al. 2022)

18.3 Therapeutic Microbiota Modulation Against COVID-19

18.3.1 Dietary Intervention

Dietary intervention has long been a convenient and safe approach against various diseases, of which dietary nutrients are capable of preventing disease and reducing disease severity. For patients with COVID-19, acute inflammation is occurred accompanied with excess production of pro-inflammatory cytokines, suggesting that intake of nutrients with anti-inflammatory and anti-oxidant effects may fasten disease recovery. Indeed, several dietary components involving omega-3 polyunsaturated fatty acids, vitamins, zinc, plant-based polyphenols (e.g. flavonoids and phenolic acids), polysaccharides, and a panoply of herbs from traditional Chinese medicine, were reported to be beneficial to COVID-19 patients (Iddir et al. 2020). On the other hand, dietary fibres are known to be protective against gut barrier disruption which can restrict bacterial translocation into the systemic circulation, whereas diets with high fat and protein contents are associated with mucosal barrier dysfunction (Camilleri et al. 2019). A multi-centre retrospective study with more than 7300 subjects found that the disease outcome of COVID-19 patients with pre-existing type 2 diabetes who are expected to have increased mortality rate could be improved by well-controlled blood glucose (Zhu et al. 2020). These data highlight the feasibility of a low glycaemic index diet with green vegetables and fruits to improve outcome in hospitalised patients. Hence, it is plausible that COVID-19 patients can benefit from strengthened immunity and reduced inflammation and oxidative stress via appropriate dietary intervention, thereby alleviating disease severity and accelerating recovery.

18.3.2 Prebiotics

Prebiotics refer to a group of dietary fibres such as fructans and galactans that can only be digested by gut commensal microbes but not the host. These prebiotics can stimulate the growth of probiotics for health benefits. For instance, plant-based fibres promote the growth of probiotics *Lactobacillus* and *Bifidobacterium*, meanwhile limiting the expansion of *Clostridium* or other opportunistic pathogenic bacteria (Iddir et al. 2020). In general, many prebiotic fibres are metabolised and degraded by gut microbes to generate SCFAs (e.g. acetate, propionate, and butyrate) as end products. SCFAs are immunomodulatory metabolites capable of enhancing effector activities of B cells and $CD8^+$ T cells (Trompette et al. 2018) and producing anti-inflammatory cytokines (Alameddine et al. 2019). Given the importance of SCFAs, dietary prebiotics have been considered as a crucial initiator of SCFA synthesis by promoting the growth of SCFA-producing bacteria. *F. prausnitzii* is a key producer of SCFAs but its depletion in COVID-19 patients has been consistently reported in multiple studies (Yeoh et al. 2021; Zuo et al. 2020). To restore its abundance, different nutrients derived from plant-based fibres were identified to have the ability to stimulate the growth of *F. prausnitzii* (Benus et al. 2010), thereby rebalancing the dysbiotic microbiota and dysregulated metabolites in the gut. Nevertheless, it is noteworthy to pinpoint that there is still a lack of interventional studies to demonstrate the therapeutic efficacy of supplementing prebiotics or other dietary nutrients to patients with COVID-19 (Xavier-Santos et al. 2022). Based on the current evidence, it is most likely that dietary and prebiotic intervention may act as an adjunct to current therapeutics against SARS-CoV-2 infection.

18.3.3 Probiotics

Probiotic supplementation is one of the most well acknowledged approaches of microbiota modulation to confer health benefits. Administrating probiotics particularly *Lactobacillus* or *Bifidobacterium* has long been associated with a variety of beneficial effects such as improvement of immunity and restoration of microbial balance. For example, a commercially used strain of *Lactobacillus rhamnosus* could promote T cell-mediated immune response in pneumococcal-infected mice (Barbieri et al. 2017) and alleviate symptoms of acute respiratory infection in children (Laursen and Hojsak 2018). For SARS-CoV-2 infection, increasing interests have emerged to use probiotics as a therapeutic strategy. Although there is very few evidence reporting the efficacy of probiotics for COVID-19 management, several trials using a single strain or a cocktail of probiotics to reduce COVID-19 severity and/or improve treatment efficacy are in progress (Table 18.1). Results of an open-label pilot study (NCT04950803) showed that oral supplementation of a probiotic formula (SIM01) for 4 weeks that aims to replenish depleted microbial species caused by SARS-CoV-2 infection, could hasten recovery, enhance immunity, and suppress serum pro-inflammatory cytokines in hospitalised COVID-19 patients accompanied with the enrichment of gut beneficial bacteria (Zhang et al. 2021). Meanwhile, therapeutic approaches that target ACE2 to restore RAS balance such as ACE inhibitors are also rapidly being developed and tested in clinical trials (Penninger et al. 2021). ACE2 could interact with gut microbes, as evidenced by the positive correlation between ACE2 expression and microbial alterations in patients with COVID-19 (Zuo et al. 2020). These findings therefore suggest the feasibility of combining pharmacological agents with probiotics against SARS-CoV-2 infection. Caution is however needed as these drugs can also upregulate ACE2 expression and may enhance viral entry into host cells (Sanders et al. 2020). To address this concern, soluble recombinant human ACE2 (rhACE2) has been emerged which can act as a competitive interceptor by binding the viral spike proteins to neutralise SARS-CoV-2, and also minimise organ injuries by rebalancing RAS and lowering circulatory concentration of angiotensin II (Penninger et al. 2021; Zoufaly et al. 2020). Interestingly, bioengineering a probiotic species *Lactobacillus paracasei* into a live vector for oral delivery of rhACE2 showed positive outcome in mice, and this approach may facilitate large-scale production of high-quality ACE2 with sufficient bioavailability in the future (Verma et al. 2019).

Table 18.1 Ongoing clinical studies of gut microbiota regarding to COVID-19[a]

Study type	Trial ID and phase[b]	Main aim	Country	Estimated participants
Observational	NCT04770649 Phase: N/A	Influence of microbiota and its function on immune system and efficacy of COVID-19 vaccine	United States	10,000
Observational	NCT04359836 Phase: N/A	Change in faecal microbiota of COVID-19 patients	United States	250
Observational	NCT04669938 Phase: N/A	Microbiota of COVID-19 patients in ICU for outcome prediction of disease severity	France	200
Observational	NCT05178238 Phase: N/A	Microbiota in COVID-19 patients with different viral loads	France	200
Observational	NCT04913142 Phase: N/A	Oral and faecal microbiota of ICU patients with or without SARS-CoV-2 infection	France	60
Observational	NCT04497402 Phase: N/A	Sex difference in microbiota of COVID-19 patients	Italy	88
Observational	NCT05150834 Phase: N/A	Change in faecal microbiota after COVID-19 vaccination	Korea	53
Interventional	NCT04941703 Phase: 1 and 2	Efficacy of combining magnesium citrate with probiotics in hospitalised COVID-19 patients Dose: 296 mL magnesium citrate + probiotics twice daily for 6 days or until discharge	United States	30
Interventional	NCT05227170 Phase: N/A	Efficacy of probiotic *Lactobacillus plantarum* 299v against PACS Dose: 2×10^9 CFU of Lp299v daily for 8 weeks	United States	80
Interventional	NCT04884776 Phase: N/A	Efficacy of a microbiome immunity formula to improve immune functions, reduce adverse events associated with COVID-19 vaccinations, and reduce hospitalisation in vulnerable subjects (patients with underlying type 2 DM and elderlies) Dose: 1×10^9 CFU of 3 *Bifidobacteria* and 3 prebiotics twice daily for 12 weeks	Hong Kong	484
Interventional	NCT04950803 Phase: N/A	Efficacy of an oral microbiome immunity formula to enhance immunity and reduce long-term complications in patients recovered from COVID-19 Dose: 1×10^9 CFU of 3 *Bifidobacteria* and 3 prebiotics daily for 3 months	Hong Kong	280

Table 18.1 (continued)

Study type	Trial ID and phase[b]	Main aim	Country	Estimated participants
Interventional	NCT04730284 Phase: N/A	Efficacy of a synbiotic formula in hospitalised COVID-19 patients Dose: 4 g tailored-made synbiotics daily for 28 days	Hong Kong	20
Interventional	NCT04813718 Phase: N/A	Efficacy of a mixture of prebiotics and probiotics Omni-Biotic Pro Vi 5 against post-COVID-19 syndrome Dose: N/A	Austria	20
Interventional	NCT04666116 Phase: N/A	Efficacy of nutritional supplement by nasopharyngeal smear to decrease viral load in hospitalised COVID-19 patients Dose: Supplement of mixture of probiotics (*Bifidobacterium longum*, *Bifidobacterium animalis* subsp. *lactis*, and *Lactobacillus rhamnosus*), vitamin D, zinc, and selenium	Spain	96
Interventional	NCT04922918 Phase: N/A	Impact of probiotics on preventing SARS-CoV-2 infection in elderly living in a nursing home Dose: 1×10^9 CFU of *Ligilactobacillus salivarius* MP101 daily for 4 months	Spain	25
Interventional	NCT04979065 Phase: N/A	Impact of a mixture of probiotics and vitamin D on preventing SARS-CoV-2 infection in obese people Dose: Supplement twice daily for 3 months	Indonesia	80
Interventional	NCT04486482 Phase: N/A	Efficacy of a glycan KB109 in COVID-19 patients in the outpatient setting Dose: KB109 for 35 days	United States	50

ICU intensive care unit

[a] The search was conducted on clinicaltrials.gov in July 2022. Completed, not yet recruiting, suspended or terminated trials were excluded

[b] FDA definitions of clinical trial phases

Although microbiota modulation could potentially be a therapeutic strategy, its efficacy remains relatively unsatisfactory and increasing evidence has suggested that microbiota modulation may be more effective as adjuvants of current treatment options. Indeed, several studies reported moderate efficacy of probiotics against acute respiratory infection, whereas probiotics as adjuvants may improve clinical outcomes (Suez et al. 2019). Currently, there are multiple clinical studies investigating the efficacy of probiotic supplementation in patients with COVID-19. Researchers in Austria are evaluating the efficacy of probiotic mixture to alleviate gastrointestinal symptoms in hospitalised COVID-19 patients (NCT04420676) and complications after discharge (NCT04813718). Combined use of prebiotics and probiotics in hospitalised COVID-19 patients is being studied by researchers in Spain (NCT04666116) and Hong Kong (NCT04730284). Studies are also ongoing to investigate whether probiotics can lower risk of SARS-CoV-2 infection by boosting immunity in uninfected elderly subjects (NCT04922918) and obese individuals (NCT04979065). Clinical studies targeting the gut microbiota as therapeutics in COVID-19 are summarised in Table 18.1.

18.3.4 Faecal Microbiota Transplantation

Faecal microbiota transplantation (FMT), also known as the stool transplant, is a therapeutic approach to modulate the gut microbiota by transferring faecal microbes from a non-disease individual (i.e. donor) into another individual (i.e. recipient). To date, FMT is the first-line treatment for recurrent *Clostridioides difficile* infection, whereas its application against other diseases including inflammatory bowel disease and colorectal cancer is being heavily investigated. For SARS-CoV-2 infection, a case report with two subjects reported that faecal microbiota transplantation (FMT) was safe for patients with recurrent *C. difficile* infection and coexisting COVID-19 (Bilinski et al. 2022), and might have a role in accelerating recovery. A larger clinical trial to examine the role of FMT in COVID-19 is now in progress (NCT04824222). Importantly, SARS-CoV-2 could be present in faecal samples of asymptomatic individuals which would be potentially transmitted and infected the recipient. Vigilant donor screening and SARS-CoV-2 testing are therefore highly recommended to perform in all donors to ensure the safety of FMT during the COVID-19 pandemic (Ianiro et al. 2020).

18.4 Future Directions

At the society level, the long-lasting COVID-19 pandemic has dramatically upended daily lives. Current pandemic control measures and practices are expected to have substantial and potentially long-term effects on the human microbiota across the globe, given strict implementation of hygiene measures, physical separation, and other measures that influence overall microbial diversity. Several studies reported that SARS-CoV-2-infected women have higher rate of caesarean sections. Initial recommendations also discouraged infected mothers from breastfeeding and participating in skin-to-skin care, all of which would undoubtedly affect the golden period of microbiota development in early life. Hence, infection control measures must be balanced with strategies that promote microbial diversity to impart optimal health outcomes and potentially modulate susceptibility of children to COVID-19.

At the individual level, the World Health Organisation (WHO) has proposed a shift from western-style diet with high contents of fats and sugars to a well-balanced and diversified diet. This is of great importance especially in elderly subjects and those with cardiovascular disease, type 2 diabetes, or other chronic diseases who would suffer from poorer outcomes with SARS-CoV-2 infection. Intake of adequate and diversified nutrients is recommended to avoid malnutrition and maintain immune homeostasis in these high-risk individuals (Volkert et al. 2019). A well-balanced diet can also benefit the gut microbiota with the enrichment of probiotics (e.g. *Lactobacillus, Bifidobacterium,* and *Streptococcus thermophilus*) and SCFAs, meanwhile lowering the abundance of opportunistic pathobionts (De Filippis et al. 2016). Notably, whether modulating the gut microbiota with dietary intervention can reduce susceptibility of SARS-CoV-2 infection and severity warrants prospective studies.

At the hospital level, antibiotics are widely prescribed to patients with COVID-19 of which up to three quarters of patients received empirical antibiotics to prevent bacterial co-infection, even though co-infection was identified in less than 5% of patients (Vaughn et al. 2021). Similarly, other studies have reported no difference in outcomes with or without the use of antibiotics in hospitalised COVID-19 patients (Yeoh et al. 2021; Zuo et al. 2020), hence indicating that antibiotics could be unessential against SARS-CoV-2 infection. Meanwhile, antibiotics could greatly alter the gut microbiota which may bring detrimental impacts to patients with COVID-19. Indeed, the gut microbiota in antibiotic-treated patients displayed further depletion of beneficial commensals including *F. prausnitzii, E. rectale*, and *L. bacterium* compared to patients without antibiotics. Caution is therefore needed when prescribing antibiotics as unnecessary use of antibiotics can cause more severe gut dysbiosis with greater depletion of beneficial bacteria as well as increased antimicrobial resistance. In a WHO guidance for COVID-19 clinical management (https://www.who.int/publications/i/item/WHO-2019-nCoV-clinical-2021-1), antibiotic therapy or prophylaxis is not recommended in patients with mild or moderate COVID-19 unless there is evidence or suspicion of bacterial infection. In addition, longer follow-up of recovered COVID-19 patients up to 12 months is needed to address questions related to the duration of dysbiosis after recovery, link between dysbiosis and PACS, and whether dysbiosis or enrichment/depletion of gut microbes predisposes recovered individuals to future health issues.

To date, although there are lots of clinical studies revealing the importance of gut microbiota in COVID-19 pathogenesis and severity, these findings are mostly derived from descriptive and associative human studies without in-depth functional investigations. Extensive mechanistic studies are required to uncover the causal relationship between the gut microbiota and SARS-CoV-2 infection. Animal experiment is the fundamental tool for mechanistic investigation of human diseases. However, mouse model that can accurately mimic SARS-CoV-2 infection in humans has been lacking. While some articles infected a transgenic mouse model expressing human ACE2 (namely K18-hACE2) with SARS-CoV-2 to assess drug efficacy (Alvarado et al. 2021) or dysbiosis-associated bacteraemia (Venzon et al. 2021), to what extent these mice can replicate viral infection in humans needs further validation. Moreover, current clinical data supporting the use of probiotics against SARS-CoV-2 infection are scarce, and numerous issues including determination of optimal strain(s), dosing regimen, and duration of intervention remain to be solved. To address these challenges, supplementing probiotics to preclinical animal models could be feasible for deciphering the efficacy and underlying mechanism, and these findings may potentially facilitate the application of probiotics in COVID-19 patients.

At the global level, vaccination has been the most effective and common way to reduce the severity of SARS-CoV-2 infection. Yet, it remains controversial how long immunity lasts from SARS-CoV-2 vaccines, and scientists around the world are racing to determine what level of neutralising antibodies or immune markers has the closest relationship to the effectiveness of COVID-19 vaccine. Recently, the gut microbiota was suggested to influence vaccine efficacy, as evidenced by the significant impairment of antibody response in healthy subjects receiving antibiotics prior to H1N1 influenza vaccination (Hagan et al. 2019). Similarly, it is most likely that the gut microbiota also plays an essential role in SARS-CoV-2 vaccine immune response and vaccine-related adverse effects. Indeed, a clinical study revealed the significant enrichment of probiotic *Bifidobacterium adolescentis* in vaccine recipients with high neutralising antibodies (Ng et al. 2022). The results also identified that *Prevotella copri* and two *Megamonas* species were enriched in recipients with fewer adverse events, indicating that these microbes may have anti-inflammatory role in host immune response. Meanwhile, a large population-based study in the United States is currently recruiting up to 10,000 participants to decipher the correlation between gut microbiota and efficacy of COVID-19 vaccine (NCT04770649). Waning immunity and SARS-CoV-2 variants will likely be a long-term challenge. In light of this, every means to prolong immunity and reduce complications are needed. The central role of gut microbiota in immunity against SARS-CoV-2 infection and microbiota modulation to improve SARS-CoV-2 vaccine efficacy are low-hanging fruit that should be seriously considered.

References

Alameddine J, Godefroy E, Papargyris L, et al. Faecalibacterium prausnitzii skews human DC to prime IL10-producing T cells through TLR2/6/JNK Signaling and IL-10, IL-27, CD39, and IDO-1 induction. Front Immunol. 2019;10:143.

Albrich WC, Ghosh TS, Ahearn-Ford S, et al. A high-risk gut microbiota configuration associates with fatal hyperinflammatory immune and metabolic responses to SARS-CoV-2. Gut Microbes. 2022;14:2073131.

Alvarado DM, Son J, Thackray LB, et al. Mesalamine reduces intestinal ACE2 expression without modifying SARS-CoV-2 infection or disease severity in mice. bioRxiv. 2021.

Barbieri N, Herrera M, Salva S, et al. Lactobacillus rhamnosus CRL1505 nasal administration improves recovery of T-cell mediated immunity against pneumococcal infection in malnourished mice. Benef Microbes. 2017;8:393–405.

Benus RF, van der Werf TS, Welling GW, et al. Association between Faecalibacterium prausnitzii and dietary fibre in colonic fermentation in healthy human subjects. Br J Nutr. 2010;104:693–700.

Bilinski J, Winter K, Jasinski M, et al. Rapid resolution of COVID-19 after faecal microbiota transplantation. Gut. 2022;71(1):230–2.

Camilleri M, Lyle BJ, Madsen KL, et al. Role for diet in normal gut barrier function: developing guidance within the framework of food-labeling regulations. Am J Physiol Gastrointest Liver Physiol. 2019;317:G17–39.

Carfi A, Bernabei R, Landi F, et al. Persistent symptoms in patients after acute COVID-19. JAMA. 2020;324:603–5.

Chen Y, Gu S, Chen Y, et al. Six-month follow-up of gut microbiota richness in patients with COVID-19. Gut. 2022;71:222–5.

Cheung KS, Hung IFN, Chan PPY, et al. Gastrointestinal manifestations of SARS-CoV-2 infection and virus load in Fecal samples from a Hong Kong cohort: systematic review and meta-analysis. Gastroenterology. 2020;159:81–95.

De Filippis F, Pellegrini N, Vannini L, et al. High-level adherence to a Mediterranean diet beneficially impacts the gut microbiota and associated metabolome. Gut. 2016;65:1812–21.

Hagan T, Cortese M, Rouphael N, et al. Antibiotics-driven gut microbiome perturbation alters immunity to vaccines in humans. Cell. 2019;178:1313–1328.e13.

Hashimoto T, Perlot T, Rehman A, et al. ACE2 links amino acid malnutrition to microbial ecology and intestinal inflammation. Nature. 2012;487:477–81.

Huang C, Wang Y, Li X, et al. Clinical features of patients infected with 2019 novel coronavirus in Wuhan, China. Lancet. 2020;395:497–506.

Ianiro G, Mullish BH, Kelly CR, et al. Reorganisation of faecal microbiota transplant services during the COVID-19 pandemic. Gut. 2020;69:1555–63.

Iddir M, Brito A, Dingeo G, et al. Strengthening the immune system and reducing inflammation and oxidative stress through diet and nutrition: considerations during the COVID-19 crisis. Nutrients. 2020;12:1562.

Kitamoto S, Alteri CJ, Rodrigues M, et al. Dietary L-serine confers a competitive fitness advantage to Enterobacteriaceae in the inflamed gut. Nat Microbiol. 2020;5:116–25.

Kotfis K, Skonieczna-Zydecka K. COVID-19: gastrointestinal symptoms and potential sources of SARS-CoV-2 transmission. Anaesthesiol Intensive Ther. 2020;52:171–2.

Lamers MM, Beumer J, van der Vaart J, et al. SARS-CoV-2 productively infects human gut enterocytes. Science. 2020;369:50–4.

Lau HCH, Ng SC, Yu L. Targeting the gut microbiota in coronavirus disease 2019: hype or hope? Gastroenterology. 2022;162:9–16.

Laursen RP, Hojsak I. Probiotics for respiratory tract infections in children attending day care centers—a systematic review. Eur J Pediatr. 2018;177:979–94.

Liu Q, Mak JWY, Su Q, et al. Gut microbiota dynamics in a prospective cohort of patients with post-acute COVID-19 syndrome. Gut. 2022;71:544–52.

Livanos AE, Jha D, Cossarini F, et al. Intestinal host response to SARS-CoV-2 infection and COVID-19 outcomes in patients with gastrointestinal symptoms. Gastroenterology. 2021;160:2435–2450.e34.

Ng SC, Peng Y, Zhang L, et al. Gut microbiota composition is associated with SARS-CoV-2 vaccine immunogenicity and adverse events. Gut. 2022;71:1106–16.

Nyberg T, Ferguson NM, Nash SG, et al. Comparative analysis of the risks of hospitalisation and death associated with SARS-CoV-2 omicron (B.1.1.529) and delta (B.1.617.2) variants in England: a cohort study. Lancet. 2022;399:1303–12.

Penninger JM, Grant MB, Sung JJY. The role of angiotensin converting enzyme 2 in modulating gut microbiota, intestinal inflammation, and coronavirus infection. Gastroenterology. 2021;160:39–46.

Ren Z, Wang H, Cui G, et al. Alterations in the human oral and gut microbiomes and lipidomics in COVID-19. Gut. 2021;70:1253–65.

Sanders JM, Monogue ML, Jodlowski TZ, et al. Pharmacologic treatments for coronavirus disease 2019 (COVID-19): a review. JAMA. 2020;323:1824–36.

Shang J, Ye G, Shi K, et al. Structural basis of receptor recognition by SARS-CoV-2. Nature. 2020;581:221–4.

Shkoporov AN, Hill C. Bacteriophages of the human gut: the "known unknown" of the microbiome. Cell Host Microbe. 2019;25:195–209.

Shuai H, Chan JF, Hu B, et al. Attenuated replication and pathogenicity of SARS-CoV-2 B.1.1.529 Omicron. Nature. 2022;603:693–9.

Suez J, Zmora N, Segal E, et al. The pros, cons, and many unknowns of probiotics. Nat Med. 2019;25:716–29.

Trompette A, Gollwitzer ES, Pattaroni C, et al. Dietary fiber confers protection against flu by shaping Ly6c(−) patrolling monocyte hematopoiesis and CD8(+) T cell metabolism. Immunity. 2018;48:992–1005.e8.

Vaughn VM, Gandhi TN, Petty LA, et al. Empiric antibacterial therapy and community-onset bacterial coinfection in patients hospitalized with coronavirus disease 2019 (COVID-19): a multi-hospital cohort study. Clin Infect Dis. 2021;72:e533–41.

Venzon M, Bernard-Raichon L, Klein J, et al. Gut microbiome dysbiosis during COVID-19 is associated with increased risk for bacteremia and microbial translocation. Res Sq. 2021.

Verma A, Xu K, Du T, et al. Expression of human ACE2 in Lactobacillus and beneficial effects in diabetic retinopathy in mice. Mol Ther Methods Clin Dev. 2019;14:161–70.

Volkert D, Beck AM, Cederholm T, et al. ESPEN guideline on clinical nutrition and hydration in geriatrics. Clin Nutr. 2019;38:10–47.

Xavier-Santos D, Padilha M, Fabiano GA, et al. Evidences and perspectives of the use of probiotics, prebiotics, synbiotics, and postbiotics as adjuvants for prevention and treatment of COVID-19: a bibliometric analysis and systematic review. Trends Food Sci Technol. 2022;120:174–92.

Yeoh YK, Zuo T, Lui GC, et al. Gut microbiota composition reflects disease severity and dysfunctional immune responses in patients with COVID-19. Gut. 2021;70:698–706.

Zang R, Gomez Castro MF, McCune BT, et al. TMPRSS2 and TMPRSS4 promote SARS-CoV-2 infection of human small intestinal enterocytes. Sci Immunol. 2020;5:eabc3582.

Zhang L XZ, Mak JWY, Chan FKL. Ng SC. SIM01 as a novel microbiome replacement therapy for COVID-19: an open-label pilot study. Asian Pacific Digestive Week. Virtual, 2021:PP-0464.

Zhou J, Li C, Liu X, et al. Infection of bat and human intestinal organoids by SARS-CoV-2. Nat Med. 2020;26:1077–83.

Zhu L, She ZG, Cheng X, et al. Association of blood glucose control and outcomes in patients with COVID-19 and pre-existing type 2 diabetes. Cell Metab. 2020;31:1068–1077.e3.

Zoufaly A, Poglitsch M, Aberle JH, et al. Human recombinant soluble ACE2 in severe COVID-19. Lancet Respir Med. 2020;8:1154–8.

Zuo T, Zhang F, Lui GCY, et al. Alterations in gut microbiota of patients with COVID-19 during time of hospitalization. Gastroenterology. 2020;159:944–955.e8.

Zuo T, Liu Q, Zhang F, et al. Depicting SARS-CoV-2 faecal viral activity in association with gut microbiota composition in patients with COVID-19. Gut. 2021;70:276–84.

MIX
Papier aus verantwortungsvollen Quellen
Paper from responsible sources
FSC® C105338

If you have any concerns about our products,
you can contact us on
ProductSafety@springernature.com

In case Publisher is established outside the EU,
the EU authorized representative is:
Springer Nature Customer Service Center GmbH
Europaplatz 3, 69115 Heidelberg, Germany

Printed by Libri Plureos GmbH
in Hamburg, Germany